Advances in Reproductive Health

A Clinical Guide to Contraception

nova
Medicine & Health
New York

Obstetrics and Gynecology Advances

More information about this series can be found at
https://novapublishers.com/product-category/series/obstetrics-and-gynecology-advances/

Sexology Research and Issues

More information about this series can be found at
https://novapublishers.com/product-category/series/sexology-research-and-issues/

Llanos Belmonte Andújar
Ana Fuentes Rozalén
Editors

Advances in Reproductive Health

A Clinical Guide to Contraception

nova
Medicine & Health
New York

DOI: https://doi.org/10.52305/ROIH5688

Library of Congress Cataloging-in-Publication Data

Library of Congress Control Number: 2025949526
ISBN: 979-8-90134-038-7 (Hardcover)
ISBN: 979-8-90134-126-1 (eBook)

Published by Nova Science Publishers, Inc. † New York

Contents

Preface

The term *contraception* refers to the use of drugs or techniques by individuals or couples to control their fertility at a given time. A contraceptive is any action intended to prevent or reduce the likelihood of pregnancy during vaginal intercourse.

Family planning is understood as the range of supplies and services that allow individuals and couples to have the number of children they desire and to decide when and how often to have them. This includes, among others, modern contraceptive methods such as birth control pills, intrauterine devices (IUDs), injectables, male and female condoms, as well as natural methods and permanent surgical options.

Family planning services encompass not only access to contraceptive methods, but also medical care, personalized counseling, education, and information related to sexual and reproductive health, as well as follow-up or removal when needed.

According to the 1994 International Conference on Population and Development held in Cairo:

> "Reproductive health is a state of complete physical, mental and social well-being and not merely the absence of disease or infirmity, in all matters relating to the reproductive system and to its functions and processes. Reproductive health therefore implies that people are able to have a satisfying and safe sex life and that they have the capability to reproduce and the freedom to decide if, when and how often to do so. Implicit in this last condition are the right of men and women to be informed and to have access to safe, effective, affordable and acceptable methods of family planning of their choice, as well as other methods of their choice for regulation of fertility which are not against the law, and the right of access to appropriate health-care services that will enable women to go safely through pregnancy and childbirth. Reproductive health includes sexual health, the purpose of which is the enhancement of life and personal relations."

Family planning and access to modern contraception are essential not only for the well-being and autonomy of women, but also for the health and development of communities. These interventions provide global benefits such as reducing pregnancy-related health risks, lowering infant mortality rates, preventing HIV/AIDS, reducing adolescent pregnancies, slowing population growth, and promoting empowerment through better education and informed decision-making.

For this reason, it is essential to incorporate modern contraceptive methods into contraceptive counseling for anyone who requests it, in order to guarantee comprehensive sexual and reproductive health care that respects fundamental rights.

In line with the third edition of the WHO's *Selected Practice Recommendations for Contraceptive Use* (2018), users must receive adequate, understandable, and accessible information that allows them to make informed and voluntary choices. This information must include relative effectiveness, proper use, how each method works, common side effects, health risks and benefits, warning signs, return to fertility after discontinuation, and protection against sexually transmitted infections (STIs).

It is also critical that individuals be counseled both on methods that require user compliance and on alternatives that are less user-dependent, so that each woman can choose the method that best fits her circumstances. For methods requiring medical procedures (e.g., sterilization, implants, IUDs, diaphragms, cervical caps), trained health providers and equipped facilities must be available, with appropriate supplies and up-to-date evaluation tools.

We must also acknowledge that lack of access to effective contraception has serious consequences. Unintended pregnancies remain one of the main causes of abortion worldwide. The figures vary greatly depending on the country and the laws that regulate them. Globally, it is estimated that around 73 million abortions occur each year, and many of these procedures are performed in unsafe conditions, especially in countries where access to safe services is limited. This can have serious consequences for women's health, such as infections, hemorrhages, medical complications, and even death in cases of unsafe abortions, posing significant risks to women's physical and mental health. Ensuring access to safe contraception and comprehensive sexuality education is therefore a key strategy to prevent unsafe abortions and safeguard women's well-being and lives.

These are the reasons behind the creation of this book, which aims to provide healthcare professionals with a clear, practical, and up-to-date guide to the counseling and management of the various contraceptive methods available today. This work is intended as a useful tool to help implement international recommendations on sexual and reproductive health, contributing to a more equitable, informed, and healthy society.

Acknowledgments

To all those brave men and women throughout history who have taken small but significant steps to ensure that today we have all the contraceptive options detailed in this book, that make life easier for many women and, in some cases, even save their lives.

May the day come when all women on this planet have access to these methods and can decide for themselves, with adequate information, how many children they want to have, when to have them, and with whom.

Chapter 1

Contraceptive Counselling: Anamnesis and Physical Examination in Contraception

M. M. Pérez Haro[1,2,*], MD
S. Rico Cardenal[3], MD
G. Serrano García[1], MD, PhD
A. M. Fuentes Rozalén[4], MD
and M. T. Gómez García[1,5], PhD

[1]Obstetrics and Gynaecology Department, Albacete University Hospital Complex, Albacete, Spain
[2]Instituto Bernabeu of Albacete, Spain
[3]Obstetrics and Gynaecology Department, Hospital of Villarrobledo, Villarrobledo, Albacete, Spain
[4]Instituto Bernabeu of Alicante, Spain
[5]Medical Science Department, School of Medicine of Albacete, University of Castilla-La Mancha, Spain

Abstract

Contraceptive counselling is a person-centred clinical process aimed at providing accurate information and support in choosing the most appropriate contraceptive method. This process requires a thorough medical history and, in certain cases, a targeted physical examination, with the aim of ensuring safety, efficacy, and satisfaction. The use of evidence-based clinical guidelines, such as the World Health Organization (WHO) Medical Eligibility Criteria (MEC), the U.S. Medical Eligibility Criteria for Contraceptive Use (CDC, 2024), or the UK Medical Eligibility Criteria for Contraceptive Use (UKMEC, 2019), is essential to optimise care.

Keywords: eligibility criteria, WHO, CDC, contraception, medical history, physical examination, contraceptive counselling, sexual and reproductive health

* Corresponding Author's Email: mmar.perezh@gmail.com

In: Advances in Reproductive Health
Editors: Llanos Belmonte Andujar and Ana Fuentes Rozalen
ISBN: 979-8-90134-038-7

Introduction

Modern contraception is a cornerstone of sexual and reproductive health, significantly contributing to the reduction of unintended pregnancies, maternal morbidity, and the promotion of reproductive autonomy. High-quality contraceptive counselling is essential to encourage rational and sustained use of contraceptive methods (WHO, 2015).

Principles of Contraceptive Counselling

The key pillars of adequate contraceptive counselling include:

1. Person-centred approach: Care should be tailored to individual needs, values, and preferences, fostering a trusting therapeutic relationship (Dehlendorf, Krajewski & Borrero, 2014). It should also consider the patient's medical history, risk factors, age, and frequency of sexual activity (Moreno Gómez, 2015; Dehlendorf et al., 2016).
2. Counselling principles:
    - Provide complete, up-to-date, and balanced information on the different contraceptive methods.
    - Promote informed decision-making.
    - Ensure accessibility and equity.
    - Consider the sociocultural context, educational level, and health literacy of each patient.
3. Support tools: Visual aids, comparative efficacy charts, digital apps, WHO guidelines (WHO, 2015), Centers for Disease Control and Prevention (CDC) (Figures 1 and 2) (Nguyen et al., 2024), the American College of Obstetricians and Gynecologists (ACOG) (Kottke et al., 2022), and other scientific bodies focused on women's health and reproductive care.

Anamnesis in Contraception

One of the main tools available to us—an essential pillar in prescribing contraception—is a detailed anamnesis. A thorough medical history, considering the following aspects, ensures appropriate prescription, minimises risks associated with contraceptive use, facilitates adherence, and maximises effectiveness.

A contraceptive-focused medical history should explore (Nguyen et al., 2024; WHO, 2015; Curtis et al., 2016):

1. *Gynaecological and obstetric history:*
    - Age at menarche, cycle characteristics (duration, frequency, amount of bleeding, presence of dysmenorrhoea)
    - History of pregnancies, miscarriages, births, and any complications
    - Reproductive intentions (number of children, desired timing)

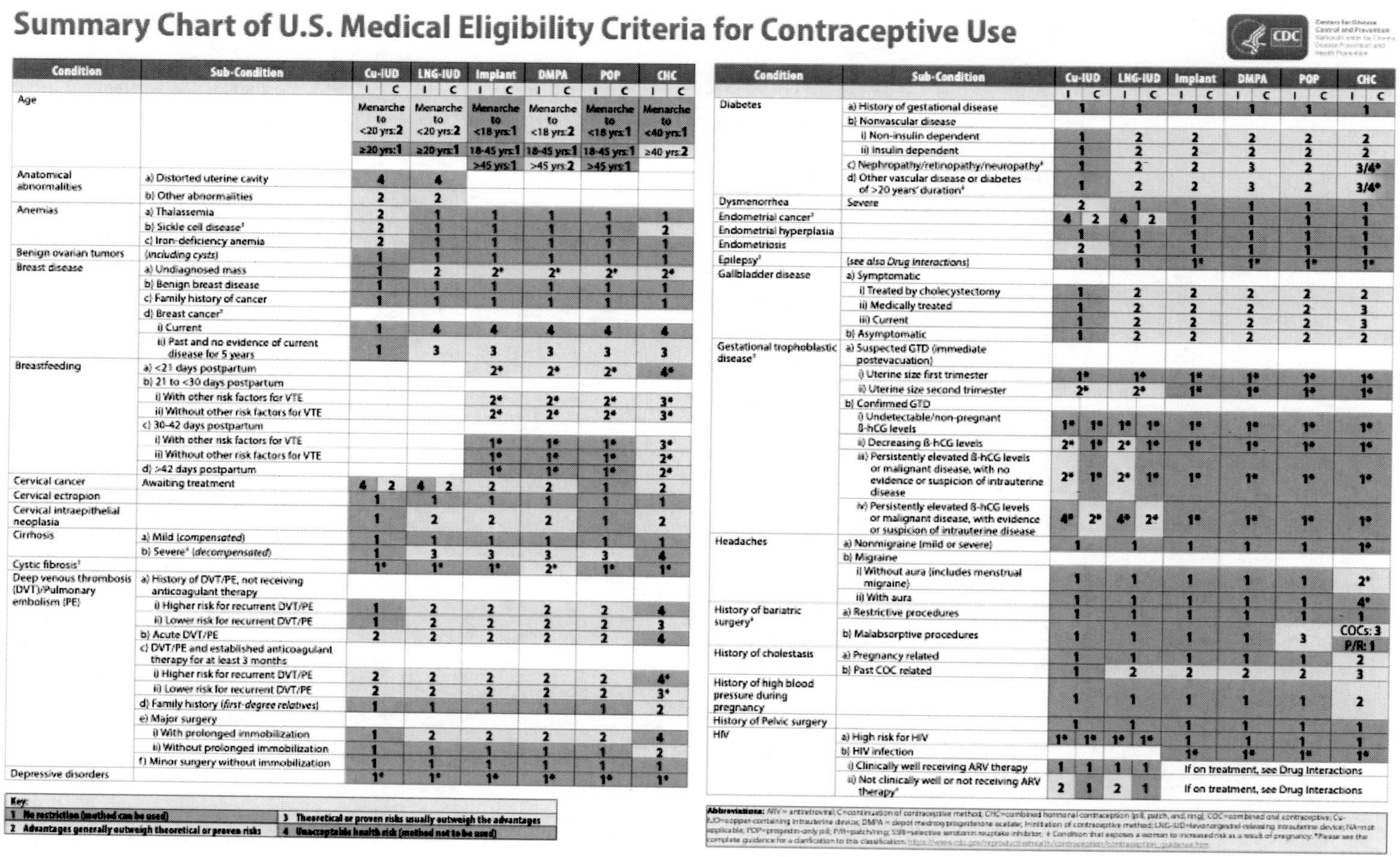

Summary Chart of U.S. Medical Eligibility Criteria for Contraceptive Use

CDC Centers for Disease Control and Prevention

Condition	Sub-Condition	Cu-IUD	LNG-IUD	Implant	DMPA	POP	CHC
Age		Menarche to <20 yrs: 2; ≥20 yrs: 1	Menarche to <20 yrs: 2; ≥20 yrs: 1	Menarche to <18 yrs: 1; 18-45 yrs: 1; >45 yrs: 1	Menarche to <18 yrs: 2; 18-45 yrs: 1; >45 yrs: 2	Menarche to <18 yrs: 1; 18-45 yrs: 1; >45 yrs: 1	Menarche to <40 yrs: 1; ≥40 yrs: 2
Anatomical abnormalities	a) Distorted uterine cavity	4	4				
	b) Other abnormalities	2	2				
Anemias	a) Thalassemia	2	1	1	1	1	1
	b) Sickle cell disease‡	2	1	1	1	1	2
	c) Iron-deficiency anemia	2	1	1	1	1	1
Benign ovarian tumors	(including cysts)	1	1	1	1	1	1
Breast disease	a) Undiagnosed mass	1	2	2*	2*	2*	2*
	b) Benign breast disease	1	1	1	1	1	1
	c) Family history of cancer	1	1	1	1	1	1
	d) Breast cancer‡						
	i) Current	1	4	4	4	4	4
	ii) Past and no evidence of current disease for 5 years	1	3	3	3	3	3
Breastfeeding	a) <21 days postpartum			2*	2*	2*	4*
	b) 21 to <30 days postpartum						
	i) With other risk factors for VTE			2*	2*	2*	3*
	ii) Without other risk factors for VTE			2*	2*	2*	3*
	c) 30-42 days postpartum						
	i) With other risk factors for VTE			1*	1*	1*	3*
	ii) Without other risk factors for VTE			1*	1*	1*	2*
	d) >42 days postpartum			1*	1*	1*	2*
Cervical cancer	Awaiting treatment	I: 4, C: 2	I: 4, C: 2	2	2	1	2
Cervical ectropion		1	1	1	1	1	1
Cervical intraepithelial neoplasia		1	2	2	2	1	2
Cirrhosis	a) Mild (compensated)	1	1	1	1	1	1
	b) Severe‡ (decompensated)	1	3	3	3	3	4
Cystic fibrosis‡		1*	1*	1*	2*	1*	1*
Deep venous thrombosis (DVT)/Pulmonary embolism (PE)	a) History of DVT/PE, not receiving anticoagulant therapy						
	i) Higher risk for recurrent DVT/PE	1	2	2	2	2	4
	ii) Lower risk for recurrent DVT/PE	1	2	2	2	2	3
	b) Acute DVT/PE	2	2	2	2	2	4
	c) DVT/PE and established anticoagulant therapy for at least 3 months						
	i) Higher risk for recurrent DVT/PE	2	2	2	2	2	4*
	ii) Lower risk for recurrent DVT/PE	2	2	2	2	2	3*
	d) Family history (first-degree relatives)	1	1	1	1	1	2
	e) Major surgery						
	i) With prolonged immobilization	1	2	2	2	2	4
	ii) Without prolonged immobilization	1	1	1	1	1	2
	f) Minor surgery without immobilization	1	1	1	1	1	1
Depressive disorders		1*	1*	1*	1*	1*	1*

Condition	Sub-Condition	Cu-IUD	LNG-IUD	Implant	DMPA	POP	CHC
Diabetes	a) History of gestational disease	1	1	1	1	1	1
	b) Nonvascular disease						
	i) Non-insulin dependent	1	2	2	2	2	2
	ii) Insulin dependent	1	2	2	2	2	2
	c) Nephropathy/retinopathy/neuropathy‡	1	2	2	3	2	3/4*
	d) Other vascular disease or diabetes of >20 years' duration‡	1	2	2	3	2	3/4*
Dysmenorrhea	Severe	2	1	1	1	1	1
Endometrial cancer‡		I: 4, C: 2	I: 4, C: 2	1	1	1	1
Endometrial hyperplasia		1	1	1	1	1	1
Endometriosis		2	1	1	1	1	1
Epilepsy‡	(see also Drug Interactions)	1	1	1*	1*	1*	1*
Gallbladder disease	a) Symptomatic						
	i) Treated by cholecystectomy	1	2	2	2	2	2
	ii) Medically treated	1	2	2	2	2	3
	iii) Current	1	2	2	2	2	3
	b) Asymptomatic	1	2	2	2	2	2
Gestational trophoblastic disease‡	a) Suspected GTD (immediate postevacuation)						
	i) Uterine size first trimester	1*	1*	1*	1*	1*	1*
	ii) Uterine size second trimester	2*	2*	1*	1*	1*	1*
	b) Confirmed GTD						
	i) Undetectable/non-pregnant ß-hCG levels	I: 1*, C: 1*	I: 1*, C: 1*	1*	1*	1*	1*
	ii) Decreasing ß-hCG levels	I: 2*, C: 1*	I: 2*, C: 1*	1*	1*	1*	1*
	iii) Persistently elevated ß-hCG levels or malignant disease, with no evidence or suspicion of intrauterine disease	I: 2*, C: 1*	I: 2*, C: 1*	1*	1*	1*	1*
	iv) Persistently elevated ß-hCG levels or malignant disease, with evidence or suspicion of intrauterine disease	I: 4*, C: 2*	I: 4*, C: 2*	1*	1*	1*	1*
Headaches	a) Nonmigraine (mild or severe)	1	1	1	1	1	1*
	b) Migraine						
	i) Without aura (includes menstrual migraine)	1	1	1	1	1	2*
	ii) With aura	1	1	1	1	1	4*
History of bariatric surgery‡	a) Restrictive procedures	1	1	1	1	1	1
	b) Malabsorptive procedures	1	1	1	1	3	COCs: 3; P/R: 1
History of cholestasis	a) Pregnancy related	1	1	1	1	1	2
	b) Past COC related	1	2	2	2	2	3
History of high blood pressure during pregnancy		1	1	1	1	1	2
History of Pelvic surgery		1	1	1	1	1	1
HIV	a) High risk for HIV	I: 1*, C: 1*	I: 1*, C: 1*	1	1	1	1
	b) HIV infection			1*	1*	1*	1*
	i) Clinically well receiving ARV therapy	I: 1, C: 1	I: 1, C: 1	If on treatment, see Drug Interactions			
	ii) Not clinically well or not receiving ARV therapy*	I: 2, C: 1	I: 2, C: 1	If on treatment, see Drug Interactions			

Key:

1	No restriction (method can be used)	3	Theoretical or proven risks usually outweigh the advantages
2	Advantages generally outweigh theoretical or proven risks	4	Unacceptable health risk (method not to be used)

Abbreviations: ARV = antiretroviral; C=continuation of contraceptive method; CHC=combined hormonal contraception (pill, patch, and ring); COC=combined oral contraceptive; Cu-IUD=copper-containing intrauterine device; DMPA = depot medroxyprogesterone acetate; I=initiation of contraceptive method; LNG-IUD=levonorgestrel-releasing intrauterine device; NA=not applicable; POP=progestin-only pill; P/R=patch/ring; SSRI=selective serotonin reuptake inhibitor; ‡ Condition that exposes a woman to increased risk as a result of pregnancy. *Please see the complete guidance for a clarification to this classification: [illegible]

Figure 1. Centers for Disease Control and Prevention (CDC). (2024). *U.S. Medical Eligibility Criteria for Contraceptive Use – Summary Chart*. U.S. Department of Health and Human Services. Retrieved from https://www.cdc.gov/contraception/media/pdfs/2024/07/us-mec-summary-chart-color-508.pdf. Public domain.

Summary Chart of U.S. Medical Eligibility Criteria for Contraceptive Use

CDC Centers for Disease Control and Prevention

Condition	Sub-Condition	Cu-IUD		LNG-IUD		Implant		DMPA		POP		CHC	
		I	C	I	C	I	C	I	C	I	C	I	C
Hypertension	a) Adequately controlled hypertension	1*		1*		1*		2*		1*		3*	
	b) Elevated blood pressure levels *(properly taken measurements)*												
	i) Systolic 140-159 or diastolic 90-99	1*		1*		1*		2*		1*		3*	
	ii) Systolic ≥160 or diastolic ≥100[‡]	1*		2*		2*		3*		2*		4*	
	c) Vascular disease	1*		2*		2*		3*		2*		4*	
Inflammatory bowel disease	*(Ulcerative colitis, Crohn's disease)*	1		1		1		2		2		2/3*	
Ischemic heart disease[‡]	Current and history of	1		2	3	2	3	3		2	3	4	
Known thrombogenic mutations[‡]		1*		2*		2*		2*		2*		4*	
Liver tumors	a) Benign												
	i) Focal nodular hyperplasia	1		2		2		2		2		2	
	ii) Hepatocellular adenoma[‡]	1		3		3		3		3		4	
	b) Malignant[‡] (hepatoma)	1		3		3		3		3		4	
Malaria		1		1		1		1		1		1	
Multiple risk factors for atherosclerotic cardiovascular disease	(e.g., older age, smoking, diabetes, hypertension, low HDL, high LDL, or high triglyceride levels)	1		2		2*		3*		2*		3/4*	
Multiple sclerosis	a) With prolonged immobility	1		1		1		2		1		3	
	b) Without prolonged immobility	1		1		1		2		1		1	
Obesity	a) Body mass index (BMI) ≥30 kg/m²	1		1		1		1		1		2	
	b) Menarche to <18 years and BMI ≥ 30 kg/m²	1		1		1		2		1		2	
Ovarian cancer[‡]		1		1		1		1		1		1	
Parity	a) Nulliparous	2		2		1		1		1		1	
	b) Parous	1		1		1		1		1		1	
Past ectopic pregnancy		1		1		1		1		2		1	
Pelvic inflammatory disease	a) Past												
	i) With subsequent pregnancy	1	1	1	1	1		1		1		1	
	ii) Without subsequent pregnancy	2	2	2	2	1		1		1		1	
	b) Current	4	2*	4	2*	1		1		1		1	
Peripartum cardiomyopathy[‡]	a) Normal or mildly impaired cardiac function												
	i) <6 months	2		2		1		1		1		4	
	ii) ≥6 months	2		2		1		1		1		3	
	b) Moderately or severely impaired cardiac function	2		2		2		2		2		4	
Postabortion	a) First trimester	1*		1*		1*		1*		1*		1*	
	b) Second trimester	2*		2*		1*		1*		1*		1*	
	c) Immediate postseptic abortion	4		4		1*		1*		1*		1*	
Postpartum *(nonbreastfeeding women)*	a) <21 days					1		1		1		4	
	b) 21 days to 42 days												
	i) With other risk factors for VTE					1		1		1		3*	
	ii) Without other risk factors for VTE					1		1		1		2	
	c) >42 days					1		1		1		1	
Postpartum *(in breastfeeding or non-breastfeeding women, including cesarean delivery)*	a) <10 minutes after delivery of the placenta												
	i) Breastfeeding	1*		2*									
	ii) Nonbreastfeeding	1*		1*									
	b) 10 minutes after delivery of the placenta to <4 weeks	2*		2*									
	c) ≥4 weeks	1*		1*									
	d) Postpartum sepsis	4		4									

Condition	Sub-Condition	Cu-IUD		LNG-IUD		Implant		DMPA		POP		CHC	
		I	C	I	C	I	C	I	C	I	C	I	C
Pregnancy		4*		4*		NA*		NA*		NA*		NA*	
Rheumatoid arthritis	a) On immunosuppressive therapy	2	1	2	1	1		2/3*		1		2	
	b) Not on immunosuppressive therapy	1		1		1		2		1		2	
Schistosomiasis	a) Uncomplicated	1		1		1		1		1		1	
	b) Fibrosis of the liver[‡]	1		1		1		1		1		1	
Sexually transmitted diseases (STDs)	a) Current purulent cervicitis or chlamydial infection or gonococcal infection	4	2*	4	2*	1		1		1		1	
	b) Vaginitis *(including trichomonas vaginalis and bacterial vaginosis)*	2	2	2	2	1		1		1		1	
	c) Other factors relating to STDs	2*	2	2*	2	1		1		1		1	
Smoking	a) Age <35	1		1		1		1		1		2	
	b) Age ≥35, <15 cigarettes/day	1		1		1		1		1		3	
	c) Age ≥35, ≥15 cigarettes/day	1		1		1		1		1		4	
Solid organ transplantation[‡]	a) Complicated	3	2	3	2	2		2		2		4	
	b) Uncomplicated	2		2		2		2		2		2*	
Stroke[‡]	History of cerebrovascular accident	1		2		2	3	3		2	3	4	
Superficial venous disorders	a) Varicose veins	1		1		1		1		1		1	
	b) Superficial venous thrombosis (acute or history)	1		1		1		1		1		3*	
Systemic lupus erythematosus[‡]	a) Positive (or unknown) antiphospholipid antibodies	1*	1*	3*		3*		3*	3*	3*		4*	
	b) Severe thrombocytopenia	3*	2*	2*		2*		3*	2*	2*		2*	
	c) Immunosuppressive therapy	2*	1*	2*		2*		2*	2*	2*		2*	
	d) None of the above	1*	1*	2*		2*		2*	2*	2*		2*	
Thyroid disorders	Simple goiter/ hyperthyroid/hypothyroid	1		1		1		1		1		1	
Tuberculosis[‡] *(see also Drug interactions)*	a) Nonpelvic	1	1	1	1	1*		1*		1*		1*	
	b) Pelvic	4	3	4	3	1*		1*		1*		1*	
Unexplained vaginal bleeding	(suspicious for serious condition) before evaluation	4*	2*	4*	2*	3*		3*		2*		2*	
Uterine fibroids		2		2		1		1		1		1	
Valvular heart disease	a) Uncomplicated	1		1		1		1		1		2	
	b) Complicated[‡]	1		1		1		1		1		4	
Vaginal bleeding patterns	a) Irregular pattern without heavy bleeding	1		1	1	2		2		2		1	
	b) Heavy or prolonged bleeding	2*		1*	2*	2*		2*		2*		1*	
Viral hepatitis	a) Acute or flare	1		1		1		1		1		3/4*	2
	b) Carrier/Chronic	1		1		1		1		1		1	1
Drug Interactions													
Antiretrovirals used for prevention (PrEP) or treatment of HIV	Fosamprenavir (FPV) All other ARVs are 1 or 2 for all methods.	1/2*	1*	1/2*	1*	2*		2*		2*		3*	
Anticonvulsant therapy	a) Certain anticonvulsants (phenytoin, carbamazepine, barbiturates, primidone, topiramate, oxcarbazepine)	1		1		2*		1*		3*		3*	
	b) Lamotrigine	1		1		1		1		1		3*	
Antimicrobial therapy	a) Broad spectrum antibiotics	1		1		1		1		1		1	
	b) Antifungals	1		1		1		1		1		1	
	c) Antiparasitics	1		1		1		1		1		1	
	d) Rifampin or rifabutin therapy	1		1		2*		1*		3*		3*	
SSRIs		1		1		1		1		1		1	
St. John's wort		1		1		2		1		2		2	

Updated in 2020. This summary sheet only contains a subset of the recommendations from the U.S. MEC. For complete guidance, see [illegible]. Most contraceptive methods do not protect against sexually transmitted diseases (STDs). Consistent and correct use of the male latex condom reduces the risk of STDs and HIV.

CS314239-A

Figure 2. Centers for Disease Control and Prevention (CDC). (2024). *U.S. Medical Eligibility Criteria for Contraceptive Use – Summary Chart*. U.S. Department of Health and Human Services. Retrieved from https://www.cdc.gov/contraception/media/pdfs/2024/07/us-mec-summary-chart-color-508.pdf. Public domain.

Table 1. Examinations and tests required before initiating contraceptive methods

Contraceptive Method	Physical Examination Required	Additional Tests Required	Remarks
Combined oral contraceptives (COCs)	Blood pressure	None routinely	Do not initiate if hypertension is uncontrolled. Pelvic exam and cervical smear are not required.
Progestogen-only contraceptives (pill or injectables)	Blood pressure (optional)	None routinely	Safe for most women. Pelvic exam and cervical smear are not required.
Subdermal implant	Basic general assessment (BMI, blood pressure)	Pregnancy test (if in doubt)	No gynaecological examination or laboratory tests required.
Copper intrauterine device (Cu-IUD)	Speculum examination, bimanual palpation	Pregnancy test, STI screening (if at risk)	No need for prior cervical cancer screening. STI screening if <25 years or risk factors present.
Hormonal intrauterine device (LNG-IUD)	Speculum examination, bimanual palpation	Pregnancy test, STI screening (if at risk)	Can be used in nulliparous women (as with Cu-IUD).
Contraceptive patch	Blood pressure	None routinely	Pelvic examination not required.
Vaginal ring	Blood pressure	None routinely	No prior vaginal examination required.
Male/female condom	None	None	No examination required. Promote use in all women at risk of STIs.
Natural methods (rhythm, basal temperature, etc.)	General assessment (BMI, blood pressure)	None	Requires accurate education on the method.
Emergency contraception (levonorgestrel, ulipristal, Cu-IUD)	None	Pregnancy test (if pregnancy suspected)	Cu-IUD is the most effective. Assess for STI if IUD is chosen and STI risk exists. Requires written informed consent.
Tubal ligation	Complete pre-surgical evaluation, including full gynaecological exam with transvaginal ultrasound	Preoperative tests (per local protocol)	Permanent and irreversible method. Requires written informed consent.
Vasectomy (in male partner)	Physical examination of male genitalia	Postoperative semen analysis (to confirm azoospermia)	Permanent method. Requires written informed consent.

2. *Medical history:*
   - Chronic conditions (hypertension, diabetes mellitus, lupus, epilepsy, liver diseases, and other conditions that may represent a contraindication to the use of certain contraceptive methods)
   - History of venous thromboembolism, migraine with aura
   - Hormone-sensitive cancers
3. *Sexual history:*
   - Number of partners, type of sexual practices
   - Previous or current sexually transmitted infections (STIs)
   - Risk of STI exposure
4. *Family history:*
   - Hereditary thrombophilias
   - Family history of breast cancer, cardiovascular events
5. *Regular medication and habits:*
   - CYP450 enzyme-inducing drugs (which may interact with hormonal contraceptives and thereby affect their effectiveness, or conversely, be affected in their efficacy by the contraceptives themselves when prescribed for other medical conditions).
   - Use of tobacco, alcohol, and drugs
   - Mental health and psychosocial factors:
   - Depression, anxiety, eating disorders
   - Reproductive coercion, gender-based violence

Physical Examination

Physical examination is not essential in most cases to initiate contraceptive methods (WHO, 2015). Based on clinical need, it may include (Table 1):

1. *General assessment*: Body Mass Index (BMI), blood pressure (especially when using combined hormonal contraceptives)
2. *Gynaecological examination*:
   - Only in cases of intrauterine device (IUD) placement, suspected pathology, or collection of cervicovaginal swabs to rule out STIs in certain cases.
   - Speculum examination, bimanual palpation, sample collection if STI testing is required.
3. *Additional tests:*
   - Only when clinically indicated
   - Pregnancy test, serologies, cervical cancer screening according to national protocols
4. *Informed consent*. All contraceptive methods require informed consent, either verbal or written, especially in the case of IUDs, tubal ligation, subdermal implants, or vasectomy.

Choice of Contraceptive Method

The choice of contraceptive method should be based on three main pillars:

1. Efficacy (typical use vs. perfect use) (Trussell, 2011; (Trussell 2011; Centers for Disease Control and Prevention 2014) (Figure 3))
2. Contraindications according to WHO MEC (WHO, 2015; Nguyen et al., 2024)
3. Patient preferences and lifestyle (Cohen et al., 2024).

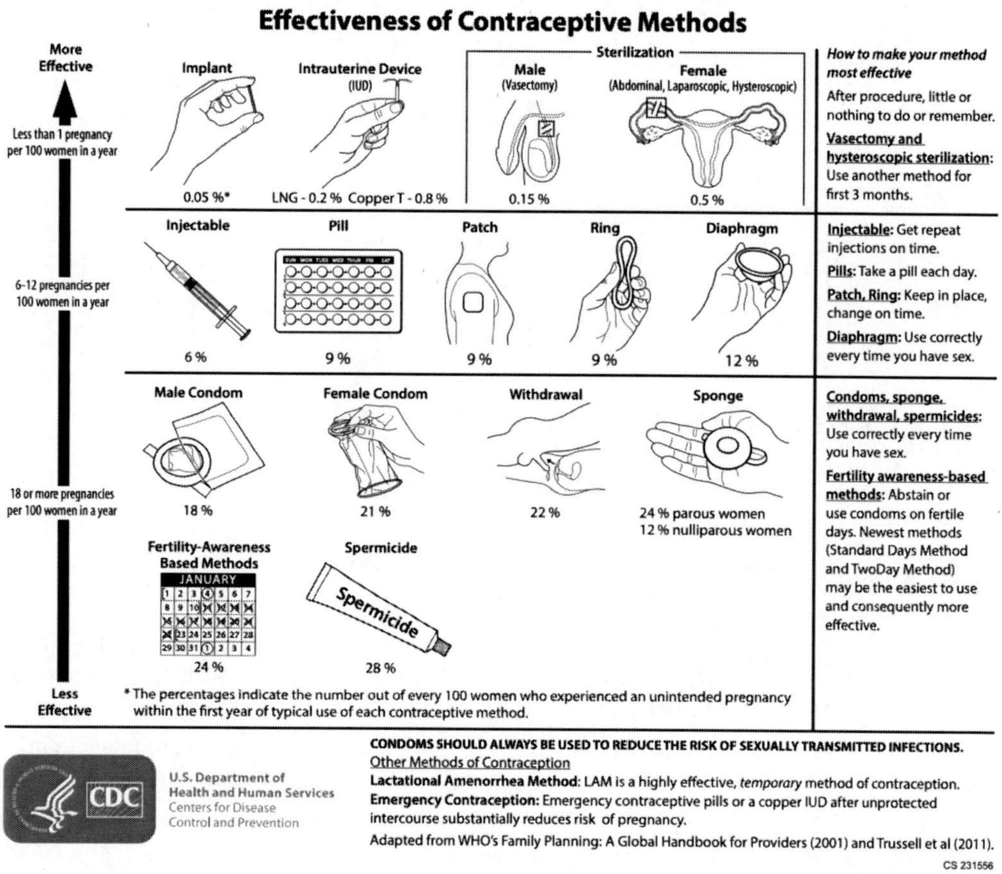

Figure 3. *Effectiveness of Contraceptive Methods*. Centers for Disease Control and Prevention, Morbidity and Mortality Weekly Report. Adapted from WHO and Trussell (2011). Public domain.

Classification of Methods According to Contraceptive Effectiveness

Contraceptive methods are classified by effectiveness into three groups based on failure rates during the first year of typical and perfect use. This classification is essential in counselling, as it helps align the method with patient expectations, capabilities, and needs (Figure 3).

- *High effectiveness*:
  - Includes methods with a failure rate of less than 1% with typical use, due to their minimal dependence on user behaviour (Trussell 2011; CDC 2014). This group includes:
  - Long-acting reversible contraception (LARC): copper or hormonal intrauterine devices (IUDs, levonorgestrel) and subdermal etonogestrel implants.
  - Permanent methods: tubal ligation and vasectomy.
- *Moderate effectiveness*:
  - Methods that require correct and consistent use, with failure rates of 6–9% with typical use. Their effectiveness largely depends on the user's adherence (WHO 2015; Nguyen et al. 2024; Curtis et al. 2024)
  - Combined oral contraceptives
  - Transdermal patches
  - Vaginal rings
- *Low effectiveness:*
  - Methods that are highly dependent on behavior and correct use each time. Typical-use failure rates exceed 10%, and are higher among adolescents and less experienced couples (Sundaram et al. 2017; Nguyen et al. 2024).
  - Male and female condoms
  - Natural methods (calendar, basal temperature, cervical mucus)
  - Withdrawal
  - Spermicides

Contraindications and Medical Evaluation: WHO MEC

The assessment of the patient's medical and personal conditions is an essential component in the selection of a contraceptive method. For this purpose, the Medical Eligibility Criteria (MEC) developed by the World Health Organization (WHO) are used (Table 2). These criteria provide a classification based on the balance of risks and benefits for each method and clinical condition (WHO 2015).

Classification of the WHO Medical Eligibility Criteria

Table 2. World Health Organization. *Medical eligibility criteria for contraceptive use.* 5th ed. Geneva: World Health Organization; 2015. Example: A woman with severe hypertension (>160/100 mmHg) is Category 4 for combined hormonal contraceptives and Category 2 for copper IUD, making the IUD the preferred option in this context

Category	Clinical meaning
Category 1	No restriction for use
Category 2	Advantages outweigh potential or proven risks
Category 3	Not recommended unless no other method is available. The risk generally outweighs the benefit.
Category 4	Unacceptable risk; method contraindicated

Conditions to Evaluate

The WHO has defined more than 80 medical conditions and personal characteristics that should be assessed when selecting a contraceptive method (World Health Organization. Reproductive Health and Research and World Health Organization 2015; Nguyen et al. 2024). Among the most relevant are:

- Cardiovascular diseases: hypertension, ischemic heart disease, heart failure, DVT, stroke
- Metabolic disorders: diabetes (with or without complications), obesity, dyslipidaemia
- Gynaecological conditions: abnormal bleeding, fibroids, gestational trophoblastic disease, cervical cancer
- Personal factors: age, smoking, postpartum, breastfeeding, nulliparity.
- Infections: HIV, STIs, pelvic tuberculosis.
- Concomitant medication: enzyme inducers (e.g. antiepileptics, rifampicin).

Evaluation by Type of Contraceptive Method

The WHO MEC provides specific guidance for each contraceptive method:

1. *Combined hormonal methods (COCs, patch, ring):*
   Contraindicated (Category 4) in women with:
    - Severe hypertension (>160/100 mmHg)
    - History of deep vein thrombosis or pulmonary embolism (DVT/PE)
    - Migraine with aura.
    - Age >35 and smoker

   Use with caution (Category 2 or 3):
    - Uncomplicated diabetes.
    - Breastfeeding (from 6 months).
    - Resolved liver disease.
2. *Progestogen-only methods (minipill, implant, injectables):*
    - Generally safe in women with cardiovascular risk
    - Suitable from immediate postpartum in breastfeeding women
    - Contraindicated: in women with a history of breast cancer (category 4)
3. *Intrauterine devices (copper or hormonal):*
    - Contraindicated (Category 4) in:
    - Current pregnancy.
    - Pelvic inflammatory disease.
    - Untreated cervical cancer.
    - Permitted (Category 2) in:
    - Nulliparous women.
    - Adolescents.
    - HIV-positive women without active pelvic inflammatory disease, PID (WHO 2021).
4. *Emergency contraception:*
    - Oral methods (levonorgestrel, ulipristal) can be used in almost all conditions (Category 1 or 2).

- Copper IUD is highly effective but contraindicated in active STI or PID (Category 4).

Patient Preferences and Lifestyle

Besides medical criteria and efficacy, method choice should also respect personal preferences, cultural context, and life circumstances. A patient-centered approach enhances adherence and satisfaction.

1. *Adolescents:* Adolescents have specific needs regarding contraception. (Allen, Kaunitz, and Bartz 2019). It is essential to:
    - Ensure confidentiality and privacy, key aspects to facilitate access to reproductive health services.
    - Integrate into comprehensive sex education.
    - Prioritise highly effective, low-maintenance methods (e.g., LARC), which have been shown to significantly reduce rates of unintended pregnancy in this population.
2. *Postpartum and breastfeeding:* Postpartum contraception must take into account thromboembolic risks and the impact on breastfeeding: (World Health Organization. Reproductive Health and Research and World Health Organization 2015; Nguyen et al. 2024).
    - Combined hormonal methods are contraindicated in the first 6 weeks postpartum if breastfeeding (WHO category 4), and its use should be deferred until 6 months if exclusively breastfeeding.
    - Recommended: progestogen-only methods (mini-pill, implants, injectables) or LARC (copper or hormonal IUD, subdermal implant).
3. *Women with disabilities:* Women with disabilities often face physical, cognitive, or access-related barriers that hinder the use and follow-up of contraceptive methods. (Gerancher 2017). Contraceptive counselling should:
    - Tailor counselling to autonomy, caregiver support, and cognitive/physical ability.
    - Prefer low-maintenance methods (e.g., LARC), especially in cases of cognitive or motor impairment.
    - Adapt informed consent and educational materials to accessible formats.
4. *Vulnerable populations* (migrants, victims of violence, ethnic minorities, homeless, incarcerated, mental illness). They require an approach based on sexual and reproductive rights (World Health Organization 2014):
    - Ensure non-coercive, culturally competent care based on sexual and reproductive rights.
    - Facilitate access to effective methods without unnecessary delays or visits.
    - Train professionals in intercultural skills and work with community mediators.

Conclusion

Contraceptive counselling is a crucial clinical intervention in sexual and reproductive health. Its main goal is to ensure informed, safe, and effective contraceptive choices tailored to each individual.

Its proper implementation helps reduce unplanned pregnancies, improve reproductive autonomy, and ensure continuous and satisfactory use of the chosen method.

1. *A person-centred approach* is key, requiring adaptation of information and clinical support to the individual's needs, values, social context, and life stage. Shared decision-making is essential.
2. *Thorough anamnesis* is the foundation of prescribing contraception and must explore medical, gynaecological, sexual, family, and psychosocial history—especially conditions that may contraindicate certain methods.
3. *Physical examination* is not usually mandatory but may be indicated depending on the method or context. For example, blood pressure should be checked before starting combined hormonal contraception; pelvic exams may be necessary before IUD insertion.
4. *Method selection should be based on:*
   - Contraceptive effectiveness: prioritising low-failure methods such as LARC or definitive contraceptive methods.
   - Medical eligibility criteria: according to guidelines such as those from the WHO (2015), the CDC (2024), and the UKMEC (2019), which allow for the assessment of the risks and benefits of using each method under various clinical conditions
   - Lifestyle and personal preferences: taking into account specific situations such as adolescence, postpartum, disability, or social vulnerability, where safe, effective, and accessible methods should be prioritized.
5. *Postpartum contraception* requires specific attention: combined methods are contraindicated in the first 6 weeks if breastfeeding, whereas progestogen-only and LARC methods are appropriate soon after delivery or after several weeks, depending on the circumstances.
6. It is crucial to address structural, social, and access-related barriers that may hinder the proper use of contraceptive methods, especially among adolescents, women with disabilities, or groups in vulnerable situations. Respect for sexual and reproductive rights must guide all clinical decisions.

In conclusion, contraceptive counselling should not be limited to a mere prescription, but rather understood as a comprehensive process of care, active listening, and clinical support based on the best available evidence. Incorporating tools such as the MEC and prioritising a trusting therapeutic relationship is key to improving reproductive health outcomes.

References

Centers for Disease Control and Prevention, CDC. 2014. 'Appendix D: Contraceptive Effectiveness'. Morbidity and Mortality Weekly Report (MMWR). 2014. https://www.cdc.gov/mmwr/preview/mmwrhtml/rr6304a5.htm?utm_source=chatgpt.com.

Cohen, Mandy K, Charlotte K Kent, Tong Yang, Alexander J Gottardy, Maureen A Leahy, Stephen R Spriggs, Armina Velarde, et al. 2024. 'Morbidity and Mortality Weekly Report U.S. Medical Eligibility Criteria for Contraceptive Use, 2024 Recommendations and Reports Centers for Disease Control and Prevention MMWR Editorial and Production Staff (Serials) MMWR Editorial Board'.

Curtis, Kathryn M., Tara C. Jatlaoui, Naomi K. Tepper, Lauren B. Zapata, Leah G. Horton, Denise J. Jamieson, and Maura K. Whiteman. 2016. 'U.S. Selected Practice Recommendations for Contraceptive Use, 2016'. *MMWR. Recommendations and Reports: Morbidity and Mortality Weekly Report. Recommendations and Reports* 65 (4): 1–66. https://doi.org/10.15585/MMWR.RR6504A1.

Curtis, Kathryn M., Antoinette T. Nguyen, Naomi K. Tepper, Lauren B. Zapata, Emily M. Snyder, Kendra Hatfield-Timajchy, Katherine Kortsmit, Megan A. Cohen, and Maura K. Whiteman. 2024. 'U.S. Selected Practice Recommendations for Contraceptive Use, 2024'. *MMWR. Recommendations and Reports* 73 (3): 1–77. https://doi.org/10.15585/MMWR.RR7303A1.

Dehlendorf, Christine, Edith Fox, Lauren Sobel, and Sonya Borrero. 2016. 'Patient-Centered Contraceptive Counseling: Evidence to Inform Practice'. *Current Obstetrics and Gynecology Reports* 5 (1): 55–63. https://doi.org/10.1007/s13669-016-0139-1.

Gerancher, Karen R. 2017. 'Counseling Adolescents About Contraception'. *Obstetrics and Gynecology* 130 (2): 486–87. https://doi.org/10.1097/AOG.0000000000002228.

Kottke, Melissa, Lisa Goldthwaite, Kavita Arora, and Jennifer Villavicencio. 2022. 'Patient-Centered Contraceptive Counseling.' *Obstetrics and Gynecology* 139 (2): 350–53. https://doi.org/10.1097/AOG.0000000000004659.

Moreno Gómez, Ana I. 2015. 'Consejo Contraceptivo'. http://www.msssi.gob.es/profesionales/saludPublica/prevPromocion/.

Nguyen, Antoinette T., Kathryn M. Curtis, Naomi K. Tepper, Katherine Kortsmit, Anna W. Brittain, Emily M. Snyder, Megan A. Cohen, Lauren B. Zapata, and Maura K. Whiteman. 2024a. 'U.S. Medical Eligibility Criteria for Contraceptive Use, 2024.' *MMWR Recommendations and Reports* 73 (4): 1–126. https://doi.org/10.15585/MMWR.RR7304A1.

Organisation Mondiale de la Santé. 2014. 'Ensuring Human Rights in the Provision of Contraceptive Information and Services'. *Oms*, 34. www.who.int.

Sundaram, Aparna, Barbara Vaughan, Kathryn Kost, Akinrinola Bankole, Lawrence Finer, Susheela Singh, and James Trussell. 2017. 'Contraceptive Failure in the United States: Estimates from the 2006–2010 National Survey of Family Growth'. *Perspectives on Sexual and Reproductive Health* 49 (1): 7–16. https://doi.org/10.1363/PSRH.12017/FULL.

Trussell, James. 2011. 'Contraceptive Failure in the United States'. *Contraception* 83 (5): 397–404. https://doi.org/10.1016/j.contraception.2011.01.021.

World Health Organization. Reproductive Health and Research, and World Health Organization. 2015. 'Medical Eligibility Criteria for Contraceptive Use, 5th Ed. 2015: Geneva,' 276.

World Health Organization. 2021. 'Consolidated Guidelines on HIV Prevention, Testing, Service Delivery and Monitoring: Recommendations for a Public Health Approach.' *World Health Organization*, 592.

Chapter 2

Pharmacokinetics and Pharmacodynamics of Contraceptive Hormones

E. González Mirasol[1,2,*], PhD
A. M. Fuentes Rozalén[3], MD
Ll. Belmonte Andújar[1,2], PhD
M. T. Gómez García[1,2], PhD
and M. Moreno Palmero[1], MD
[1]Obstetrics and Gynaecology Department, Albacete University Hospital Complex, Albacete, Spain
[2]Medical Science Department, School of Medicine of Albacete, University of Castilla-La Mancha, Spain
[3]Instituto Bernabeu of Alicante, Spain

Abstract

This chapter will discuss the pharmacokinetic and pharmacodynamic aspects of contraceptive hormones. The main pharmacokinetic characteristics of contraceptive hormones and their routes of administration will be reviewed, with special interest in those that involve a clinically important modification, and that may be related to the appearance of side effects. Likewise, modifications related to obesity will be reviewed. We will study the mode of action of contraceptive hormones, both at the ovulatory level, on the cervical mucus and the endometrium, as well as their most striking metabolic effects.

Keywords: hormonal contraception, estrogen, progestogens, ethinylestradiol, estradiol, estrona, estetrol, leconorgestrol, desogestrel, dienogest, etonogestrel, pharmacokinetics, pharmacodynamics, metabolic effects

Introduction

Different types of estrogens and progestogens are used in contraception, either in combination as combined hormonal contraceptives (CHCs) or as progestins alone. Estrogens are 18-carbon

* Corresponding Author's Email: mgleze@gmail.com

In: Advances in Reproductive Health
Editors: Llanos Belmonte Andujar and Ana Fuentes Rozalen
ISBN: 979-8-90134-038-7

steroids, without a side chain and with an A-ring of phenolic nature. The natural estrogens are estrone, 17ß-estradiol (E2), estriol and estetrol, present in fetal development. (Alemany 2021), and those currently used in contraception are ethinylestradiol, estradiol and estetrol.

Progestogens constitute a more numerous group. Progesterone, the natural progestogen, is not used in contraception; therefore, all those used are synthetic. For a molecule to have progestogenic activity, it must have a 3-keto group and a double bond between C4 and C5 in the A-ring. (Capozzi, Scambia, and Lello 2022). The earliest contraceptive progestogens were derived from testosterone, including 19-norderivates (such as norethindrone), gonanes (such as levonorgestrel, desogestrel, etonogestrel, norgestimate, or gestodene) and non-ethinylated derivatives (such as dienogest). Other progestogens are derived from progesterone, such as pregnanes (such as medroxyprogesterone acetate, cyproterone acetate, and chlormadinone acetate) and 19-norpregnanes (such as nomegestrol acetate and nestorone). Finally, drospirenone is derived from spironolactone.

For these hormones to act, they must reach the target cells and bind to their specific receptors. Their effects will depend on the amount of hormone and the number and availability of receptors.

Pharmacokinetics is the discipline that studies the processes that determine how and in what quantity a hormone reaches its target cells. This includes its absorption, distribution in the body, metabolism and elimination. It analyzes what the body does to the drug. (Harvey et al. 2020).

Absorption is the process by which a drug moves from the site of administration into the bloodstream. When the oral route is used, hormones are initially transformed by intestinal and bacterial enzymes, and then, after absorption, reach the liver where they undergo further metabolism before passing into the systemic blood, along with these metabolites. The fraction of active drug that reaches circulation is called bioavailability (Fotherby 1996), and depends on intestinal absorption and first-pass hepatic metabolism. (A. B. Edelman, Cherala, y Stanczyk 2010). *Distribution* refers to the movement of the drug from the blood to the different body tissues, influenced by factors such as body mass, blood flow and binding to plasma proteins. Distribution equilibrium is reached when drug entry and exit into the tissues are equalized, and the concentration in the tissues reflects the plasma concentration (Le 2022). While distribution occurs, the processes of metabolism and excretion are also taking place, making it a dynamic and complex process. *Metabolism* consists of the chemical transformation of the drug, mainly in the liver, by means of enzymes that carry out chemical reactions such as oxidation, reduction, hydrolysis, conjugation, sulfation, and glucuronidation, generating metabolites that can modify the original activity of the drug. *Excretion* is the elimination of the drug and its metabolites from the body, mainly by the renal route (urine) and, to a lesser extent, by the biliary route. The reabsorption of drugs eliminated by the bile into the intestine is known as enterohepatic circulation.

Finally, *pharmacodynamics* studies the mechanisms of action and the effects that the drug exerts on the organism, both desired and adverse, as a result of the interaction between the hormone and its receptor. (Ruiz-Gayo y Fernández-Alonso 2013), and can be summarized by what the drug does to the body (Harvey et al. 2020).

Pharmacokinetics

There is great variability between and within individuals in the pharmacokinetic parameters of estrogens and progestogens. (Kuhl 1990; Lobo y Stanczyk 1994).

Estrogens

Ethinylestradiol (EE)

Ethinylestradiol (EE) is rapidly and completely absorbed after oral administration, reaching peak serum concentrations approximately 1 to 2 hours after ingestion. During the absorption process and first-pass hepatic metabolism, EE undergoes extensive metabolization, resulting in a mean oral bioavailability of about 45%, with considerable interindividual variability, with values ranging from 20% to 80%. Regarding its distribution, EE bonds in a high percentage (about 98%) nonspecifically to serum albumin and does not bind directly to sex hormone binding globulin (SHBG), although it induces an increase in serum concentrations of this protein, a relevant phenomenon in the context of combined contraception. The metabolism of EE occurs mainly by aromatic hydroxylation mediated by the hepatic cytochrome P450 system, generating hydroxylated and methylated metabolites found in serum both in free and conjugated form (glucuronides or sulfates). EE presents enterohepatic circulation, which allows its intestinal reabsorption after biliary excretion, contributing to a second peak in plasma levels between 10 and 14 hours after oral administration. The elimination of EE is mainly through urine (Kuhl 1990; Lobo y Stanczyk 1994; Sitruk-Ware y Nath 2013; Stanczyk, Archer, y Bhavnani 2013; Stanczyk, Winer, et al. 2024).

EE tends to accumulate in various tissues, especially in adipose tissue and myometrium (Kuhl 1990). Its half-life ranges from 10 to 20 hours, although there is variability in its determination according to the sources. (Lobo y Stanczyk 1994; Sitruk-Ware y Nath 2013; Stanczyk, Archer, y Bhavnani 2013).

Estradiol

When E2 is administered orally, it has a very short half-life, but this is prolonged when it is used in micronized formulations or conjugated in the form of estradiol valerate. These two products have similar pharmacodynamics and pharmacokinetics and are therefore considered the same from a clinical point of view. Estradiol valerate is metabolized to valeric acid and 17ß-estradiol, which in turn is transformed into estrone and estrone sulfate (Sitruk-Ware y Nath 2013; Stanczyk 2024). After oral administration, estradiol valerate absorption is complete, with first hepatic step, which results in estradiol, estrone and estriol, whereby 95% of the orally administered dose is metabolized before entering the systemic circulation, with a bioavailability of 3%. Estradiol circulates bound to SHBG (38%), and albumin (60%). Estradiol and its metabolites are excreted mainly in the urine, and approximately 10% is excreted in the feces (Zeun et al. 2009).

Estetrol

The most recent synthetic estrogen used in contraception is estetrol (E4), which is the estrogen naturally produced in the human fetal liver during pregnancy. After oral administration it is rapidly absorbed, reaching the maximum concentration within one hour, with a half-life of 24-32 hours, which is longer than that of E4 (Gérard et al. 2022). The Cmax of estetrol is reduced by approximately 50% after food intake. E4 has a high oral bioavailability, between 70 and 90% (Fruzzetti et al. 2021; Gemzell-Danielsson et al. 2022); although it is reduced to 50% when combined with drospirenone (Lee y Syed 2022). It has a long half-life in humans, with a mean of 28-32 hours, which is about twice as long as E2. (Fruzzetti et al. 2021; Gemzell-Danielsson et al. 2022; Gérard et al. 2022). It is metabolized at the liver level, by glucuronidation, mainly by the enzyme uridine 5'-diphospho-glucuronosyltransferase to form glucuronide and sulfate conjugates that are excreted in the urine, and by direct sulfation at an unconfirmed site (Fruzzetti et al. 2021; Gérard et al. 2022; Lee y Syed 2022). E4 is not transformed into hydroxylated metabolites, precursors of quinone estrogens, which are capable of reacting with DNA and causing genotoxic damage, a mechanism implicated in the development of breast cancer (Stanczyk 2024). Estetrol (E4) is not metabolized by cytochrome P450 (CYP450) enzymes. Consequently, unlike estradiol (E2) and ethinylestradiol (EE), it does not present clinically significant interactions of inhibition or induction with cytochrome P450 liver enzymes or with other drugs metabolized by this pathway (Fruzzetti et al. 2021; Gemzell-Danielsson et al. 2022; Gérard et al. 2022; Paton 2022; Stanczyk, Winer, et al. 2024; Slíva 2024). E4 shows moderate protein binding (about 50%) in human plasma (Fruzzetti et al. 2021; Gemzell-Danielsson et al. 2022; Gérard et al. 2022; Lee y Syed 2022). It does not appear to enter the enterohepatic circulation (Fruzzetti et al. 2021; Gérard et al. 2022). E4 is excreted in the urine (Fruzzetti et al. 2021; Gérard et al. 2022) and in the feces (Lee y Syed 2022).

Progestogens

In general terms, the metabolism of these compounds varies significantly among individuals, which is reflected in a remarkable diversity of side effects at both the individual and population level. Thus, the same dose may generate different responses in different individuals (Fotherby 1996; Capozzi, Scambia, y Lello 2022).

Table 1. Main pharmacokinetic parameters of some pro progestogens

	LNG	DSG	GTD	DNG	DRSP	NET	MPAo	MPAim
Bioavailability	97-99%	74%	96-100%	90%	76%	64%	5-15%	100%
FPH	no	Sí	no					
Union to SHBG	47%	38-57%		no	no	36%		no
Union to albumin	50%	40-58%		90%	95-97%	61%		80%
Metabolism P450	si	si	Sí	si	Sí			
Elimination:								
Urine	40-68%				38%			
Stool	16-48%				44%			
Average life	20h			10h				

LNG: levonorgestrel; DSG: desogestrel; GTD: gestodene; DNG: dienogest; DRSP: drospirenone; NET: noretisterone; MPAo: oral medroxyprogesterone acetate; MPAim: intramuscular medroxyprogesterone acetate. FPH: first pass hepatic.

We will not give a detailed description of the pharmacokinetics of each of the progestogens. In Table 1, we present here a summary of the main pharmacokinetic data of the main progestogens, and a more detailed description can be found in the following studies: (Kuhnz, Gansau, y Fuhrmeister 1992; Fotherby 1996; Kuhl 1990; Lobo y Stanczyk 1994; Krattenmacher 2000; Schindler et al. 2008; Sitruk-Ware y Nath 2010; 2013; Xin et al. 2016; Chiara Del Savio et al. 2020; Hofmann et al. 2020; Bick et al. 2021; Capozzi, Scambia, y Lello 2022; Stanczyk, McGough, et al. 2024; Lee y Syed 2022).

Peculiarities of the Different Routes of Administration

Since we have different routes of administration of hormonal contraceptives, it is important to consider the pharmacokinetic differences, and to what extent they may affect the variability of hormone levels, bioavailability and side effects.

Oral Route

COCs are subject to hepatic first-pass metabolism, which may reduce the bioavailability of their active ingredients, a matter of primary interest to pharmacologists, who are responsible for designing the various preparations, and this is beyond the scope of this presentation. After each daily administration, plasma hormone concentrations show peaks and valleys. Throughout the cycle, EE concentrations increase from the first day of pill-taking until day 7, to remain *stable* until day 21 of pill-taking, and decrease in the week of rest. *Progestogen* increases from day 1, and its levels remain stable until day 21, declining in the rest week *(Rodriguez et al. 2024).* The area under the curve (AUC) of EE is intermediate compared to other routes: higher than vaginal, but lower than transdermal (van den Heuvel et al. 2005). Comparing the different levonorgestrel (LNG)-based contraceptive methods, the combined oral contraceptive showed the highest systemic exposure, followed comparably by the single progestin pill and the implant; and finally, intrauterine systems (IUS) recorded the lowest exposure, in decreasing order: IUS-LNG 20, IUS-LNG 12 and IUS-LNG 8, differences that were accentuated at the end of the recommended use periods (Reinecke et al. 2018; Hofmann et al. 2020). A new modification has been introduced in the composition of the pills used in the oral route, which allows their prolonged release, resulting in a decrease in the peaks typical of the oral route but without reducing the total exposure of the hormones (Grandi 2025), which translates into better control of the cycle without modifying its tolerance (Biskupska-Bodova et al. 2025).

Transdermal Route

Transdermal patch administration avoids hepatic first-pass metabolism and provides more stable and sustained plasma drug levels without the fluctuations of the oral route (Abrams et al. 2002; van den Heuvel et al. 2005). After application to the skin, pharmacological levels in plasma reach steady state at approximately 48 hours and remain stable during the week of use, and remain stable for up to 10 days after application of the patch (Abrams et al. 2002; Devineni et al. 2007). Its absorption is not modified in conditions like those found in a gym (sauna, jacuzzi, treadmill and other aerobic exercises) and in a cold-water bath. Nor is its pharmacokinetics modified depending on the site of application: abdomen, buttock, arm or torso (Abrams et al. 2002). With the patch, the exposure to EE is higher than with the oral route (van den Heuvel et al. 2005; Devineni et al. 2007) and vaginal (van den Heuvel et al. 2005), and there is an increase in SHBG levels with respect to the oral route (Devineni et al. 2007), although the possible effect of this is unknown. Continuous use does not modify pharmacokinetics with respect to conventional use (Lavelanet, Rybin, y White 2017).

Vaginal Route

The vaginal ring releases low and constant doses of EE and progestogen, which are absorbed through the vagina, thus avoiding hepatic first-pass metabolism. Six rings have been designed with only progestogens, and seven with combined estrogens and progestogens (Taylor et al. 2020).

The vaginal route has the lowest EE exposure (van den Heuvel et al. 2005; Roumen 2007), with less daily variability of serum EE and progestogen levels, which may translate into better cycle control, with less irregular bleeding than with the other routes (Bjarnadóttir, Tuppurainen, y Killick 2002; López-Picado, Lapuente, y Lete 2017).

Subcutaneous Route (Implant)

Subcutaneous implants are used for progestogen-only contraception. Administered by subcutaneous implants, the bioavailability of etonogestrel is very high, 99% after insertion and 94% after two years. Its concentration reaches its maximum three months after implantation, and remains there during the second and third year, before decreasing at the end of the third year. Effective concentrations are reached 8 hours after insertion (Mäkäräinen et al. 1998), and 6 days after withdrawal, progestogens levels are undetectable (Wenzl et al. 1998; Bennink 2000). The mean concentration at the end of the first week is equivalent to the equilibrium concentration provided by the oral route with EE/DSG, decreasing thereafter, while the Cmax of ENG with ring is 40% compared to the oral route (Timmer y Mulders 2000). ENG circulates tightly bound to serum proteins, mainly albumin, and not to SHBG. It is metabolized by hydroxylation and conjugation to the glucuronide and sulfate form. The elimination half-life is 25 hours. Excretion of ~0.2% occurs in breast milk (Goldstuck y Le 2018).

Comparisons Between Different Routes of Administration

Two meta-analyses have summarized the information to compare whether the pharmacokinetic peculiarities of the different routes of hormone administration, which we have seen, translate into clinical changes (López-Picado, Lapuente, y Lete 2017; Vleskó et al. 2024). In one of them (López-Picado, Lapuente, y Lete 2017) a lower number of pregnancies is found with the vaginal route, although the difference is not significant by little, studying the percentage of pregnancies); while in the other (Vleskó et al. 2024), comparing the Pearl index, no differences are found.

The vaginal route has less irregular bleeding than the oral route (López-Picado, Lapuente, y Lete 2017), but more leucorrea (Vleskó et al. 2024); whereas the patch is associated with increased breast discomfort (Vleskó et al. 2024). Nausea and vomiting are less with the vaginal route compared to the oral or patch, and there are no differences in headaches or dysmenorrhea (López-Picado, Lapuente, y Lete 2017; Vleskó et al. 2024).

Pharmacokinetic Modifications with Obesity

In obese women, several modifications of the pharmacokinetics of contraceptive hormones occur:

- The time to reach Cmax is shortened by increased gastric vascularization (Tasset y Edelman 2025), while Cmax and AUC (Westhoff et al. 2010; A. B. Edelman et al. 2013; Luo et al. 2019), and mean EE and LNG levels are lower (Westhoff et al. 2010). Even so, these parameters are similar among obese women taking CHC with 30 µg EE and 150 µg LNG compared to normal-weight women taking them with 20 µg EE and 100 µg LNG (A. B. Edelman et al. 2014). Etonogestrel concentrations are unchanged in obese women using Implanon (Taylor et al. 2020).
- Steroidal compounds have a larger volume of distribution (Tasset y Edelman 2025).
- There is a decrease in SHBG, which increases the free fraction and concentrations of LNG and competition with transporter proteins for serum lipoproteins (Luo et al. 2019; Hofmann et al. 2020; Tasset y Edelman 2025).
- There is an alteration in metabolism, due to the appearance of fatty liver and the presence of inflammatory cytokines (Luo et al. 2019; Tasset y Edelman 2025).
- Increased elimination of drugs due to increased renal filtration (Tasset y Edelman 2025).

However, no correlation was found between these pharmacokinetic variations and a lower ovarian activity (A. B. Edelman et al. 2013), or higher follicular activity (Westhoff et al. 2010), nor a higher frequency of ovulations (Westhoff et al. 2014).

Nevertheless, it is important that we consider whether these pharmacokinetic differences may translate into increased failure in obese women. There are two observational studies of the same group, one a retrospective cohort study (Holt, Cushing-Haugen, y Daling 2002), and the other a case-control study (Holt et al. 2005), which report that the failure rate with CHC is higher among women in the upper weight quartile compared to women in the other quartiles when the lower doses are used, but not with the 50 µg EE contraceptives, and that the failure rate with CHC is higher among women in the lower weight quartiles when the lower doses are used, but not with the 50 µg EE contraceptives.

In 2015, a review was published to assess contraceptive failure linked to obesity with 8 phase 3 studies (7 using the oral route and one transdermal) that were in the existing database at the US FDA that concluded that there is a 30-40% higher risk of failure among obese women, with respect to non-obese women. However, this relative difference is quite small when considered on an individual basis, with a Pearl Index of 3.14 among women with BMI >30, compared to 2.53 among women with BMI >30 (Yamazaki et al. 2015).

The Cochrane also has a systematic review on the influence of weight on the effectiveness of contraceptives, with the latest update published in 2016, without demonstrating a clear association between higher BMI or weight and the effectiveness of hormonal contraceptives, although they acknowledge that there are few studies conducted. In the 12 studies they locate, most did not show more pregnancies in overweight or obese women. In two of five studies using birth control pills, differences were found between BMI groups. In one, overweight women had a higher risk of pregnancy, while the other found a lower pregnancy rate. The overall quality of the evidence was considered low for the purposes of this review (Lopez et al. 2016).

No relationship in contraceptive failure as a function of obesity with etonogestrel implant or LNG IUD (Lopez et al. 2016), with E4/DRSP (Jensen et al. 2022), nor with E2 (von Stockum et al. 2023).

The data suggest that there is no loss of UA efficacy with obesity, although the data are not conclusive at this time (Festin et al. 2017; A. Edelman et al. 2024). Increasing the drug dose neither modifies its pharmacokinetics nor alters the delay in ovulation (A. Edelman et al. 2025). In conclusion, there is no clear evidence of clinically important reduced contraceptive efficacy in obese women. The U.S. Medical Eligibility Criteria for Contraceptive Use of 2024 does not state that obesity is a contraindication for CHC (Nguyen 2024). Definitive data are not available whether bariatric surgery alters the pharmacokinetics of contraceptives, but it appears that at least after Roux-en-Y gastric bypass the pharmacokinetics of EE and LNG are not altered (Moreira De Brito et al. 2021).

Pharmacodynamics

Contraceptive hormones exert their action by binding to different types of receptors, modulating gene transcription in the nucleus, as classically thought, and simultaneously activating various signaling pathways at the cell membrane level.

Actions of Estrogens on Their Receptors

Estrogens act by binding to three types of receptors: the alpha and beta estrogen receptors, and the G protein-coupled oestrogen receptor (GPER). The alpha and beta receptors are hormone-inducible transcription factors, very similar to each other. and differ mainly in their location in different organs, or even in different tissues of the same organ. The alpha receptors are in the uterus, ovarian theca cells, breast, liver and in the muscle cells of the uterine arteries; whereas the beta receptors are found in the bone marrow, brain, ovarian granulosa cells, and in the endothelial cells of the endometrial vessels (Stanczyk, Winer, et al. 2024). E2 has an equal affinity for ER alpha and beta. In relation to the affinity of E2, estrone has 10% affinity for ER alpha and 2% for ER beta; and E3, 10% with ER alpha, and 35% with ER beta. The binding affinity of EE for ER alpha was twice that of E2, but only half for ER beta; and E4 has minimal affinity for ER alpha and beta (3-4%) (Zhu et al. 2006).

Although alpha and beta receptors act at the nuclear level in DNA activation, part of the alpha receptors also participate in intracellular signaling cascades called membrane-initiated steroid signaling (Cheskis et al. 2007; Stanczyk, Winer, et al. 2024), together with GPER, participating in a large set of actions throughout the organism (Prossnitz y Barton 2023; Bartkowiak-Wieczorek et al. 2024).

Stetrol is not involved in this membrane signaling linked to the alpha-receptor (Gérard et al. 2022). E4 can activate the nuclear ER alpha but instead antagonizes the membrane ER, unlike other estrogens. Precisely because of this fact, it has agonist activity in the uterus, in the brain (flushing, inhibition of ovulation, etc.) and in the bones, mixed agonist and antagonist activities in the breast and an almost neutral character in the liver (Douxfils et al. 2022), so it is considered as a selective estrogen receptor modulator. The action of these membrane alpha receptors in the vascular system is responsible for most of the beneficial effects of E4 on the vascular system including enhancement of nitric oxide production, vasodilation and prevention of atherosclerosis, neointimal proliferation and hypertension. In mammary tumor tissue, it acts as an estrogen antagonist in the presence of E2 (Fruzzetti et al. 2021; Gérard et al. 2022; Lee y Syed 2022; Paton 2022), and may decrease the proliferation of mammary epithelial cells (Gallez et al. 2021; Frisendahl, Kallner, y Gemzell-Danielsson 2024), so its potential use in breast cancer patients is being studied (Battipaglia et al. 2024).

Actions of Progestogens on the Different Receptors

Progestogens exert modulatory effects on the endometrium and exhibit antigonadotrophic action. Their activity is due both to genomic interactions with progestin receptors (PR-A and PR-B) and to rapid non-genomic actions on the cell surface. In most tissues, the action of progestogens depends on estrogens, since estrogens induce the expression of gestagen receptors, while progestogens reduce the expression of estrogen receptors (Capozzi, Scambia, y Lello 2022).

In addition, progestogens can interact with different types of receptors (estrogenic, androgenic, glucocorticoid and mineralocorticoid), acting as agonists or antagonists depending on the context. All progestogens share progestogenic, antigonadotrophic and antiestrogenic activity. Let us look at some of the peculiarities of these progestins that may have clinical influence. Nestorone does not bind to androgen receptors, but does bind to the glucocorticoid receptor, although without any clinical repercussions. It has a high contraceptive efficacy as it is the most potent progestin, with the highest anti-ovulatory activity of the existing progestogens (Sitruk-Ware y Nath 2013). Nomegestrol acetate is a derivative of 19-norprogesterone. It is a potent antigonadotropic in women, with a high progestational action, although less than that of nesterone and trimegestone. It is a potent agonist of PRG receptors to which it binds with high affinity. It has no androgenic, estrogenic or glucocorticoid action (Sitruk-Ware y Nath 2010; 2013). It has mild to moderate anti-androgenic properties (Burke 2013). Dienogest has a potent anti-androgenic action, which is 40% of that of cyproterone; and direct anti-proliferative and anti-inflammatory effect on the endometrium (Sitruk-Ware y Nath 2010; 2013). Drospirenone has antiandrogenic, antimineralcorticoid and antigonadotropic activity, without androgenic, estrogenic, glucocorticoid or antiglucocorticoid activity (Krattenmacher 2000; Schindler et al. 2008; Chiara Del Savio et al. 2020; Capozzi, Scambia, y Lello 2022).

Mechanism of Action

Combined Hormonal Contraception

Estrogens and progestins inhibit ovulation, but progestogen is considered to be the main factor involved in this inhibition, which is enhanced by estrogen (Stanczyk, Winer, et al. 2024). Progestogen blocks LH secretion and the LH peak, thus preventing ovulation, and estrogen blocks FSH, thus preventing the appearance of a dominant follicle, as evidenced by the absence of follicular growth on ultrasound and the low levels of estradiol and progesterone (Rivera, Yacobson, y Grimes 1999; Taylor et al. 2020). Ovulation inhibition is achieved by interfering with GnRh secretion in the hypothalamus. There is also a direct suppressive effect on the gonadotropin-producing cells of the pituitary gland. Therefore, there is suppression of the amplitude without reduction of the frequency of the FSH and LH pulse (Lobo y Stanczyk 1994; Rivera, Yacobson, y Grimes 1999). These effects are independent of the estrogen or progestogen used, or their doses (Rossmanith, Steffens, y Schramm 1997; I. Duijkers et al. 2021; Paton 2022). There is also evidence of direct ovarian effects including inhibition of follicular development and atresia, which are achieved even at a dose lower than that required to achieve anovulation (Lobo y Stanczyk 1994).

There are also changes in the cervical mucus, with a reduction in its quantity, increase in its thickness and reduction in its thinning, all of which impede the penetration of spermatozoa (Lobo y Stanczyk 1994; Rivera, Yacobson, y Grimes 1999), effect that persists with lower doses (Rossmanith, Steffens, y Schramm 1997).

Effects on the endometrium include suppression of the glands, resulting in a decidualized reaction with atrophic changes and a nearly denuded endometrium (Lobo y Stanczyk 1994; Rivera, Yacobson, y Grimes 1999). This endometrial atrophy is revealed by ultrasound measurement of endometrial thickness, which is less than 8 mm even with low-dose ACHO (20 μg EE with 500 μg norestisterone; or 20 μg EE with 150 μg DSG) (Rossmanith, Steffens, y Schramm 1997). Given the potent effect on ovulation inhibition, it is unlikely that endometrial changes play an important role, if any, in the observed contraceptive efficacy of combined oral contraceptives (Rivera, Yacobson, y Grimes 1999). In response to this atrophying action of gestagen, estrogen stabilizes the endometrium (Taylor et al. 2020).

Oral Contraception with Progestogens (POP)

Different levels of ovulation inhibition are achieved, depending on the preparation used. Studies with norgestrel report a high variability of ovulation inhibition, ranging from 14 to 84% (McCann y Potter 1994; Glasier et al. 2022). When levonorgestrel is used at a dose of 30 μg, 28% of women have ovulation (C. F. Rice et al. 1999), and it is necessary to increase it up to 115 μg/day to achieve ovulation inhibition, although follicular activity may persist (I. J. M. Duijkers et al. 2022). However, 75 μg Desogestrel is sufficient to inhibit ovulation, although follicular activity and growth may persist (C. Rice et al. 1996; C. F. Rice et al. 1999). In short, depending on the progestagen and the dose used, 40% of women with progestagen-only pill could ovulate. In other cases, there is follicular activity, but the corpus luteum does not form, or there are signs of luteal insufficiency (Rivera, Yacobson, y Grimes 1999; Taylor et al. 2020)

Traditionally, action on cervical mucus has been considered important for the action of POP. The volume of cervical mucus is greatly reduced in the middle of the cycle, its viscosity and cellular content is increased, and its molecular structure is altered, making sperm penetration and motility more difficult (McCann y Potter 1994; C. Rice et al. 1996; Rivera, Yacobson, y Grimes 1999; Han et al. 2022, 075). Even among ovulating women, some mucus alteration is observed and no user is considered as unprotected mucus (Insler test ≥ 9) (Han et al. 2022, 075). With the first preparations, this effect appeared 2-4 h after oral intake and persisted for 22-24h, which required being very careful with the intake, without delays (Taylor et al. 2020).

It is thought that the effects at the endometrial level could be one of the methods of action of POP. When the endometrium is studied in POP users, a series of histological alterations are found. In some cases, there is normal endometrial secretory activity; but in most cases, different types of abnormalities are identified, such as atrophy, proliferative activity, which may be suppressed, or irregular secretory activity (McCann y Potter 1994; Bastianelli et al. 2020). With prolonged use, the endometrium atrophies, the glands become small and scanty, lined by a low columnar epithelium with abundant stroma, and the superficial vessels are thin-walled and ectatic (Bastianelli et al. 2020).

Progestogen Intrauterine Device (IUD-LNG)

With the three existing models of this device, FSH is at normal levels and ovarian follicles can be found (Apter et al. 2014; Goldstuck y Le 2018). After Mirena insertion there are initially serum levels of ~200pg/ml, which is around the threshold for ovulation inhibition, which is why up to 40% of users do not ovulate. As serum LNG levels decrease over time, so does ovulation inhibition (Xiao et al. 1990), and ovulation may occur even in amenorrheic women. With Jaydess and Kyleena the LH peak is not suppressed, and 95% of cycles are ovulatory (Apter et al. 2014; Goldstuck y Le 2018).

The contraceptive efficacy of LNG-IUD is maintained even with very low serum levels of levonorgestrel, since intrauterine release rates of LNG as low as 3μg/day are sufficient to produce changes in cervical mucus and endometrium. The nature of the cervical mucus is altered, with decreased viscosity and increased cellularity, which prevents the passage of spermatozoa, as evidenced by a decrease in the Insler score (Apter et al. 2014; Han, Taub, y Jensen 2017; Goldstuck y Le 2018). Of all the progestogens the alteration of cervical mucus as a mechanism of action of LNG-IUD is the one that has been best demonstrated (Han, Taub, y Jensen 2017). With the use of progestogen-releasing IUDs, there is alteration of the structure and function of the endometrium. The endometrial glands are atrophic, and the stroma is decidualized, this change being more marked at the beginning of their use. Leukocytic infiltrates with plasma cells, and foci of hemorrhagic infarction, necrobiosis or necrosis, and scarring are seen, and areas of calcification can be found after 3 years of use. Rarely, some proliferative activity may appear, and occasionally, microscopic and edematous superficial micropapillae were observed (Silverberg et al. 1986; Critchley et al. 1998; Goldstuck y Le 2018; Bastianelli et al. 2020). With Jaydess and Kyleena, all endometrium also has this effect of progestogens (Apter et al. 2014). No relationship between endometrial changes and the occurrence of bleeding during IUD use (Critchley et al. 1998).

Alteration of tubal motility and function has been described (Goldstuck y Le 2018), although the degree of involvement of these changes in contraceptive efficacy is unknown.

Progestogen Implant

With Norplant (levonorgestrel-releasing implant), about half of the women could ovulate, but in these women there are no normal cycles, but often altered cycles, with insufficient corpus luteum (McCann y Potter 1994; Rivera, Yacobson, y Grimes 1999; Taylor et al. 2020). With other implants, ovulation is inhibited in 80% of the cycles in the first year, decreasing to 50% at the end of 5 years, although it seems that many of these ovulations are dysfunctional (Mäkäräinen et al. 1998; Croxatto 2002). The Implanon implant consistently blocks ovulation. At 3 years of use, the release rate of ENG is ~ 25-30 μg/day and this invariably produces serum ENG levels of >90pg/ml, which is the approximate level of ovulation inhibition, and only in less than 3% of cycles is progesterone detected. However, FSH secretion is not inhibited, so follicular development occurs, with estradiol secretion (Mäkäräinen et al. 1998; Bennink 2000; Croxatto 2002).

Cervical mucus thickens, increases in viscosity and decreases in quantity, forming a barrier that prevents the passage of sperm (Bennink 2000; Croxatto 2002; Han, Taub, y Jensen 2017; Taylor et al. 2020).

With progestogen implants, the endometrium is inactive or weakly proliferative in 50% of users, menstrual type in 15% and suggestive of endometrial alteration in 25% (Bennink 2000; Croxatto 2002). At the end of the first year, endometrial thickness is significantly reduced, when the endometrium becomes inactive or weakly proliferative. Long-term administration induces a variety of changes ranging from an atrophic picture to evidence of endometrial detachment and some proliferation. Occasionally there may be secretory changes (Bastianelli et al. 2020). The endometrial effect appears more marked in implants with etonogestrel (Mäkäräinen et al. 1998).

Medroxyprogesterone Acetate Depot Injection

It is somewhat different from other progestogens, since the circulating levels of hormone it produces are sufficient to block the LH peak, thus inhibiting ovulation, although as it does not suppress follicular growth and estradiol production are at levels similar to an early follicular phase of the natural cycle (Lobo y Stanczyk 1994; Rivera, Yacobson, y Grimes 1999; Taylor et al. 2020). As with the other progestogens, cervical mucus becomes thin and thick, making sperm penetration unlikely (Rivera, Yacobson, y Grimes 1999). Endometrial changes initially consist of a gestational-type glandular hyperplasia with a markedly decidualized stroma. Over time, this picture develops into endometrial atrophy, characterized by a reduced density of dilated, thin-walled superficial vessels and microvessels (Bastianelli et al. 2020).

Metabolic Effects

Effects on Carbohydrate Metabolism

High and medium doses of oral hormonal contraceptives with EE may decrease glucose tolerance and increase insulin resistance, especially those containing androgenic gestagens (Cree et al. 2024), although at low doses these effects are usually mild and transitory, with no relevant clinical impact in non-diabetic women (Bastianelli et al. 2017; Inka Wiegratz y Kuhl 2006; Lopez, Grimes, y Schulz 2019; Silva-Bermudez et al. 2020). Contraceptives combining estradiol (Ågren et al. 2011; Burke 2013) or E4/DRSP (Gérard et al. 2022; Lee y Syed 2022) have minimal or no impact on carbohydrate metabolism. In general, progestogens can induce insulin resistance, compensated by an increase in insulin secretion, but blood levels of glucose, insulin or C-peptide are not altered (Crook et al. 1993; Inka Wiegratz y Kuhl 2006).

Etonogestrel implant is not associated with changes in blood glucose levels (Cristina A. F. Guazzelli et al. 2011).

In any case, follow-up studies have shown that hormonal contraceptives do not increase the risk of developing diabetes mellitus, even in patients with impaired carbohydrate metabolism or a history of gestational diabetes. In practice, even insulin-dependent diabetic patients can take the new contraceptive formulations, after weighing the beneficial contraceptive effects against the risk of thrombosis they present. No differences in metabolic changes depending on vaginal or oral administration (Mohamed, El-Sherbiny, y Mostafa 2011).

Prolonged use also does not impair carbohydrate metabolism, and observed changes in glucose tolerance or insulin resistance are usually mild and reversible over time (Lopez, Grimes, y Schulz 2019; I Wiegratz et al. 2010).

Effects on the Liver

Estrogens influence the synthesis of DNA, RNA, liver enzymes and plasma proteins, and can alter the transport of biliary components, as can some progestogens. Although combined hormonal contraceptives are not hepatotoxic and do not cause hepatic necrosis, their use is associated with a slightly increased risk of gallstones in the early years, especially in predisposed women, although this effect is usually not clinically relevant. Even in experimental animals, a decrease in hepatic fibrosis has been shown with the intake of CHC (Soria-Jasso et al. 2019). In most studies, no changes in transaminase levels are observed (Cristina A. F. Guazzelli et al. 2011; Özcan et al. 2024); and if they increase, they do so moderately and without reaching clearly abnormal levels (Kowalska et al. 2018).

The high concentration of steroids in the portal vein after oral administration of CHC significantly impacts the synthesis of various liver proteins, such as sexual hormone binding globulin (SHBG), corticosteroid binding globulin, thyroid binding globulin, angiotensinogen and coagulation factors (A. B. Edelman, Cherala, y Stanczyk 2010). Ethinylestradiol, especially orally, markedly increases SHBG synthesis, an effect that is much smaller when administered vaginally (Roumen y Mishell 2012), or transdermally (Devineni et al. 2007), whereas MPA intramuscularly decreases it (Avenant et al. 2024).

On the other hand, combined oral contraceptives containing estetrol have a much more limited impact on liver function and plasma protein levels compared to preparations based on ethinylestradiol and levonorgestrel or drospirenone (Fruzzetti et al. 2021; Paton 2022).

Effect on Coagulation Factors

The relationship between the use of combined hormonal contraceptives and the risk of thrombosis has been extensively studied. CHCs modify most of the proteins involved in the coagulation and fibrinolysis systems (Douxfils, Morimont, y Bouvy 2020), so the relationship between these changes and thrombosis is investigated.

Estrogens increase the activity of several coagulation factors (I, II, VII, VIII, IX, X, XI and XII) by approximately 30 to 50%; and decrease protein S (Samsioe 1994; I. Wiegratz et al. 2004; Inka Wiegratz y Kuhl 2006; Sitruk-Ware y Nath 2011; Douxfils, Morimont, y Bouvy 2020). As a consequence of decreased protein S activity, the development of acquired resistance to activated protein C (APC), a prothrombotic state, is favored (Douxfils, Morimont, y Bouvy 2020). However, these effects are partially compensated by the increase in antithrombin III, protein C and fibrinolytic activity, maintaining a certain hemostatic balance (Samsioe 1994; I. Wiegratz et al. 2004; Sitruk-Ware y Nath 2011; Farris et al. 2017; Inka Wiegratz y Kuhl 2006).

Ethinylestradiol is primarily responsible for these alterations (Sitruk-Ware y Nath 2010), although the dose and type of progestogen also play a role (Stanczyk, Archer, y Bhavnani 2013). Lower dose ethinylestradiol preparations have similar, but smaller magnitude changes (Farris et al. 2017). Attempts have been made to associate the thrombotic risk mainly with resistance to activated protein C induced by the estrogenic component, which would be attenuated by decreased estrogenic activity and increased androgenic activity of contraceptive preparations (Inka Wiegratz y Kuhl 2006; Douxfils, Morimont, y Bouvy 2020; Gemzell-Danielsson et al. 2022; Gérard et al. 2022; Skeith y Bates 2024). In addition, other mechanisms such as upregulation of the thrombin receptor and altered venous flow may contribute to thrombotic risk (Inka Wiegratz y Kuhl 2006). No significant effects on platelet aggregation have been observed (Samsioe 1994). There is no direct correlation between changes in coagulation factors and the risk of thrombosis, and these parameters are not predictive of thrombosis risk (Sitruk-Ware y Nath 2010).

After discontinuation of CHC, hemostatic parameters usually normalize in 4 to 8 weeks (Robinson et al. 1991), which justifies discontinuing their use before this time in case of major surgery. However, resistance to activated protein C seems to recover immediately after cessation of their use (Inka Wiegratz y Kuhl 2006).

Contraceptives with estradiol have a lower impact on clotting factors and APC resistance compared to those containing ethinylestradiol (Junge et al. 2011; Burke 2013; Lete et al. 2015; Haverinen et al. 2022); and it appears that it may be even lower with estetrol (Fruzzetti et al. 2021; Douxfils et al. 2020; Gemzell-Danielsson et al. 2022; Gérard et al. 2022; Lee y Syed 2022; Morimont et al. 2022) resulting in a lower thrombotic risk (Reed et al. 2021; Bauerfeind et al. 2024; Douxfils et al. 2024; Didembourg et al. 2025).

Medroxyprogesterone acetate has been shown to increase thrombin receptor, thrombin-induced tissue factor production and procoagulatory activity in the vascular wall, possibly due to its glucocorticoid activity (Sitruk-Ware y Nath 2011). The remaining progestogens do not produce changes in coagulation factors or protein C resistance, regardless of the way by which they are administered (Samsioe 1994; Chiara Del Savio et al. 2020; Blanco-Molina et al. 2012; Skeith y Bates 2024).

Actions on Lipid Metabolism

Ethinylestradiol increases VLDL secretion and stimulates apolipoprotein A synthesis, which raises HDL levels (Silva-Bermudez et al. 2020). With increased VLDL, an increase in LDL values can be seen, without clinical impact (Silva-Bermudez et al. 2020; Staudt et al. 2024), although reduced endothelial lipoprotein lipase activity and increased hepatic LDL uptake together lead to a net decrease in LDL levels (Inka Wiegratz y Kuhl 2006). The effects of progestogens on lipids vary according to their androgenic activity: progestins such as LNG and NET can counteract the dose-dependent increase in triglycerides and HDL induced by EE, whereas three-phase combinations with levonorgestrel do not significantly alter HDL, LDL or apoprotein levels (Inka Wiegratz y Kuhl 2006; Staudt et al. 2024). Desogestrel has a slightly favorable effect on the lipid profile, while gestodene is neutral (Sitruk-Ware y Nath 2011), and medroxyprogesterone acetate can slightly reduce triglycerides and HDL and increase LDLv (Inka Wiegratz y Kuhl 2006). For its part, drospirenone associated with EE increases HDL without substantially modifying LDL (Sitruk-Ware y Nath 2011). Overall, estrogens, alone or combined with progestins, induce a favorable lipid profile, mainly by reducing LDL and increasing HDL, which explains part of their cardiovascular protective effect.

EE combined with different progestogens can increase triglycerides (Silva-Bermudez et al. 2020; Inka Wiegratz y Kuhl 2006), although these changes are usually mild and do not significantly affect the lipid profile after one year of use (Stanczyk, Archer, y Bhavnani 2013).

CHCs with natural estrogens do not change LDL and HDL levels (Ågren et al. 2011); or increase HDL and decrease LDL (Sitruk-Ware y Nath 2011; Junge et al. 2011; Bastianelli et al. 2017; Silva-Bermudez et al. 2020). On the other hand, nomegestrol acetate shows no relevant effects on lipid profile (Sitruk-Ware y Nath 2010; Burke 2013). Comparing ring versus oral, there is no difference in lipid metabolism (Cristina Aparecida Falbo Guazzelli et al. 2012)

Contraceptives with estetrol (E4) and drospirenone (DRSP) have minimal impact on LDL levels, while slightly increasing HDL and triglyceride (TG) levels, although to a lesser extent than EE/DRSP formulations, suggesting minimal impact on lipid metabolism (Mawet et al. 2015; Fruzzetti et al. 2021; Gérard et al. 2022; Lee y Syed 2022).

With etonogestrel implantation there is a decrease in TG and LDL levels, with no change in HDL levels (Cristina A. F. Guazzelli et al. 2011). With the vaginal route, there is also a decrease in LDL (Mohamed, El-Sherbiny, y Mostafa 2011).

Despite these lipid alterations, low-dose combined hormonal contraceptives have not been shown to increase the risk of atherogenesis in women. Even in primate studies, although less favorable lipid profiles are observed, there is less atherosclerotic plaque formation (Inka Wiegratz y Kuhl 2006). In conclusion, CHC-induced lipid changes do not translate into increased cardiovascular risk in current clinical practice.

Effects on Bones

Estrogens favor bone maintenance, due to their antiabsorptive (inhibiting bone resorption by suppressing osteoclast formation) and anabolic (favoring bone formation) effects, and by reducing the rate of bone remodeling by modulating the activity of osteoclasts and osteoblasts (Nappi et al. 2012; Hadji, Colli, y Regidor 2019). In turn, progestogens, at physiological doses, have osteoanabolic activity; but at supraphysiological doses, they can inhibit osteoblastic differentiation (Nappi et al. 2012; Rocca et al. 2021). During puberty, estrogens have a biphasic effect on periosteal bone. In early puberty, low estrogen levels stimulate bone accumulation, whereas, in late puberty, their higher concentrations inhibit periosteal bone apposition. The exact concentration of estradiol associated with this change and the role of growth hormone (GH) and other factors are still under investigation (Trémollieres 2013).

The evidence on the impact of CHCs on bone mass is inconclusive because most studies are observational designs with contradictory results; conducted with great variability in preparations, doses and user profiles (age, baseline bone mass status). Bone mineral density (BMD) is an indicator of bone strength. Bone mass develops gradually during childhood, and undergoes rapid growth during puberty and adolescence (Rocca et al. 2021).

Early studies on the use of CHC in adolescents indicated that their use may hinder optimal bone mass acquisition, especially when initiated a few years after menarche and before reaching peak bone mass (Martins, Curtis, y Glasier 2006; Sarfati y de Vernejoul 2009; Nappi et al. 2012; Trémollieres 2013; Bastianelli et al. 2017). These data are confirmed by a Canadian study (Brajic et al. 2018) that showed that adolescent girls aged 16 to 19 years who used CHC had lower bone mineral density gain at the femoral neck, hip, and lumbar spine compared to non-users. However, in women aged 20 to 24 years, the use of CHC was associated with a more favorable evolution of BMD in the femoral neck. Two meta-analyses in adolescents (Goshtasebi et al. 2019; Lim, Said, y Latthe 2025) have related a smaller increase or slowing of bone accumulation and a reduction in bone formation markers in CHC users versus nonusers, although the difference was small, and with high heterogeneity between studies. Regarding progestogens, in general they do not affect bone mass, except for medroxyprogesterone acetate, which can be associated with a slight annual reduction (1-2%) in BMD in adolescents, an effect that is reversible upon discontinuation of treatment (Guilbert et al. 2009; Nappi et al. 2012; Lopez et al. 2014; Rocca et al. 2021). However, this effect does not contraindicate its use or limit its duration, and neither routine BMD monitoring nor the systematic use of calcium or estrogen supplementation is recommended

In adult women, the use of combined hormonal contraceptives, including estradiol-containing preparations (E2-NOMAC), does not produce significant differences in bone mass compared to non-users (Martins, Curtis, y Glasier 2006; Sarfati y de Vernejoul 2009; Nappi et al. 2012; Burke 2013; Rocca et al. 2021). Nor have negative effects on bone density been observed in athletes (Redinger y Baker 2022), or in women with premature ovarian failure, where there may even be a protective effect (Bastianelli et al. 2017). Medroxyprogesterone acetate may be associated with a slight decrease in bone mineral density in adults, but this effect is small, reversible after discontinuation of treatment and does not exceed one standard deviation (Guilbert et al. 2009; Sarfati y de Vernejoul 2009; Nappi et al. 2012; Rocca et al. 2021). Other oral progestogens and implants, such as Implanon, do not adversely affect bone mass, as ovarian estradiol production is sufficient for its maintenance (Bennink 2000; Sarfati y de Vernejoul 2009; Nappi et al. 2012; Rocca et al. 2021). Changes are also not observed with the levonorgestrel IUD (LNG-IUD) (Nappi et al. 2012; Rocca et al. 2021).

During perimenopause, the data are somewhat contradictory: some studies show no change in BMD, while others suggest that HC can reduce age-associated bone loss, even with low doses of ethinyl estradiol, pointing to a possible beneficial effect at this stage (Nappi et al. 2012; Trémollieres 2013; Bastianelli et al. 2017; Kim et al. 2022).

The effects of combined hormonal contraceptives on the risk of bone fracture have been evaluated in several systematic reviews, based on observational studies, in the absence of clinical trials.The available evidence based on these studies of varying quality, indicates that the use of CHCs is not associated with an increased risk of fracture in women of any age, although data specific to adolescents and women in perimenopause remain limited (Martins, Curtis, y Glasier 2006; Lopez et al. 2015). Two more recent studies, support these data. In the first, there is a reduction in fractures, mainly between the ages of 18 and 25 years, and with no differences found between 45 and 55 years (Dombrowski et al. 2017); and in the second, neither the use of contraceptives, nor their duration is related to the occurrence of fractures (Farahmand et al. 2024). In summary, current scientific evidence indicates that CHCs do not increase the risk of bone fractures in the general population.

With respect to other hormonal methods, the levonorgestrel-releasing IUD has been associated in some studies with a reduction in fracture risk (Lopez et al. 2015; Hadji, Colli, y Regidor 2019). In contrast, the data on medroxyprogesterone acetate are less conclusive, ranging from no risk (Sarfati y de Vernejoul 2009)), to an increased risk, especially with prolonged use and in young women or women older than 50 years, although the absolute magnitude of this risk is small (Lopez et al. 2015).

Effects on Blood Pressure

With the first contraceptives, an increase in arterial hypertension was found in 5% of CHC users (Woods 1988). With current contraceptives, a slight increase in blood pressure (BP)may occur, but generally does not reach pathological levels (Stanczyk, Archer, y Bhavnani 2013; Takeda et al. 2021; Cameron, Blyler, y Bello 2023; Staudt et al. 2024; de Souza et al. 2024; Piersol y Buckman 2025), with a greater impact on CHC with gestodene (de Souza et al. 2024); whereas with drospirenone there is a decrease in BP (Krattenmacher 2000; de Souza et al. 2024). This response seems to be greater during exercise, since after exertion, diastolic BP remains higher in oral contraceptive users, possibly due to greater sympathetic activity (Takeda et al. 2021), although it is not yet clear whether this may contribute to the development of long-term hypertension. Contraceptives with estradiol or estetrol do not increase BP (Cameron, Blyler, y Bello 2023). Progestogens do not increase BP (Cameron, Blyler, y Bello 2023; Singer et al. 2025).

No significant increase in the incidence of arterial hypertension has been observed in women using modern combined hormonal contraceptives. Although in isolated cases there may be an idiosyncratic reaction with the development of hypertension, which justifies the need for regular clinical control (Bhullar, Rabinovich-Nikitin, y Kirshenbaum 2024).

Mineralcorticoid Effect

Ethinylestradiol increases hepatic production of angiotensinogen, which elevates the substrate available for renin. This promotes the formation of angiotensin I and II, increasing aldosterone levels. In response, a negative feedback mechanism is activated that reduces renin concentration, although its activity remains elevated. These changes tend to attenuate with prolonged use of EE (Inka Wiegratz y Kuhl 2006). As for the progestogens, most of them (levonorgestrel, norethisterone acetate, 3-ketodesogestrel and cyproterone acetate) lack significant mineralocorticoid and antimineralocorticoid activity at contraceptive doses. Gestodene also has no relevant activity in this regard (Inka Wiegratz y Kuhl 2006; Singer et al. 2025). However, drospirenone stands out for its potent antimineralocorticoid effect, promoting sodium excretion without affecting potassium excretion, and elevating plasma and urinary renin and aldosterone activity (Krattenmacher 2000; Singer et al. 2025). The combination of estetrol with drospirenone also does not stimulate the renin-angiotensin-aldosterone system (Gérard et al. 2022).

Antiandrogenic Effect

Contraceptives containing progestogens with higher androgenic activity may cause androgenic side effects, such as acne or hirsutism, especially in predisposed women. In these cases, the use of combinations of EE with progestogens with anti-androgenic action is recommended. However, the clinical improvement on acne or hirsutism with these preparations is only slightly superior to that of other estrogen-dominant contraceptives (Inka Wiegratz y Kuhl 2006).

All currently used ACHOs have an anti-androgenic effect, because of:

- *Reduction of androgen synthesis*: They decrease ovarian and adrenal production of androgens and their precursors (effect observed with NET, LNG, NGM, DG and GSD).
- *Increased SHBG:* EE increases hepatic production of sex hormone binding globulin, which reduces the free fraction of androgens. This effect can be counteracted by androgenic progestogens, so the final SHBG level depends on both the dose of EE and the properties of the progestogen. Preparations with anti-androgenic progestins (CPA, DNG, DSR, CMA) significantly elevate SHBG, although they have little effect on androgen synthesis.
- *5α-reductase inhibition*: Some contraceptives inhibit this enzyme, decreasing the conversion of testosterone to dihydrotestosterone, a more potent androgen (Krattenmacher 2000; Rabe et al. 2000).

Taken together, these mechanisms explain the usefulness of hormonal contraceptives in the management of hyperandrogenic disorders, although the clinical difference between the various preparations is usually modest, except in the cases of drospirenone and cyproterone acetate, which have the greatest antiandrogenic efficacy.

Conclusion

For decades, EE has been the estrogen used, so that the analysis of the effects of contraception, its benefits and risks, is based on the use of this estrogen. However, the progressive reduction of its dose and the incorporation of new progestogens have transformed this scenario, providing new pharmacological profiles that may offer specific clinical advantages.

Finally, the emergence of innovative compounds such as estetrol opens promising avenues for maintaining contraceptive efficacy with a less intense systemic burden, which could translate into a lower incidence of thrombotic events and an improved cardiovascular profile.

References

Abrams, Larry S., Donna M. Skee, Jaya Natarajan, Frankie A. Wong, y Gary D. Anderson. 2002. "Pharmacokinetics of a Contraceptive Patch (Evra/Ortho Evra) Containing Norelgestromin and Ethinyloestradiol at Four Application Sites." *British Journal of Clinical Pharmacology* 53 (2): 141-46. https://doi.org/10.1046/j.0306-5251.2001.01532.x.

Ågren, Ulla M., Marjatta Anttila, Kristiina Mäenpää-Liukko, Maija-Liisa Rantala, Hilkka Rautiainen, Werner F. Sommer, y Ellen Mommers. 2011. "Effects of a Monophasic Combined Oral Contraceptive Containing Nomegestrol Acetate and 17β-Oestradiol Compared with One Containing Levonorgestrel and Ethinylestradiol on Haemostasis, Lipids and Carbohydrate Metabolism." *The European Journal of Contraception & Reproductive Health Care: The Official Journal of the European Society of Contraception* 16 (6): 444-57. https://doi.org/10.3109/13625187.2011.604450.

Alemany, Marià. 2021. "Estrogens and the Regulation of Glucose Metabolism." *World Journal of Diabetes* 12 (10): 1622-54. https://doi.org/10.4239/wjd.v12.i10.1622.

Apter, Dan, Kristina Gemzell-Danielsson, Brian Hauck, Kimberly Rosen, y Christian Zurth. 2014. "Pharmacokinetics of Two Low-Dose Levonorgestrel-Releasing Intrauterine Systems and Effects on Ovulation Rate and Cervical Function: Pooled Analyses of Phase II and III Studies." *Fertility and Sterility* 101 (6): 1656-1662.e1-4. https://doi.org/10.1016/j.fertnstert.2014.03.004.

Avenant, Chanel, Mandisa Singata-Madliki, Alexis J. Bick, Donita Africander, Yusentha Balakrishna, Karl-Heinz Storbeck, Johnson M. Moliki, et al. 2024. "The Injectable Contraceptives Depot Medroxyprogesterone Acetate and Norethisterone Enanthate Substantially and Differentially Decrease Testosterone and Sex Hormone Binding Globulin Levels: A Secondary Study from the WHICH Randomized Clinical Trial." *PloS One* 19 (8): e0307736. https://doi.org/10.1371/journal.pone.0307736.

Bartkowiak-Wieczorek, Joanna, Agnieszka Jaros, Anna Gajdzińska, Paulina Wojtyła-Buciora, Igor Szymański, Julian Szymaniak, Wojciech Janusz, Iga Walczak, Gabriela Jonaszka, y Agnieszka Bienert. 2024. "The Dual Faces of Oestrogen: The Impact of Exogenous Oestrogen on the Physiological and Pathophysiological Functions of Tissues and Organs." *International Journal of Molecular Sciences* 25 (15): 8167. https://doi.org/10.3390/ijms25158167.

Bastianelli, Carlo, Manuela Farris, Vincenzina Bruni, Elena Rosato, Ivo Brosens, y Giuseppe Benagiano. 2020. "Effects of Progestin-Only Contraceptives on the Endometrium." *Expert Review of Clinical Pharmacology*, septiembre. https://doi.org/10.1080/17512433.2020.1821649.

Bastianelli, Carlo, Manuela Farris, Elena Rosato, Ivo Brosens, y Giuseppe Benagiano. 2017. "Pharmacodynamics of Combined Estrogen-Progestin Oral Contraceptives: 1. Effects on Metabolism."

Expert Review of Clinical Pharmacology 10 (3): 315-26. https://doi.org/10.1080/17512433.2017.1271708.

Battipaglia, Christian, Alessandro D. Genazzani, Rossella E. Nappi, y Antonio La Marca. 2024. "Insights on Estetrol, the Native Estrogen: From Contraception to Hormone Replacement Therapy." *Minerva Obstetrics and Gynecology*, septiembre. https://doi.org/10.23736/S2724-606X.24.05594-5.

Bauerfeind, Anja, Sophia von Stockum, Tanja Boehnke, y Klaas Heinemann. 2024. "Venous Thromboembolic Risk of Estradiol Valerate-Dienogest Compared with Ethinyl Estradiol-Levonorgestrel Combined Oral Contraceptives." *Obstetrics and Gynecology* 143 (3): 431-34. https://doi.org/10.1097/AOG.0000000000005509.

Bennink, H. J. 2000. "The Pharmacokinetics and Pharmacodynamics of Implanon, a Single-Rod Etonogestrel Contraceptive Implant." *The European Journal of Contraception & Reproductive Health Care: The Official Journal of the European Society of Contraception* 5 Suppl 2 (septiembre):12-20.

Bhullar, Sukhwinder K., Inna Rabinovich-Nikitin, y Lorrie Kirshenbaum. 2024. "Oral Hormonal Contraceptives and Cardiovascular Risks in Females." *Canadian Journal of Physiology and Pharmacology*, mayo. https://doi.org/10.1139/cjpp-2024-0041.

Bick, Alexis J., Renate Louw-du Toit, Salndave B. Skosana, Donita Africander, y Janet P. Hapgood. 2021. "Pharmacokinetics, Metabolism and Serum Concentrations of Progestins Used in Contraception." *Pharmacology & Therapeutics* 222 (junio):107789. https://doi.org/10.1016/j.pharmthera.2020.107789.

Biskupska-Bodova, Kristina, Joanna Sójka-Kupny, Tamás Nyirády, Anne E. Burke, Alicyoy Angulo, y Pedro Antonio Regidor. 2025. "A Randomised Double-Blind Trial to Determine the Bleeding Profile of the Prolonged-Release Contraceptive Dienogest 2 Mg/Ethinylestradiol 0.02 Mg versus an Immediate-Release Formulation of Drospirenone 3 Mg/Ethinylestradiol 0.02 Mg." *The European Journal of Contraception & Reproductive Health Care: The Official Journal of the European Society of Contraception* 30 (1): 3-12. https://doi.org/10.1080/13625187.2024.2398433.

Bjarnadóttir, Ragnheidur I., Marjo Tuppurainen, y Stephen R. Killick. 2002. "Comparison of Cycle Control with a Combined Contraceptive Vaginal Ring and Oral Levonorgestrel/Ethinyl Estradiol." *American Journal of Obstetrics and Gynecology* 186 (3): 389-95. https://doi.org/10.1067/mob.2002.121103.

Blanco-Molina, M. A., M. Lozano, A. Cano, I. Cristobal, L. P. Pallardo, y I. Lete. 2012. "Progestin-Only Contraception and Venous Thromboembolism." *Thrombosis Research* 129 (5): e257-262. https://doi.org/10.1016/j.thromres.2012.02.042.

Brajic, Tatjana S., Claudie Berger, Katharina Schlammerl, Heather Macdonald, Shirin Kalyan, David A. Hanley, Jonathan D. Adachi, Christopher S. Kovacs, Jerilynn C. Prior, y CaMos Research Group. 2018. "Combined Hormonal Contraceptives Use and Bone Mineral Density Changes in Adolescent and Young Women in a Prospective Population-Based Canada-Wide Observational Study." *Journal of Musculoskeletal & Neuronal Interactions* 18 (2): 227-36.

Burke, Anne. 2013. "Nomegestrol Acetate-17b-Estradiol for Oral Contraception." *Patient Preference and Adherence* 7:607-19. https://doi.org/10.2147/PPA.S39371.

Cameron, Natalie A., Ciantel A. Blyler, y Natalie A. Bello. 2023. "Oral Contraceptive Pills and Hypertension: A Review of Current Evidence and Recommendations." *Hypertension (Dallas, Tex.: 1979)* 80 (5): 924-35. https://doi.org/10.1161/HYPERTENSIONAHA.122.20018.

Capozzi, Anna, Giovanni Scambia, y Stefano Lello. 2022. "Clinical Pharmacology of Progestins." *Minerva Obstetrics and Gynecology* 74 (4): 364-76. https://doi.org/10.23736/S2724-606X.21.04881-8.

Cheskis, Boris J., James G. Greger, Sunil Nagpal, y Leonard P. Freedman. 2007. "Signaling by Estrogens." *Journal of Cellular Physiology* 213 (3): 610-17. https://doi.org/10.1002/jcp.21253.

Chiara Del Savio, Maria, Riccardo De Fata, Fabio Facchinetti, y Giovanni Grandi. 2020. "Drospirenone 4 Mg-Only Pill (DOP) in 24+4 Regimen: A New Option for Oral Contraception." *Expert Review of Clinical Pharmacology* 13 (7): 685-94. https://doi.org/10.1080/17512433.2020.1783247.

Cree, Julia M. E., Niamh M. Brennan, Sally D. Poppitt, y Jennifer L. Miles-Chan. 2024. "The Effect of the Oral Contraceptive Pill on Acute Glycaemic Response to an Oral Glucose Bolus in Healthy Young Women: A Randomised Crossover Study." *Nutrients* 16 (20): 3490. https://doi.org/10.3390/nu16203490.

Critchley, H. O., H. Wang, R. L. Jones, R. W. Kelly, T. A. Drudy, A. E. Gebbie, C. H. Buckley, A. S. McNeilly, y A. F. Glasier. 1998. "Morphological and Functional Features of Endometrial Decidualization Following

Long-Term Intrauterine Levonorgestrel Delivery." *Human Reproduction (Oxford, England)* 13 (5): 1218-24. https://doi.org/10.1093/humrep/13.5.1218.

Crook, D., I. F. Godsland, M. Worthington, C. V. Felton, A. J. Proudler, y J. C. Stevenson. 1993. "A Comparative Metabolic Study of Two Low-Estrogen-Dose Oral Contraceptives Containing Desogestrel or Gestodene Progestins." *American Journal of Obstetrics and Gynecology* 169 (5): 1183-89. https://doi.org/10.1016/0002-9378(93)90279-r.

Croxatto, Horacio B. 2002. "Mechanisms That Explain the Contraceptive Action of Progestin Implants for Women." *Contraception* 65 (1): 21-27. https://doi.org/10.1016/s0010-7824(01)00294-3.

Devineni, Damayanthi, Donna Skee, Nicole Vaccaro, Joseph Massarella, Luc Janssens, Katherine D. LaGuardia, y Albert T. Leung. 2007. "Pharmacokinetics and Pharmacodynamics of a Transdermal Contraceptive Patch and an Oral Contraceptive." *Journal of Clinical Pharmacology* 47 (4): 497-509. https://doi.org/10.1177/0091270006297919.

Didembourg, Marie, Médéa Locquet, Lucie Raskin, Babel Tsague Tchimchoua, Jean-Michel Dogné, Charlotte Beaudart, y Jonathan Douxfils. 2025. "Lower Reporting of Venous Thromboembolisms Events with Natural Estrogen-Based Combined Oral Contraceptives Compared to Ethinylestradiol-Containing Pills: A Disproportionality Analysis of the Eudravigilance Database." *Contraception* 142 (febrero):110727. https://doi.org/10.1016/j.contraception.2024.110727.

Dombrowski, S., L. Jacob, P. Hadji, y K. Kostev. 2017. "Oral Contraceptive Use and Fracture Risk-a Retrospective Study of 12,970 Women in the UK." *Osteoporosis International: A Journal Established as Result of Cooperation between the European Foundation for Osteoporosis and the National Osteoporosis Foundation of the USA* 28 (8): 2349-55. https://doi.org/10.1007/s00198-017-4036-x.

Douxfils, Jonathan, Christine Klipping, Ingrid Duijkers, Virginie Kinet, Marie Mawet, Catherine Maillard, Maud Jost, Jan Rosing, y Jean-Michel Foidart. 2020. "Evaluation of the Effect of a New Oral Contraceptive Containing Estetrol and Drospirenone on Hemostasis Parameters." *Contraception* 102 (6): 396-402. https://doi.org/10.1016/j.contraception.2020.08.015.

Douxfils, Jonathan, Laure Morimont, y Céline Bouvy. 2020. "Oral Contraceptives and Venous Thromboembolism: Focus on Testing That May Enable Prediction and Assessment of the Risk." *Seminars in Thrombosis and Hemostasis* 46 (8): 872-86. https://doi.org/10.1055/s-0040-1714140.

Douxfils, Jonathan, Laure Morimont, Ulysse Gaspard, Wulf H. Utian, y Jean-Michel Foidart. 2022. "Estetrol Is Not a SERM but a NEST and Has a Specific Safety Profile on Coagulation." *Thrombosis Research*, septiembre, S0049-3848(22)00387-5. https://doi.org/10.1016/j.thromres.2022.09.007.

Douxfils, Jonathan, Lucie Raskin, Marie Didembourg, Nathalie Donis, Jean-Michel Dogné, Laure Morimont, y Charlotte Beaudart. 2024. "Are Natural Estrogens Used in Contraception at Lower Risk of Venous Thromboembolism than Synthetic Ones? A Systematic Literature Review and Meta-Analysis." *Frontiers in Endocrinology* 15:1428597. https://doi.org/10.3389/fendo.2024.1428597.

Duijkers, Ingrid J. M., Christine Klipping, Tanja Rautenberg, Barbara S. Schug, Prithi S. Kochhar, Hermann Osterwald, y Michael Oettel. 2022. "Effect on Ovarian Activity and Ovulation Inhibition of Different Oral Dosages of Levonorgestrel." *Contraception* 110 (junio):6-15. https://doi.org/10.1016/j.contraception.2022.01.018.

Duijkers, Ingrid, Christine Klipping, Virginie Kinet, Maud Jost, Adriana Bastidas, y Jean-Michel Foidart. 2021. "Effects of an Oral Contraceptive Containing Estetrol and Drospirenone on Ovarian Function." *Contraception* 103 (6): 386-93. https://doi.org/10.1016/j.contraception.2021.03.003.

Edelman, Alison B., Ganesh Cherala, Myrna Y. Munar, Barent Dubois, Martha McInnis, Frank Z. Stanczyk, y Jeffrey T. Jensen. 2013. "Prolonged Monitoring of Ethinyl Estradiol and Levonorgestrel Levels Confirms an Altered Pharmacokinetic Profile in Obese Oral Contraceptives Users." *Contraception* 87 (2): 220-26. https://doi.org/10.1016/j.contraception.2012.10.008.

Edelman, Alison B., Ganesh Cherala, Myrna Y. Munar, Martha McInnis, Frank Z. Stanczyk, y Jeffrey T. Jensen. 2014. "Correcting Oral Contraceptive Pharmacokinetic Alterations Due to Obesity: A Randomized Controlled Trial." *Contraception* 90 (5): 550-56. https://doi.org/10.1016/j.contraception.2014.06.033.

Edelman, Alison B., Ganesh Cherala, y Frank Z. Stanczyk. 2010. "Metabolism and Pharmacokinetics of Contraceptive Steroids in Obese Women: A Review." *Contraception* 82 (4): 314-23. https://doi.org/10.1016/j.contraception.2010.04.016.

Edelman, Alison, Jon D. Hennebold, Kise Bond, Jeong Y. Lim, Ganesh Cherala, Steven W. Blue, Shawn P. Kraft, David W. Erikson, David Archer, y Jeffery Jensen. 2025. "Double Dosing Ulipristal Acetate Emergency Contraception for Individuals with Obesity: A Randomised Crossover Trial." *BMJ Sexual & Reproductive Health* 51 (1): 27-35. https://doi.org/10.1136/bmjsrh-2024-202401.

Edelman, Alison, Jeffrey T. Jensen, Jill Brown, Michael Thomas, David F. Archer, Courtney A. Schreiber, Stephanie Teal, Carolyn Westhoff, Clint Dart, y Diana L. Blithe. 2024. "Emergency Contraception for Individuals Weighing 80 Kg or Greater: A Randomized Trial of 30 Mg Ulipristal Acetate and 1.5 Mg or 3.0 Mg Levonorgestrel." *Contraception* 137 (septiembre):110474. https://doi.org/10.1016/j.contraception.2024.110474.

Farahmand, Maryam, Maryam Rahmati, Marzieh Saei Ghare Naz, Mina Amiri, Mahsa Noroozzadeh, Mahbanoo Farhadi-Azar, Fereidoun Azizi, y Fahimeh Ramezani Tehrani. 2024. "Fracture Incidence in Women: The Impact of Reproductive Characteristics." *BMC Public Health* 24 (1): 3409. https://doi.org/10.1186/s12889-024-20890-2.

Farris, Manuela, Carlo Bastianelli, Elena Rosato, Ivo Brosens, y Giuseppe Benagiano. 2017. "Pharmacodynamics of Combined Estrogen-Progestin Oral Contraceptives: 2. Effects on Hemostasis." *Expert Review of Clinical Pharmacology* 10 (10): 1129-44. https://doi.org/10.1080/17512433.2017.1356718.

Festin, Mario Philip R., Alexandre Peregoudov, Armando Seuc, James Kiarie, y Marleen Temmerman. 2017. "Effect of BMI and Body Weight on Pregnancy Rates with LNG as Emergency Contraception: Analysis of Four WHO HRP Studies." *Contraception* 95 (1): 50-54. https://doi.org/10.1016/j.contraception.2016.08.001.

Fotherby, K. 1996. "Bioavailability of Orally Administered Sex Steroids Used in Oral Contraception and Hormone Replacement Therapy." *Contraception* 54 (2): 59-69. https://doi.org/10.1016/0010-7824(96)00136-9.

Frisendahl, Caroline, Helena Kopp Kallner, y Kristina Gemzell-Danielsson. 2024. "The Clinical Relevance of Having More than One Estrogen in Combined Hormonal Contraception to Address the Needs of Women." *Best Practice & Research. Clinical Obstetrics & Gynaecology* 98 (noviembre):102571. https://doi.org/10.1016/j.bpobgyn.2024.102571.

Fruzzetti, Franca, Tiziana Fidecicchi, Maria Magdalena Montt Guevara, y Tommaso Simoncini. 2021. "Estetrol: A New Choice for Contraception." *Journal of Clinical Medicine* 10 (23): 5625. https://doi.org/10.3390/jcm10235625.

Gallez, Anne, Isabelle Dias Da Silva, Vincent Wuidar, Jean-Michel Foidart, y Christel Péqueux. 2021. "Estetrol and Mammary Gland: Friends or Foes?" *Journal of Mammary Gland Biology and Neoplasia* 26 (3): 297-308. https://doi.org/10.1007/s10911-021-09497-0.

Gemzell-Danielsson, Kristina, Angelo Cagnacci, Nathalie Chabbert-Buffet, Jonathan Douxfils, Jean-Michel Foidart, Ali Kubba, Luis Ignacio Lete Lasa, et al. 2022. "A Novel Estetrol-Containing Combined Oral Contraceptive: European Expert Panel Review." *The European Journal of Contraception & Reproductive Health Care: The Official Journal of the European Society of Contraception*, julio, 1-11. https://doi.org/10.1080/13625187.2022.2093850.

Gérard, Céline, Jean-François Arnal, Maud Jost, Jonathan Douxfils, Françoise Lenfant, Coralie Fontaine, René Houtman, et al. 2022. "Profile of Estetrol, a Promising Native Estrogen for Oral Contraception and the Relief of Climacteric Symptoms of Menopause." *Expert Review of Clinical Pharmacology* 15 (2): 121-37. https://doi.org/10.1080/17512433.2022.2054413.

Glasier, Anna, Alison Edelman, Mitchell D. Creinin, Leo Han, Melissa C. Matulich, Vivian Brache, Carolyn L. Westhoff, y Agnes Hemon. 2022. "Mechanism of Action of Norgestrel 0.075 Mg a Progestogen-Only Pill. I. Effect on Ovarian Activity." *Contraception* 112 (agosto):37-42. https://doi.org/10.1016/j.contraception.2022.03.022.

Goldstuck, Norman D., y Hung P. Le. 2018. "Delivery of Progestins via the Subdermal versus the Intrauterine Route: Comparison of the Pharmacology and Clinical Outcomes." *Expert Opinion on Drug Delivery* 15 (7): 717-27. https://doi.org/10.1080/17425247.2018.1498080.

Goshtasebi, Azita, Tatjana Subotic Brajic, Delia Scholes, Tamara Beres Lederer Goldberg, Abbey Berenson, y Jerilynn C. Prior. 2019. "Adolescent Use of Combined Hormonal Contraception and Peak Bone Mineral

Density Accrual: A Meta-Analysis of International Prospective Controlled Studies." *Clinical Endocrinology* 90 (4): 517-24. https://doi.org/10.1111/cen.13932.

Grandi, Giovanni. 2025. "Hormonal Prolonged-Release in Oral Contraception: How Far Are We from Vaginal Pharmacokinetics?" *The European Journal of Contraception & Reproductive Health Care: The Official Journal of the European Society of Contraception*, abril, 1-2. https://doi.org/10.1080/13625187.2025.2485217.

Guazzelli, Cristina A. F., Flaviano Teixeira de Queiroz, Marcia Barbieri, Fernando A. Barreiros, Maria Regina Torloni, y Fabio F. Araujo. 2011. "Metabolic Effects of Contraceptive Implants in Adolescents." *Contraception* 84 (4): 409-12. https://doi.org/10.1016/j.contraception.2011.02.006.

Guazzelli, Cristina Aparecida Falbo, Fernando Augusto Barreiros, Ricardo Barbosa, Maria Regina Torloni, y Marcia Barbieri. 2012. "Extended Regimens of the Contraceptive Vaginal Ring versus Hormonal Oral Contraceptives: Effects on Lipid Metabolism." *Contraception* 85 (4): 389-93. https://doi.org/10.1016/j.contraception.2011.08.014.

Guilbert, Edith R., Jacques P. Brown, Andrew M. Kaunitz, Marie-Soleil Wagner, Jocelyn Bérubé, Louise Charbonneau, Diane Francoeur, et al. 2009. "The Use of Depot-Medroxyprogesterone Acetate in Contraception and Its Potential Impact on Skeletal Health." *Contraception* 79 (3): 167-77. https://doi.org/10.1016/j.contraception.2008.10.016.

Hadji, P., E. Colli, y P.-A. Regidor. 2019. "Bone Health in Estrogen-Free Contraception." *Osteoporosis International: A Journal Established as Result of Cooperation between the European Foundation for Osteoporosis and the National Osteoporosis Foundation of the USA* 30 (12): 2391-2400. https://doi.org/10.1007/s00198-019-05103-6.

Han, Leo, Mitchell D. Creinin, Agnes Hemon, Anna Glasier, Melissa J. Chen, y Alison Edelman. 2022. "Mechanism of Action of a 0.075 Mg Norgestrel Progestogen-Only Pill 2. Effect on Cervical Mucus and Theoretical Risk of Conception." *Contraception* 112 (agosto):43-47. https://doi.org/10.1016/j.contraception.2022.03.016.

Han, Leo, Rebecca Taub, y Jeffrey T. Jensen. 2017. "Cervical Mucus and Contraception: What We Know and What We Don't." *Contraception* 96 (5): 310-21. https://doi.org/10.1016/j.contraception.2017.07.168.

Harvey, R. A., J. R. Murillo, M. A. Clark, R. Finkel, J. A. Rey, K. Whalen, y J. R. P. Martínez. 2020. *Farmacología*. 5ª. Lippincott's illustrated reviews. Barcelona: Wolters Kluwer Health. https://elibro.net/es/ereader/bibliotecauclm/124822?page=12.

Haverinen, Annina H., Kaisu M. Luiro, Timea Szanto, Marika H. Kangasniemi, Leena Hiltunen, Susanna Sainio, Terhi T. Piltonen, Riitta Lassila, Juha S. Tapanainen, y Oskari Heikinheimo. 2022. "Combined Oral Contraceptives Containing Estradiol Valerate vs Ethinylestradiol on Coagulation: A Randomized Clinical Trial." *Acta Obstetricia Et Gynecologica Scandinavica* 101 (10): 1102-11. https://doi.org/10.1111/aogs.14428.

Heuvel, Michiel Wilhelmus van den, Antoinetta Jacoba Maria van Bragt, Ali Kafi Mohammed Alnabawy, y Marc Carel John Kaptein. 2005. "Comparison of Ethinylestradiol Pharmacokinetics in Three Hormonal Contraceptive Formulations: The Vaginal Ring, the Transdermal Patch and an Oral Contraceptive." *Contraception* 72 (3): 168-74. https://doi.org/10.1016/j.contraception.2005.03.005.

Hofmann, Birte Maria, Dan Apter, Johannes Bitzer, Isabel Reinecke, Marco Serrani, Joachim Höchel, y Martin Merz. 2020. "Comparative Pharmacokinetic Analysis of Levonorgestrel-Releasing Intrauterine Systems and Levonorgestrel-Containing Contraceptives with Oral or Subdermal Administration Route." *The European Journal of Contraception & Reproductive Health Care: The Official Journal of the European Society of Contraception* 25 (6): 417-26. https://doi.org/10.1080/13625187.2020.1815008.

Holt, Victoria L., Kara L. Cushing-Haugen, y Janet R. Daling. 2002. "Body Weight and Risk of Oral Contraceptive Failure." *Obstetrics and Gynecology* 99 (5 Pt 1): 820-27. https://doi.org/10.1016/s0029-7844(02)01939-7.

Holt, Victoria L., Delia Scholes, Kristine G. Wicklund, Kara L. Cushing-Haugen, y Janet R. Daling. 2005. "Body Mass Index, Weight, and Oral Contraceptive Failure Risk." *Obstetrics and Gynecology* 105 (1): 46-52. https://doi.org/10.1097/01.AOG.0000149155.11912.52.

Jensen, Jeffrey T., Andrew M. Kaunitz, Sharon L. Achilles, János Zatik, Steven Weyers, Terhi Piltonen, Larisa Suturina, et al. 2022. "Pooled Efficacy Results of Estetrol/Drospirenone Combined Oral Contraception

Phase 3 Trials." *Contraception*, julio, S0010-7824(22)00215-3. https://doi.org/10.1016/j.contraception.2022.07.009.

Junge, Wolfgang, Uwe Mellinger, Susanne Parke, y Marco Serrani. 2011. "Metabolic and Haemostatic Effects of Estradiol Valerate/Dienogest, a Novel Oral Contraceptive: A Randomized, Open-Label, Single-Centre Study." *Clinical Drug Investigation* 31 (8): 573-84. https://doi.org/10.2165/11590220-000000000-00000.

Kim, Soo Min, Whan Shin, Hyo Jeong Kim, Ji Soo Lee, Yong-Ki Min, y Byung-Koo Yoon. 2022. "Effects of Combination Oral Contraceptives on Bone Mineral Density and Metabolism in Perimenopausal Korean Women." *Journal of Menopausal Medicine* 28 (1): 25-32. https://doi.org/10.6118/jmm.21027.

Kowalska, Katarzyna, Milena Ściskalska, Anna Bizoń, Mariola Śliwińska-Mossoń, y Halina Milnerowicz. 2018. "Influence of Oral Contraceptives on Lipid Profile and Paraoxonase and Commonly Hepatic Enzymes Activities." *Journal of Clinical Laboratory Analysis* 32 (1): e22194. https://doi.org/10.1002/jcla.22194.

Krattenmacher, R. 2000. "Drospirenone: Pharmacology and Pharmacokinetics of a Unique Progestogen." *Contraception* 62 (1): 29-38. https://doi.org/10.1016/s0010-7824(00)00133-5.

Kuhl, H. 1990. "Pharmacokinetics of Oestrogens and Progestogens." *Maturitas* 12 (3): 171-97. https://doi.org/10.1016/0378-5122(90)90003-o.

Kuhnz, W., C. Gansau, y A. Fuhrmeister. 1992. "Pharmacokinetics of Gestodene in 12 Women Who Received a Single Oral Dose of 0.075 Mg Gestodene and, after a Wash-out Phase, the Same Dose during One Treatment Cycle." *Contraception* 46 (1): 29-40. https://doi.org/10.1016/0010-7824(92)90129-h.

Lavelanet, Antonella F., Denis Rybin, y Katharine O. White. 2017. "The Pharmacokinetics of 12-Week Continuous Contraceptive Patch Use." *Contraception* 95 (6): 578-85. https://doi.org/10.1016/j.contraception.2017.03.002.

Le, Jennifer. 2022. "Absorción de los fármacos - Farmacología clínica." Manual MSD versión para profesionales. 2022. https://www.msdmanuals.com/es-es/professional/farmacolog%C3%ADa-cl%C3%ADnica/farmacocin%C3%A9tica/absorci%C3%B3n-de-los-f%C3%A1rmacos.

Lee, Arnold, y Yahiya Y. Syed. 2022. "Estetrol/Drospirenone: A Review in Oral Contraception." *Drugs* 82 (10): 1117-25. https://doi.org/10.1007/s40265-022-01738-8.

Lete, Iñaki, Nathalie Chabbert-Buffet, Christian Jamin, Stefano Lello, Paloma Lobo, Rossella E. Nappi, y Axelle Pintiaux. 2015. "Haemostatic and Metabolic Impact of Estradiol Pills and Drospirenone-Containing Ethinylestradiol Pills vs. Levonorgestrel-Containing Ethinylestradiol Pills: A Literature Review." *The European Journal of Contraception & Reproductive Health Care: The Official Journal of the European Society of Contraception* 20 (5): 329-43. https://doi.org/10.3109/13625187.2015.1050091.

Lim, Leek Mei, Wogud Ben Said, y Pallavi Latthe. 2025. "Effects of Combined Hormonal Contraceptives (CHC) on Bone Health in Adolescent Girls. A Systematic Review." *Journal of Pediatric and Adolescent Gynecology*, marzo, S1083-3188(25)00233-5. https://doi.org/10.1016/j.jpag.2025.03.004.

Lobo, R. A., y F. Z. Stanczyk. 1994. "New Knowledge in the Physiology of Hormonal Contraceptives." *American Journal of Obstetrics and Gynecology* 170 (5 Pt 2): 1499-1507. https://doi.org/10.1016/s0002-9378(94)05011-8.

Lopez, Laureen M., Alissa Bernholc, Mario Chen, Thomas W. Grey, Conrad Otterness, Carolyn Westhoff, Alison Edelman, y Frans M. Helmerhorst. 2016. "Hormonal Contraceptives for Contraception in Overweight or Obese Women." *The Cochrane Database of Systematic Reviews* 2016 (8): CD008452. https://doi.org/10.1002/14651858.CD008452.pub4.

Lopez, Laureen M., Mario Chen, Sarah Mullins Long, Kathryn M. Curtis, y Frans M. Helmerhorst. 2015. "Steroidal Contraceptives and Bone Fractures in Women: Evidence from Observational Studies." *The Cochrane Database of Systematic Reviews*, n.º 7 (julio), CD009849. https://doi.org/10.1002/14651858.CD009849.pub3.

Lopez, Laureen M., David A. Grimes, y Kenneth F. Schulz. 2019. "Steroidal Contraceptives: Effect on Carbohydrate Metabolism in Women without Diabetes Mellitus." *The Cochrane Database of Systematic Reviews* 2019 (11). https://doi.org/10.1002/14651858.CD006133.pub5.

Lopez, Laureen M., David A. Grimes, Kenneth F. Schulz, Kathryn M. Curtis, y Mario Chen. 2014. "Steroidal Contraceptives: Effect on Bone Fractures in Women." *The Cochrane Database of Systematic Reviews*, n.º 6 (junio), CD006033. https://doi.org/10.1002/14651858.CD006033.pub5.

López-Picado, Amanda, Oihane Lapuente, y Iñaki Lete. 2017. "Efficacy and Side-Effects Profile of the Ethinylestradiol and Etonogestrel Contraceptive Vaginal Ring: A Systematic Review and Meta-Analysis." *The European Journal of Contraception & Reproductive Health Care: The Official Journal of the European Society of Contraception* 22 (2): 131-46. https://doi.org/10.1080/13625187.2017.1287351.

Luo, Dandan, Carolyn L. Westhoff, Alison B. Edelman, Melissa Natavio, Frank Z. Stanczyk, y William J. Jusko. 2019. "Altered Pharmacokinetics of Combined Oral Contraceptives in Obesity - Multistudy Assessment." *Contraception* 99 (4): 256-63. https://doi.org/10.1016/j.contraception.2018.12.009.

Mäkäräinen, L., A. van Beek, L. Tuomivaara, B. Asplund, y H. Coelingh Bennink. 1998. "Ovarian Function during the Use of a Single Contraceptive Implant: Implanon Compared with Norplant." *Fertility and Sterility* 69 (4): 714-21. https://doi.org/10.1016/s0015-0282(98)00015-6.

Martins, Summer L., Kathryn M. Curtis, y Anna F. Glasier. 2006. "Combined Hormonal Contraception and Bone Health: A Systematic Review." *Contraception* 73 (5): 445-69. https://doi.org/10.1016/j.contraception.2006.01.003.

Mawet, Marie, Catherine Maillard, Christine Klipping, Yvette Zimmerman, Jean-Michel Foidart, y Herjan J. T. Coelingh Bennink. 2015. "Unique Effects on Hepatic Function, Lipid Metabolism, Bone and Growth Endocrine Parameters of Estetrol in Combined Oral Contraceptives." *The European Journal of Contraception & Reproductive Health Care: The Official Journal of the European Society of Contraception* 20 (6): 463-75. https://doi.org/10.3109/13625187.2015.1068934.

McCann, M. F., y L. S. Potter. 1994. "Progestin-Only Oral Contraception: A Comprehensive Review." *Contraception* 50 (6 Suppl 1): S1-195.

Mohamed, Ahmed M. M., Wael S. M. El-Sherbiny, y Walaa A. I. Mostafa. 2011. "Combined Contraceptive Ring versus Combined Oral Contraceptive (30-Mg Ethinylestradiol and 3-Mg Drospirenone)." *International Journal of Gynaecology and Obstetrics: The Official Organ of the International Federation of Gynaecology and Obstetrics* 114 (2): 145-48. https://doi.org/10.1016/j.ijgo.2011.03.008.

Moreira De Brito, Claudia, Maria Edna De Melo, Marcio C. Mancini, Marco Aurelio Santo, y Cintia Cercato. 2021. "Pharmacokinetics of Oral Levonorgestrel and Ethinylestradiol in Women after Roux-En-Y Gastric Bypass Surgery." *Surgery for Obesity and Related Diseases* 17 (4): 673-81. https://doi.org/10.1016/j.soard.2020.12.007.

Morimont, Laure, Maud Jost, Ulysse Gaspard, Jean Michel Foidart, Jean Michel Dogné, y Jonathan Douxfils. 2022. "LOW THROMBIN GENERATION IN USERS OF A CONTRACEPTIVE CONTAINING ESTETROL AND DROSPIRENONE." *The Journal of Clinical Endocrinology and Metabolism*, septiembre, dgac511. https://doi.org/10.1210/clinem/dgac511.

Nappi, Carmine, Giuseppe Bifulco, Giovanni A. Tommaselli, Virginia Gargano, y Costantino Di Carlo. 2012. "Hormonal Contraception and Bone Metabolism: A Systematic Review." *Contraception* 86 (6): 606-21. https://doi.org/10.1016/j.contraception.2012.04.009.

Nguyen, Antoinette T. 2024. "U.S. Medical Eligibility Criteria for Contraceptive Use, 2024." *MMWR. Recommendations and Reports* 73. https://doi.org/10.15585/mmwr.rr7304a1.

Özcan, Ömer, Wendy P. J. den Elzen, Jacquelien J. Hillebrand, Martin den Heijer, Laura L. van Loendersloot, Johan Fischer, Henrike Hamer, Robert de Jonge, y Annemieke C. Heijboer. 2024. "The Effect of Hormonal Contraceptive Therapy on Clinical Laboratory Parameters: A Literature Review." *Clinical Chemistry and Laboratory Medicine* 62 (1): 18-40. https://doi.org/10.1515/cclm-2023-0384.

Paton, David M. 2022. "Estetrol and Drospirenone: A Novel Oral Contraceptive." *Drugs of Today (Barcelona, Spain: 1998)* 58 (1): 1-8. https://doi.org/10.1358/dot.2022.58.1.3353167.

Piersol, Kelsey L., y Jennifer F. Buckman. 2025. "Elevated Blood Pressure, Stroke Volume, and Vascular Tone in Young Women Who Use Oral Contraception." *International Journal of Psychophysiology: Official Journal of the International Organization of Psychophysiology* 211 (marzo):112557. https://doi.org/10.1016/j.ijpsycho.2025.112557.

Prossnitz, Eric R., y Matthias Barton. 2023. "The G Protein-Coupled Oestrogen Receptor GPER in Health and Disease: An Update." *Nature Reviews. Endocrinology* 19 (7): 407-24. https://doi.org/10.1038/s41574-023-00822-7.

Rabe, T., A. Kowald, J. Ortmann, y S. Rehberger-Schneider. 2000. "Inhibition of Skin 5 Alpha-Reductase by Oral Contraceptive Progestins in Vitro." *Gynecological Endocrinology: The Official Journal of the*

International Society of Gynecological Endocrinology 14 (4): 223-30. https://doi.org/10.3109/09513590009167685.

Redinger, Allen L., y Breanne S. Baker. 2022. "Oral Contraceptives and Female Rowers' Skeletal Health." *Journal of Strength and Conditioning Research*, septiembre. https://doi.org/10.1519/JSC.0000000000004308.

Reed, Suzanne, Carol Koro, Julia DiBello, Kerstin Becker, Anja Bauerfeind, Christian Franke, y Klaas Heinemann. 2021. "Prospective Controlled Cohort Study on the Safety of a Monophasic Oral Contraceptive Containing Nomegestrol Acetate (2.5mg) and 17β-Oestradiol (1.5mg) (PRO-E2 Study): Risk of Venous and Arterial Thromboembolism." *The European Journal of Contraception & Reproductive Health Care: The Official Journal of the European Society of Contraception* 26 (6): 439-46. https://doi.org/10.1080/13625187.2021.1987410.

Reinecke, Isabel, Birte Hofmann, Emir Mesic, Henk-Jan Drenth, y Dirk Garmann. 2018. "An Integrated Population Pharmacokinetic Analysis to Characterize Levonorgestrel Pharmacokinetics After Different Administration Routes." *Journal of Clinical Pharmacology* 58 (12): 1639-54. https://doi.org/10.1002/jcph.1288.

Rice, C. F., S. R. Killick, T. Dieben, y H. Coelingh Bennink. 1999. "A Comparison of the Inhibition of Ovulation Achieved by Desogestrel 75 Micrograms and Levonorgestrel 30 Micrograms Daily." *Human Reproduction (Oxford, England)* 14 (4): 982-85. https://doi.org/10.1093/humrep/14.4.982.

Rice, C., S. Killick, D. Hickling, y H. Coelingh Bennink. 1996. "Ovarian Activity and Vaginal Bleeding Patterns with a Desogestrel-Only Preparation at Three Different Doses." *Human Reproduction (Oxford, England)* 11 (4): 737-40. https://doi.org/10.1093/oxfordjournals.humrep.a019245.

Rivera, R., I. Yacobson, y D. Grimes. 1999. "The Mechanism of Action of Hormonal Contraceptives and Intrauterine Contraceptive Devices." *American Journal of Obstetrics and Gynecology* 181 (5 Pt 1): 1263-69. https://doi.org/10.1016/s0002-9378(99)70120-1.

Robinson, G. E., T. Burren, I. J. Mackie, W. Bounds, K. Walshe, R. Faint, J. Guillebaud, y S. J. Machin. 1991. "Changes in Haemostasis after Stopping the Combined Contraceptive Pill: Implications for Major Surgery." *BMJ (Clinical Research Ed.)* 302 (6771): 269-71. https://doi.org/10.1136/bmj.302.6771.269.

Rocca, Morena L., Anna R. Palumbo, Giovanna Bitonti, Caterina Brisinda, y Costantino DI Carlo. 2021. "Bone Health and Hormonal Contraception." *Minerva Obstetrics and Gynecology* 73 (6): 678-96. https://doi.org/10.23736/S2724-606X.20.04688-2.

Rodriguez, Luis A., Ellen Casey, Eric Crossley, Noelle Williams, y Yasin Y. Dhaher. 2024. "The Hormonal Profile in Women Using Combined Monophasic Oral Contraceptive Pills Varies across the Pill Cycle: A Temporal Analysis of Serum Endogenous and Exogenous Hormones Using Liquid Chromatography with Tandem Mass Spectroscopy." *American Journal of Physiology. Endocrinology and Metabolism* 327 (1): E121-33. https://doi.org/10.1152/ajpendo.00418.2023.

Rossmanith, W. G., D. Steffens, y G. Schramm. 1997. "A Comparative Randomized Trial on the Impact of Two Low-Dose Oral Contraceptives on Ovarian Activity, Cervical Permeability, and Endometrial Receptivity." *Contraception* 56 (1): 23-30. https://doi.org/10.1016/s0010-7824(97)00070-x.

Roumen, Frans J M E. 2007. "The contraceptive vaginal ring compared with the combined oral contraceptive pill: a comprehensive review of randomized controlled trials." *Contraception* 75 (6): 420-29. https://doi.org/10.1016/j.contraception.2007.01.013.

Roumen, Frans J. M. E., y Daniel R. Mishell. 2012. "The Contraceptive Vaginal Ring, NuvaRing(®), a Decade after Its Introduction." *The European Journal of Contraception & Reproductive Health Care: The Official Journal of the European Society of Contraception* 17 (6): 415-27. https://doi.org/10.3109/13625187.2012.713535.

Ruiz-Gayo, Mariano, y Marisol Fernández-Alonso. 2013. *Fundamentos de farmacología básica y clinica.* 2ªEd. Madrid: Médica Panamericana.

Samsioe, G. 1994. "Coagulation and Anticoagulation Effects of Contraceptive Steroids." *American Journal of Obstetrics and Gynecology* 170 (5 Pt 2): 1523-27. https://doi.org/10.1016/s0002-9378(94)05014-3.

Sarfati, Julie, y Marie-Christine de Vernejoul. 2009. "Impact of Combined and Progestogen-Only Contraceptives on Bone Mineral Density." *Joint Bone Spine* 76 (2): 134-38. https://doi.org/10.1016/j.jbspin.2008.09.014.

Schindler, Adolf E., Carlo Campagnoli, René Druckmann, Johannes Huber, Jorge R. Pasqualini, Karl W. Schweppe, y Jos H. H. Thijssen. 2008. "Classification and Pharmacology of Progestins." *Maturitas* 61 (1-2): 171-80. https://doi.org/10.1016/j.maturitas.2008.11.013.

Silva-Bermudez, Lina S., Freddy J. K. Toloza, Maria C. Perez-Matos, Russell J. de Souza, Laura Banfield, Andrea Vargas-Villanueva, y Carlos O. Mendivil. 2020. "Effects of Oral Contraceptives on Metabolic Parameters in Adult Premenopausal Women: A Meta-Analysis." *Endocrine Connections* 9 (10): 978-98. https://doi.org/10.1530/EC-20-0423.

Silverberg, S. G., M. Haukkamaa, H. Arko, C. G. Nilsson, y T. Luukkainen. 1986. "Endometrial Morphology during Long-Term Use of Levonorgestrel-Releasing Intrauterine Devices." *International Journal of Gynecological Pathology: Official Journal of the International Society of Gynecological Pathologists* 5 (3): 235-41. https://doi.org/10.1097/00004347-198609000-00005.

Singer, Adrian, Katharina Tropschuh, Marc von Gernler, Claire Decrinis, y Petra Stute. 2025. "The Impact of Progestogens on RAAS - a Systematic Review." *BMC Women's Health* 25 (1): 81. https://doi.org/10.1186/s12905-025-03587-5.

Sitruk-Ware, Regine, y Anita Nath. 2010. "The Use of Newer Progestins for Contraception." *Contraception* 82 (5): 410-17. https://doi.org/10.1016/j.contraception.2010.04.004.

———. 2011. "Metabolic Effects of Contraceptive Steroids." *Reviews in Endocrine & Metabolic Disorders* 12 (2): 63-75. https://doi.org/10.1007/s11154-011-9182-4.

———. 2013. "Characteristics and metabolic effects of estrogen and progestins contained in oral contraceptive pills." *Best practice & research. Clinical endocrinology & metabolism* 27 (1): 13-24. https://doi.org/10.1016/j.beem.2012.09.004.

Skeith, Leslie, y Shannon M. Bates. 2024. "Estrogen, Progestin, and beyond: Thrombotic Risk and Contraceptive Choices." *Hematology. American Society of Hematology. Education Program* 2024 (1): 644-51. https://doi.org/10.1182/hematology.2024000591.

Slíva, Jiří. 2024. "Estrogenic Treatment and Liver Functions." *Ceska Gynekologie* 89 (6): 501-3. https://doi.org/10.48095/cccg2024501.

Soria-Jasso, Luis E., Raquel Cariño-Cortés, Víctor Manuel Muñoz-Pérez, Elizabeth Pérez-Hernández, Nury Pérez-Hernández, y Eduardo Fernández-Martínez. 2019. "Beneficial and Deleterious Effects of Female Sex Hormones, Oral Contraceptives, and Phytoestrogens by Immunomodulation on the Liver." *International Journal of Molecular Sciences* 20 (19): 4694. https://doi.org/10.3390/ijms20194694.

Souza, Ingrid Soares de, Gabriel Zorello Laporta, Juliana Zangirolami-Raimundo, Isabel Cristina Esposito Sorpreso, Heloisa Carla Lopes Silva Dos Santos, José Maria Soares Júnior, y Rodrigo Daminello Raimundo. 2024. "Association between the Use of Oral Contraceptives and the Occurrence of Systemic Hypertension: A Systematic Review with Statistical Comparison between Randomized Clinical Trial Interventions." *European Journal of Obstetrics & Gynecology and Reproductive Biology: X* 22 (junio):100307. https://doi.org/10.1016/j.eurox.2024.100307.

Stanczyk, Frank Z. 2024. "Metabolism of Endogenous and Exogenous Estrogens in Women." *The Journal of Steroid Biochemistry and Molecular Biology* 242 (septiembre):106539. https://doi.org/10.1016/j.jsbmb.2024.106539.

Stanczyk, Frank Z, David F Archer, y Bhagu R Bhavnani. 2013. "Ethinyl estradiol and 17β-estradiol in combined oral contraceptives: pharmacokinetics, pharmacodynamics and risk assessment." *Contraception*, enero. https://doi.org/10.1016/j.contraception.2012.12.011.

Stanczyk, Frank Z., Alexandra McGough, Laura Chagam, y Regine Sitruk-Ware. 2024. "Metabolism of Progestogens Used for Contraception and Menopausal Hormone Therapy." *Steroids* 207 (julio):109427. https://doi.org/10.1016/j.steroids.2024.109427.

Stanczyk, Frank Z., Sharon A. Winer, Jean-Michel Foidart, y David F. Archer. 2024. "Comparison of Estrogenic Components Used for Hormonal Contraception." *Contraception* 130 (febrero):110310. https://doi.org/10.1016/j.contraception.2023.110310.

Staudt, Anna, Sophia J. Kiechl, Nina Gande, Christoph Hochmayr, Benoît Bernar, Katharina Stock, Ralf Geiger, et al. 2024. "Influence of Oral Contraceptives on Lipid Profile and Trajectories in Healthy Adolescents—Data From the EVA-Tyrol Study." *Journal of Adolescent Health* 75 (3): 479-86. https://doi.org/10.1016/j.jadohealth.2024.04.017.

Stockum, Sophia von, Anja Bauerfeind, Kerstin Becker, Christian Franke, Franca Fruzzetti, Joaquim Calaf, Christoph Keck, y Klaas Heinemann. 2023. "NOMAC-E2 Shows a Better Contraceptive Effectiveness than LNG Combined Oral Contraceptives in Women under 25: Real-World PRO-E2 Study." *Gynecological Endocrinology: The Official Journal of the International Society of Gynecological Endocrinology* 39 (1): 2162036. https://doi.org/10.1080/09513590.2022.2162036.

Takeda, Ryosuke, Sarah L. Hissen, Abigail S. L. Stickford, y Qi Fu. 2021. "Impact of Oral Contraceptives on Sympathetic Neural and Cardiovascular Responses during Static Handgrip to Fatigue in Healthy Women." *Clinical Autonomic Research: Official Journal of the Clinical Autonomic Research Society* 31 (6): 779-81. https://doi.org/10.1007/s10286-021-00834-1.

Tasset, Julia, y Alison Edelman. 2025. "Considerations for Hormonal Contraception and People with Larger Bodies." *Best Practice & Research. Clinical Obstetrics & Gynaecology* 99 (febrero):102577. https://doi.org/10.1016/j.bpobgyn.2025.102577.

Taylor, Hugh S., Lubna Pal, Emre Seli, y Marc A. Fritz. 2020. *Speroff's clinical gynecologic endocrinology and infertility*. Ninth edition. Philadelphia: Wolters Kluwer.

Timmer, C. J., y T. M. Mulders. 2000. "Pharmacokinetics of Etonogestrel and Ethinylestradiol Released from a Combined Contraceptive Vaginal Ring." *Clinical Pharmacokinetics* 39 (3): 233-42. https://doi.org/10.2165/00003088-200039030-00005.

Trémollieres, Florence. 2013. "Impact of Oral Contraceptive on Bone Metabolism." *Best Practice & Research. Clinical Endocrinology & Metabolism* 27 (1): 47-53. https://doi.org/10.1016/j.beem.2012.09.002.

Vleskó, Gábor, Fanni Adél Meznerics, Péter Hegyi, Brigitta Teutsch, Márkó Unicsovics, Zoltán Sipos, Péter Fehérvári, Nándor Ács, Szabolcs Várbíró, y Márton Keszthelyi. 2024. "Comparison of Combined Parenteral and Oral Hormonal Contraceptives: A Systematic Review and Meta-Analysis of Randomized Trials." *Journal of Clinical Medicine* 13 (2): 575. https://doi.org/10.3390/jcm13020575.

Wenzl, R., A. van Beek, P. Schnabel, y J. Huber. 1998. "Pharmacokinetics of Etonogestrel Released from the Contraceptive Implant Implanon." *Contraception* 58 (5): 283-88. https://doi.org/10.1016/s0010-7824(98)00110-3.

Westhoff, Carolyn L., Isabel Reinecke, Keith Bangerter, y Martin Merz. 2014. "Impact of Body Mass Index on Suppression of Follicular Development and Ovulation Using a Transdermal Patch Containing 0.55-Mg Ethinyl Estradiol/2.1-Mg Gestodene: A Multicenter, Open-Label, Uncontrolled Study over Three Treatment Cycles." *Contraception* 90 (3): 272-79. https://doi.org/10.1016/j.contraception.2014.04.018.

Westhoff, Carolyn L, Anupama H Torgal, Elizabeth R Mayeda, Malcolm C Pike, y Frank Z Stanczyk. 2010. "Pharmacokinetics of a combined oral contraceptive in obese and normal-weight women." *Contraception* 81 (6): 474-80. https://doi.org/10.1016/j.contraception.2010.01.016.

Wiegratz, I., J. H. Lee, E. Kutschera, U. H. Winkler, y H. Kuhl. 2004. "Effect of Four Oral Contraceptives on Hemostatic Parameters." *Contraception* 70 (2): 97-106. https://doi.org/10.1016/j.contraception.2004.03.004.

Wiegratz, I, S Stahlberg, T Manthey, N Sänger, K Mittmann, E Palombo-Kinne, U Mellinger, E Lange, y H Kuhl. 2010. "Effects of combined oral contraceptive ethinylestradiol (30 microg) and dienogest (2 mg) on carbohydrate metabolism during 1 year of conventional or extended-cycle use." *Hormone and metabolic research = Hormon- und Stoffwechselforschung = Hormones et métabolisme* 42 (5): 358-63. https://doi.org/10.1055/s-0030-1248263.

Wiegratz, Inka, y Herbert Kuhl. 2006. "Metabolic and Clinical Effects of Progestogens." *The European Journal of Contraception & Reproductive Health Care: The Official Journal of the European Society of Contraception* 11 (3): 153-61. https://doi.org/10.1080/13625180600772741.

Woods, J. W. 1988. "Oral Contraceptives and Hypertension." *Hypertension (Dallas, Tex.: 1979)* 11 (3 Pt 2): II11-15. https://doi.org/10.1161/01.hyp.11.3_pt_2.ii11.

Xiao, B. L., L. Y. Zhou, X. L. Zhang, M. C. Jia, T. Luukkainen, y H. Allonen. 1990. "Pharmacokinetic and Pharmacodynamic Studies of Levonorgestrel-Releasing Intrauterine Device." *Contraception* 41 (4): 353-62. https://doi.org/10.1016/0010-7824(90)90035-t.

Xin, X., Y. Wu, X. Liu, C. Sun, T. Geng, y L. Ding. 2016. "Pharmacokinetics of Oral Combination Contraceptive Drugs Containing Ethinyl Estradiol and Levonorgestrel in Healthy Female Chinese Volunteers." *Drug Research* 66 (2): 100-106. https://doi.org/10.1055/s-0035-1554631.

Yamazaki, Michiyo, Kate Dwyer, Mahboob Sobhan, Daniel Davis, Myong-Jin Kim, Lisa Soule, Gerald Willett, y Chongwoo Yu. 2015. "Effect of Obesity on the Effectiveness of Hormonal Contraceptives: An Individual Participant Data Meta-Analysis." *Contraception* 92 (5): 445-52. https://doi.org/10.1016/j.contraception.2015.07.016.

Zeun, Susan, Ming Lu, Alkaz Uddin, Brian Zeiler, Dennis Morrison, y Hartmut Blode. 2009. "Pharmacokinetics of an Oral Contraceptive Containing Oestradiol Valerate and Dienogest." *The European Journal of Contraception & Reproductive Health Care: The Official Journal of the European Society of Contraception* 14 (3): 221-32. https://doi.org/10.1080/13625180902850039.

Zhu, Bao Ting, Gui-Zhen Han, Joong-Youn Shim, Yujing Wen, y Xiang-Rong Jiang. 2006. "Quantitative Structure-Activity Relationship of Various Endogenous Estrogen Metabolites for Human Estrogen Receptor Alpha and Beta Subtypes: Insights into the Structural Determinants Favoring a Differential Subtype Binding." *Endocrinology* 147 (9): 4132-50. https://doi.org/10.1210/en.2006-0113.

Chapter 3

Coitus Interruptus

G. Serrano García[13], MD
L. M. Gómez Muñoz[2], MD
M. M. Pérez Haro[1,3], MD
S. Rico Cardenal[4], MD
and C. Aparicio Martínez[2], MD

[1]Obstetrics and Gynecology Department, University and Hospital of Albacete, Albacete, Spain
[2]Obstetrics and Gynaecology Department, Hospital of Tomelloso, Tomelloso, Ciudad Real, Spain
[3]Instituto Bernabeu of Alicante, Spain
[4]Obstetrics and Gynaecology Department, Hospital of Villarrobledo, Villarrobledo, Albacete, Spain

Abstract

Coitus interruptus, or withdrawal, is one of the oldest known contraceptive methods, used since ancient times despite some religious prohibitions. It involves the male partner withdrawing the penis before ejaculation to prevent sperm from entering the female reproductive tract. The method's success depends on the male's control over ejaculation and the timing of withdrawal.

Physiologically, male sexual response occurs in four phases: excitement, plateau, ejaculation (emission and expulsion phases), and resolution. Effectiveness varies widely, with typical use resulting in a 78% success rate, meaning 22 out of 100 couples may experience unintended pregnancy within a year. Factors such as the presence of sperm in pre-ejaculatory fluid, frequency of sex, and fertility influence efficacy.

Epidemiologically, withdrawal is a common temporary contraceptive method globally, with usage rates varying by region from 2% to 11.6% in some countries, and generally being low in Europe and South America.

Psychosocially, coitus interruptus can encourage communication between partners but may also cause frustration or reduced pleasure. Gender dynamics may lead to unequal decision-making, placing women at higher risk of unwanted pregnancy. Additionally, it offers no protection against sexually transmitted infections and is morally opposed in some cultures and religions.

Keywords: coitus interruptus, withdrawal, contraception, ejaculation

In: Advances in Reproductive Health
Editors: Llanos Belmonte Andujar and Ana Fuentes Rozalen
ISBN: 979-8-90134-038-7

Introduction

Coitus interruptus, also known as withdrawal, is a method of contraception that has been widely used throughout human history, since records began to the present day. Although during ancient times the use of contraceptives was not generally recommended according to the religious beliefs of the time, there is evidence that this method was employed during the Middle Ages and the following eras. Some studies conclude that the only useful methods of birth control during the 18th century were abortion, coitus interruptus and abstinence (McKeown, Thomas 1955). Therefore, coitus interruptus is probably the oldest known method of birth control.

Physiological Basis

Coitus interruptus consists of withdrawing the penis from the vagina before ejaculation to prevent the deposition of sperm in the female genital tract. From a physiological point of view, the male sexual response consists of four phases (Masters, W.H.; Johnson, V.E., 1966) (Figure 1):

- *Excitation:* in this phase vasodilation occurs in the penis and leads to erection. In Cowper's glands, the production of pre-seminal fluid begins, the main function of which is to lubricate the urethra, but sometimes this fluid may contain motile sperm in sufficient concentration to fertilise an egg (Killick et al. 2011).
- *Plateau:* increases sensitivity, heart rate and muscle tension. Sperm and other secretions accumulate in the prostatic urethra prior to ejaculation.
- *Ejaculation*: consists of two phases. Firstly, the emission phase which is controlled by the sympathetic nervous system, initiating contraction of the vas deferens and prostate, causing semen to move from the testicles and seminal vesicles into the urethra. Secondly, the expulsion phase, when the muscles around the urethra contract rhythmically causing the semen to exit.
- *Resolution:* return to the basal state.

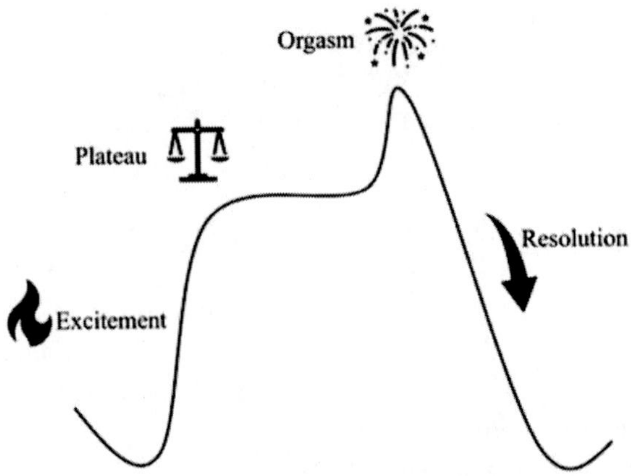

Figure 1. This graph illustrates the different phases of the sexual response cycle. Image adapted from the version by Masters and Johnson.

Its effectiveness depends exclusively on the voluntary control of the male partner and his ability to perceive the ejaculatory threshold, resulting in the withdrawal of the penis from the vagina before seminal fluid is expelled.

Contraceptive Effectiveness

The contraceptive efficacy of coitus interruptus is assessed according to the Pearl Index. This index calculates the number of unintended pregnancies that occur among 100 women using a contraceptive method during 1 year. The effectiveness of this method varies from 22% in couples who use it typically (couples who do not interrupt use for any reason) to 4% in those who use it perfectly (consistently and perfectly, without interrupting use for any reason) (Russell, J., 2011). Thus, typical efficacy is around 78%, meaning that 22 out of every 100 couples who use the method for a year will experience an unintended pregnancy. Factors influencing its efficacy include:

- Male control over ejaculation.
- Frequency of sexual intercourse.
- Age and fertility of the couple.
- The presence of sperm in pre-ejaculatory fluid.
- Combination with other methods (e.g., knowledge of the ovulatory cycle).

Epidemiological Considerations

Coitus interruptus is one of the most widely used temporary methods. According to sexual and reproductive health surveys worldwide, 8% of women in more developed countries and 3% of women in less developed countries rely on this method. This percentage may vary depending on the geographical area. In North Africa, a usage rate of 2% has been recorded, while in the rest of the continent there are hardly any data in favour of its use. In North America this percentage is 8%, with slightly less use in the United States (7.2%) than in Canada (11.6%). In Central America and the Caribbean, its use has been reported in 1% of cases, but in South America it is virtually unknown except in Colombia (2.8%), Argentina (1.6%) and Chile (0.2%). On the Asian continent, surveys report a total use of 3%, mainly in Western Asia (16%). In general, this method is rarely used among Europeans, with slightly more popular use in Northern Europe (6%) and Eastern Europe (11%). Finally, in Oceania, surveys report that 2% of Oceanian women rely on this method (Population Reference Bureau 2019).

Psychosocial and Ethical Aspects

Coitus interruptus has a number of implications for the sexual dynamics of the couple. On the one hand, it can be seen as increased sexual communication and participation of both partners during intercourse, but, on the other hand, it is also associated with frustration or decreased pleasure for the male partner when the sexual act is interrupted. It is necessary to consider that there may be situations in which the autonomy of the woman is limited by a forced choice of this method by the man, implying a gender inequality, since the woman is exposed to an increased risk of unwanted pregnancy. In addition, it is a method that does not protect against sexually transmitted diseases, which can cause public health problems in the population. In some cultures and religions, this method is morally rejected because it interferes with procreation, which is the purpose of the sexual act. Therefore, it is necessary to take these aspects into account when informing the population in order to make a free choice of this contraceptive method (Sánchez 2016).

Conclusion

- Coitus interruptus is a contraceptive method that has been widely used throughout human history.
- It is a low-cost method that is available to the entire population and has no direct side effects from its use.
- It has a low efficacy as a contraceptive method, as it depends on the voluntary control of the male partner just prior ejaculation, which can lead to unwanted pregnancies.
- It does not protect against sexually transmitted infections.
- It is necessary to inform the population beforehand about all these aspects so that they can make a free choice of this method, being aware of its advantages and limitations.

References

McKeown, Thomas, and R. G. Brown. 1955. "'Medical Evidence Related to English Population Changes in the Eighteenth Century.'" *Population Studies 9* 2: 119–41. https://doi.org/doi:10.1080/00324728.1955.10404688.

William H. Masters, Virginia E. Johnson. 1966. *Human Sexual Response*. 1981 edition. Toronto: New York: Bantam Books.

Killick, Stephen R., Christine Leary, James Trussell, and Katherine A. Guthrie. 2011. "Sperm Content of Pre-Ejaculatory Fluid." *Human Fertility* 14 (1): 48–52. https://doi.org/10.3109/14647273.2010.520798.

McKeown, Thomas, and R. G. Brown. 1955. "'Medical Evidence Related to English Population Changes in the Eighteenth Century.'" *Population Studies 9* 2: 119–41. https://doi.org/doi:10.1080/00324728.1955.10404688.

Population Reference Bureau. 2019. "Family Planning Data Sheet." *Journal of Family Medicine and Primary Care* 4 (4): 1–17. https://www.prb.org/wp-content/uploads/2019/03/fp-data-sheet-2019.pdf%0Ahttps://www.prb.org/international/geography/south-africa%0Ahttps://www.prb.org/wp-content/uploads/2019/03/fp-data-sheet-2019.pdf.

Sánchez Abellán-García, Fernando. 2016. *"Manual bioético-legal de consultas en salud."* Sociedad Española de Contracepción.

Chapter 4

Natural Contraceptive Methods

M. Moreno Palmero[1,*], MD
M. M. Castillo García[1], MD
A. Serrano Sánchez[1], MD
M. P. Mora Ábalos[1], MD
and A. Gómez Alarcón[2], MD

[1]Obstetrics and Gynecology Department, University and Hospital Complex of Albacete, Spain
[2]Obstetrics and Gynecology Department, Hospital of Almansa, Almansa, Spain

Abstract

Natural family planning using natural contraceptive methods represents a non-pharmacological alternative for fertility control based on the observation and recording of multiple biological signs related to the menstrual cycle. This chapter details the main natural family planning methods: the rhythm or calendar method, the basal body temperature method, the cervical mucus method (Billings), the symptothermal method, and the lactational amenorrhea method. Their physiological foundations, their requirements for a correct application, their efficacy rates, and their main advantages and limitations are analyzed. The review shows that, in general, all methods promise high efficacy and effectiveness when they are used appropriately and provide a high degree of bodily self-awareness. However, their main disadvantage is the lack of protection against sexually transmitted infections, especially for people who have multiple sexual partners. A detailed understanding of each of the methods is essential for adequately advising women and couples who wish to manage their fertility without resorting to hormonal or invasive contraceptive methods.

Keywords: natural contraceptive methods, natural family planning, menstrual cycle, contraceptive efficacy, ovulation, fertile window, basal body temperature, billings method, cervical mucus, rhythm method (Ogino-Knaus), symptothermal method, lactational amenorrhea, female fertility, reproductive education, body awareness; hormone-free reproductive health

---

* Corresponding Author's Email: monicampalmero@gmail.com

In: Advances in Reproductive Health
Editors: Llanos Belmonte Andujar and Ana Fuentes Rozalen
ISBN: 979-8-90134-038-7

Introduction

Natural contraceptive methods, also known as natural family planning (NFP), are based on the observation and recording of various bodily signals that allow the identification of fertile days of the menstrual cycle. This allows for avoiding sexual intercourse during these days and, consequently, preventing pregnancy without the use of hormones, devices, or other medical interventions. These methods are based on the observation of biological signs such as basal body temperature, cervical secretions, and menstrual cycle regularity (Grimes et al. 2004).

NFP methods have a long history and have been used in various forms across civilizations around the world. Since ancient times, civilizations have observed women's reproductive cycles and developed strategies to prevent pregnancy without medical intervention. For example, in Ancient Greece, methods such as observing menstrual cycles were used to regulate fertility (Riddle, 1992).

Natural contraceptive methods are strongly influenced by a philosophy of respect for the human body and its natural functioning, as they require women to understand their bodies and their natural cycles in order to make informed decisions about their fertility. Furthermore, these methods can be seen as a way to avoid external interventions, such as hormones or intrauterine devices, which can have side effects on health. The use of these mechanisms is also linked to a more ecological view of reproductive health, which seeks to respect biological processes without artificially altering them (Pallone & Bergus, 2009). These NFP methods are based on the observation and interpretation of the menstrual cycle, narrowing the fertile window and thus enabling family planning by avoiding sexual intercourse within this fertile window. Currently, there are menstrual cycle applications that analyze the cycle based on the data entered and calculate the presumed fertile window (Bettina Böttcher et al., 2024).

Efficacy and Effectiveness

The effectiveness of a contraceptive method, defined as the degree to which an intervention produces a beneficial effect under controlled and ideal conditions of adherence (Porta, 2014); in the case of a contraceptive method, it would be the degree to which it achieves its objective with strict adherence to the method, and it is one of the most important criteria that users take into account when selecting one or another. In this regard, it is important to differentiate between common contraceptive use and ideal use (Bettina Böttcher et al. 2024). The effectiveness of these methods varies considerably depending on the specific method used and adherence to it. When reviewing the different methods, pregnancy rates during the first year of typical use of NFP methods ranged from 1.8% to 33.6%, depending on the specific method. These results indicate that, although some methods can be quite effective, others have higher failure rates (Rachel Peragallo Urrutia et al. 2018). The effectiveness of natural methods depends primarily on the regularity of the woman's menstrual cycle and the willingness of both partners to closely monitor biological indicators (Ashley Jensen and Jane Wrede 2020).

NFP methods can be a valid option for many couples, but it is important to understand that their effectiveness (understood as the degree to which an intervention produces a beneficial effect under real or routine conditions (Fletcher et al., 2014)) depends mainly on consistency, knowledge of the menstrual cycle, and correct application of the different methods. Some factors that influence their success are education and training (especially for some methods, such as basal body temperature or cervical mucus); it is essential that the woman be well trained to interpret changes in her body; commitment and consistency (constant monitoring and close attention to detail); risks of incorrect application (natural methods have a relatively high failure rate if not applied correctly); and some method-specific considerations to take into account (for example, methods such as breastfeeding are only effective under specific conditions). They require adequate training on the subject, commitment, and consistency. A common disadvantage to take into account with NFP methods is that they do not present the additional effects of other types of contraceptives, such as prevention of sexually transmitted infections (STIs) in the case of barrier methods, or the beneficial non-contraceptive effects of oral contraceptives (Pallone & Bergus, 2009), (Arévalo et al., 2004a).

There are biological factors that can affect the effectiveness of these methods, among which the following can be highlighted (Arévalo et al. 2004b):

- *Menstrual cycle irregularity*: Each woman's menstrual cycle is unique and can vary from month to month. Irregular cycles can make it difficult to track fertile days and therefore disrupt methods such as the calendar or basal body temperature. Women with irregular cycles should be aware that cycle-tracking methods require more detailed monitoring and possibly be combined with other techniques to improve their effectiveness (World Health Organization, 2018).
- *A woman's age:* The frequency and regularity of ovulation may decrease as women age. This can make natural methods more difficult to follow, and the fertile window may become less predictable (Fritz & Speroff, 2011b).
- *Health conditions*: Health conditions that affect hormone levels, such as polycystic ovary syndrome or hypothyroidism, can disrupt the menstrual cycle and make it more difficult to accurately identify fertile days. Women with these conditions should take additional precautions before relying entirely on an NFP method as their sole contraceptive. Stress can also affect the menstrual cycle and ovulation, leading to more irregular cycles, which could compromise the accuracy of natural methods (Fritz & Speroff, 2011a).

Advantages and Disadvantages

A characteristic of NFP methods is that they involve both partners in understanding the menstrual cycle and in a commitment to follow the calculations and observations on both sides to ensure their effectiveness. The use of natural contraceptive methods requires open and constant communication between the couple, unlike other contraceptive methods, which are usually the responsibility of only one partner. Consistent adherence to the method is essential to reduce the risk of pregnancy, so couples must agree that using these methods will be a shared responsibility.

Natural contraceptive methods have no direct side effects on reproductive health, as they are procedures that do not involve pharmacological treatment or physical measures. This is important for women who wish to avoid the side effects of hormones, although they do not benefit from the non-contraceptive effects of hormonal contraceptives. However, it is important to remember that natural methods do not protect against STI infections, which can be a limitation for individuals with multiple sexual partners.

An additional benefit of using natural methods is that women develop greater awareness and knowledge of their menstrual cycle and overall reproductive health. This, in addition to being useful for avoiding pregnancy, also helps them better understand fertility if they wish to space their pregnancies or conceive later. Many experts believe that the body awareness gained through using NFP methods can also help women identify reproductive problems, such as polycystic ovary syndrome or endometriosis.

Any of the NFP methods can be combined with each other to increase their effectiveness. For example, some women use the basal body temperature method in conjunction with the cervical mucus monitoring method to more accurately identify their fertile days. Using both methods together synergistically allows for a more accurate assessment of fertility and reduces the risk of unintended pregnancy (Trussell, 2011).

Main natural contraceptive methods:

- *Rhythm or calendar method, Ogino-Knaus method.* This method is based on calculating the fertile days of the cycle by observing the length of past menstrual cycles. To perform this method, the patient must record her cycle for several months and avoid sexual intercourse during the fertile days of each cycle. Its effectiveness varies depending on the regularity of the menstrual cycle, ranging from 75% to 88%.
- *Basal body temperature method.* It is based on a woman measuring her body temperature every morning before getting out of bed. This method is based on the fact that, after ovulation, body temperature generally rises slightly, between 0.2°C and 0.5°C. This method maintains that sexual intercourse should be avoided from the beginning of the cycle until three days after the sustained temperature increase. Its effectiveness, with perfect use, ranges from 76% to 99%.
- *Cervical mucus method (Billings method).* It is based on observing changes in vaginal discharge throughout the menstrual cycle. During fertile days, mucus is more abundant, clear, elastic, and slippery (with a consistency similar to egg white). This method involves avoiding sexual intercourse from the moment mucus considered fertile due to its characteristics appears, until 3-4 days after the peak mucus. Its effectiveness ranges from 78% to 97%.
- *Symptothermal method.* It is based on a combination of several of the methods described above, including basal body temperature, changes in cervical mucus, and other symptoms and signs (ovulatory pain, cervical changes). It requires training to identify these multiple fertility signs and greater precision and commitment to abstaining from sexual intercourse on fertile days. It is up to 98-99% effective if used correctly.
- *Lactational amenorrhea method (LAM).* It is based on the natural infertility that occurs during the first months of exclusive breastfeeding. It has three fundamental requirements: the woman must be in amenorrhea since childbirth, be exclusively breastfed (with breastfeeding intervals no longer than 4-6 hours), and breastfeed exclusively during the first 6 months postpartum. Its effectiveness during this time, if all three requirements are met, is 98% (Pallone & Bergus, 2009), (Bettina Böttcher et al., 2024).

Rhythm or Calendar Method

The rhythm method (calendar method or Ogino-Knaus method) was developed in the 1930s by Drs. Kyusaku Ogino and Hermann Knaus. It is based on the observation that ovulation occurs approximately midway through the menstrual cycle and that the egg is viable for a short time after its release (Wilcox, Dunson, and Baird 2000). It consists of predicting the fertile days of the cycle by calculating the length of previous cycles.

Ovulation typically occurs approximately 14 days before the onset of the next menstruation. Because sperm can survive in the female reproductive tract for up to five days, and an egg remains viable for 12 to 24 hours after ovulation, the fertile window generally extends from five days before to one or two days after ovulation (Arévalo, Jennings, and Sinai 2002). The rhythm method posits that the fertile window can be estimated retrospectively by analyzing a woman's previous cycles, and abstinence and intercourse can be planned accordingly.

To correctly apply the rhythm method, it is necessary to record the duration of at least 6 to 12 consecutive menstrual cycles and identify the shortest and longest cycles, so that the fertile period can be calculated as accurately as possible. To calculate the first day of this period, 18 days should be subtracted from the number of days in the shortest cycle; and to calculate the last fertile day, 11 days would be subtracted from the number of days in the longest cycle (Wilcox, Dunson, and Baird 2000). Thus, for example, if the shortest cycle has 26 days, subtracting 18 would make the eighth day of the cycle the first day of the fertile window; and if the longest cycle is 31 days, subtracting 11 would make the twentieth day the last day of the fertile window within that cycle. This means that unprotected sexual intercourse should be avoided between days 8 and 20 of the cycle (Urrutia and Polis 2019), (Petra Frank-Herrmann et al. 2005).

The typical failure rate for the rhythm method is approximately 12–20%, i.e., 12 to 20 pregnancies per 100 women using this method for a year. The perfect success rate, under optimal conditions of use, is closer to 91%, although real-life use is often less accurate (Trussell 2011).

Its advantages include those of any NFP method: it does not involve the use of drugs or physical or hormone-releasing devices, it promotes knowledge and education about the menstrual cycle, and it has no physical side effects.

The disadvantages include its lower effectiveness compared to other, more modern natural methods (combined fertility awareness methods); for it to be an accurate procedure, menstrual cycles must be regular (it's a difficult method to follow for women who experience frequent menstrual irregularities); and, like other natural planning methods, it doesn't protect against STIs.

This method is primarily suitable for women with regular cycles and a high level of commitment who will carefully record their menstrual cycles. The reliability of the rhythm method decreases significantly in women with irregular cycles, who are breastfeeding, in perimenopause, or who have experienced recent changes in their health, stress, diet, or physical activity that could alter their ovulation pattern (World Health Organization 2018).

Basal Body Temperature (BBT) Method

The basal body temperature method is a natural family planning technique based on observing the daily variation in body temperature caused by hormonal changes during the menstrual cycle (Colombo and Masarotto 2000).

Physiologically, during the follicular phase of the menstrual cycle (prior to ovulation), progesterone levels are low, and basal body temperature remains relatively stable. After ovulation, the formation of the corpus luteum in the ovary increases progesterone production, generating a subtle temperature increase of approximately 0.2°C to 0.5°C, which is maintained until the onset of menstruation or throughout pregnancy, if conception occurs (P. Frank-Herrmann et al. 2007). Therefore, systematic daily temperature recording allows ovulation to be retrospectively identified, delimiting the end of the fertile window of the cycle.

For proper application of this method, the following are required: measure the woman's basal body temperature every morning (immediately after waking and before any physical activity), use a high-precision clinical thermometer (digital or mercury), and always measure the temperature in the same location (oral, rectal, or vaginal). Daily measurements should be recorded on a chart that visualizes temperature changes and identifies sustained temperature increases: an increase of at least 0.2°C that lasts for three consecutive days indicates that ovulation has occurred. A woman is considered to have left her fertile window once she has observed three consecutive days of elevated temperatures compared to the six previous lower measurements.

The basal body temperature method, when used correctly, is 98% effective (perfect use), while its effectiveness in typical real-life use is 80–88% (Petra Frank-Herrmann et al. 2005), (P. Frank-Herrmann et al. 2007). Its accuracy can be increased when combined with other fertility indicators, as in the symptothermal method.

As for its advantages, it is an economical, accessible, and noninvasive method that promotes detailed knowledge of the menstrual cycle, and, like other NFP methods, has no side effects.

Among the main disadvantages are: first, the fact that it does not provide prospective information, but rather retrospective information (it confirms ovulation after it has occurred); it requires daily consistency and discipline in measuring; and, as a specific characteristic of this method, there is the influence of external factors that can alter the method's effectiveness by modifying basal body temperature (fever, insomnia, stress, alcohol consumption, travel, among others).

To carry out this method rigorously, the user must be properly instructed to take measurements at the same time each day (preferably after at least three hours of continuous sleep), record any conditions that could alter the measurement, and consider this method less reliable if there are febrile illnesses or frequent sleep disturbances. In women with irregular cycles or medical conditions that affect thermoregulation, combined methods are recommended for greater contraceptive security (P. Frank-Herrmann et al. 2007), (Shacter, Gee, and Long 2007).

Cervical Mucus Method (Billings Method)

The cervical mucus method, also known as the Billings Ovulation Method, is an NFP strategy based on the systematic observation of changes in cervical mucus during the menstrual cycle.

It was developed by doctors John and Evelyn Billings in the 1950s, and has been supported by numerous clinical studies that confirm its effectiveness and scientific basis (Ecochard et al. 2015).

Cervical mucus is produced by the glands of the endocervical canal, and its quantity, consistency, and properties vary under the influence of fluctuating levels of estrogen and progesterone. During the early follicular phase, the mucus is scant, thick, and opaque, with low elasticity; whereas during the periovulatory phase, its volume progressively increases, becoming stringy, transparent, and lubricating ("egg white" mucus), which optimizes the passage of sperm through the female genital canal. Finally, in the luteal phase, the volume decreases, returning to a thick, scant mucus that forms a cervical plug. Observing these variations throughout the cycle allows a woman to identify and recognize her fertile window, as it is a reliable biomarker of her fertility status.

The Billings method is highly demanding, as it requires daily self-observation of subjective vulvar sensation (dry, wet, lubricated) and the appearance of mucus if visible, recording the characteristics of the mucus (quantity, color, elasticity, and sensation), as well as identifying the "peak of fertility," defined as the last day on which the highest quality fertile mucus is observed. To increase its effectiveness, sexual intercourse should be avoided on any day when a sensation of wetness or the presence of mucus is present, and it should be noted that the three days after peak fertility are considered the end of the fertile period, so unprotected sexual intercourse can be resumed if pregnancy is to be avoided.

Clinical studies have shown that the Billings Method, when used correctly and with proper instruction, is 97–99% effective with perfect use, and 86–90% effective with typical use (Fehring RJ, Schneider M, and Raviele K 2012). A World Health Organization multicenter trial showed that women trained in cervical mucus self-monitoring had pregnancy rates comparable to those using traditional barrier methods of contraception (World Health Organization and Johns Hopkins 2022).

Some of the advantages we could highlight about this method include the fact that it does not involve pharmacological interventions or physical devices, that it can be used both to space pregnancies and to facilitate conception, that it promotes self-knowledge of the female body, and that it is compatible with special situations such as breastfeeding and irregular cycles.

As for its disadvantages, it requires proper instruction from certified professionals, its effectiveness depends largely on adherence to established rules and correct interpretation of mucus, and, like other NFP methods, it does not protect against STIs.

The cervical mucus method is particularly useful for women with irregular cycles, during postpartum breastfeeding, and in women transitioning to menopause; in circumstances where methods based on calendar calculations are less reliable, cervical mucus monitoring may offer a more accurate natural contraceptive strategy (Padilha and Deretti 2021).

Symptothermal Method

The symptothermal method is an NFP strategy that combines the observation of multiple physiological signs of fertility; primarily changes in basal body temperature, modifications in cervical mucus, and alterations in the position and consistency of the cervix. By integrating various biological signals, this method offers one of the highest effectiveness rates among NFP procedures, both for spacing pregnancies and facilitating conception (World Health Organization and Johns Hopkins 2022). The symptothermal method is one of the most robust and scientifically validated NFP alternatives for fertility monitoring due to the wide range of variables it considers, which is why it also requires a high level of commitment, self-knowledge, and discipline for its correct application.

This method is based on the fact that the menstrual cycle is regulated by hormonal variations that impact basal body temperature (there is a characteristic temperature shift of between 0.2°C and 0.5°C during the luteal phase compared to levels during the follicular phase due to the increase in progesterone), variations in the characteristics of cervical mucus that reflect the fertile window, and peculiarities in the size and consistency of the cervix (softer, higher, and more open during the fertile period; and firmer, lower, and closed at the end of this period). The integration of all these signs allows for a more precise identification of the fertile window of the menstrual cycle.

To perform this method correctly, it requires: daily measurement of basal body temperature (preferably at the same time each morning before rising, using a high-precision basal thermometer), daily observation of cervical mucus (recording vulvar sensation and visible characteristics), and assessment of cervical position (optional, but one that can provide additional information). Using these three parameters, all observations should be systematically recorded in a dedicated chart. The fertile period extends from the appearance of the first sign of fertility (changes in mucus or cervical position) to the third day of elevated temperature. This method requires proper guidance, and initial training by certified instructors is key to success.

Scientific evidence indicates that the symptothermal method, when correctly practiced, is 98–99.6% effective (with perfect use) and 93–96% effective with typical use in determining the fertile window and avoiding an unwanted pregnancy (Petra Frank-Herrmann et al. 2005) (P. Frank-Herrmann et al. 2007). A recent meta-analysis reaffirms that dual-signal methods (basal temperature and cervical mucus) significantly reduce the rate of unintended pregnancy compared to single-signal methods (Manhart et al. 2013).

Among the advantages of the symptothermal method are its high effectiveness (comparable to barrier contraceptive methods), which increases body awareness (providing women with a high level of competence in their fertility knowledge), and promotes a healthier lifestyle, allowing couples to plan both pregnancy avoidance and conception. Like other NFP methods, it does not involve pharmacological side effects. It can also be adapted to women who are breastfeeding, postpartum, perimenopausal, and have irregular cycles (which will require closer professional support for interpretation) (Petra Frank-Herrmann et al. 2005).

Some disadvantages worth highlighting could be that it requires specific technical learning and disciplined practice, it is sensitive to factors that alter body temperature (infections, insomnia, alcohol consumption) and due to its requirements, it may be perceived as complex by some women (World Health Organization 2023).

Lactational Amenorrhea Method (LAM)

The lactational amenorrhea method (LAM) or lactational amenorrhea method or internationally known as the "Lactational Amenorrhea Method (LAM)," is a natural and temporary contraceptive method, which provides information and support to mothers to use breastfeeding as a method of NFP (Van der Wijden and Manion 2015). It was defined by scientists and fertility specialists at the Bellagio Consensus Conference in Italy in 1988, in which they established the three necessary requirements to carry out the method, with a risk of pregnancy lower than 2%, which the WHO establishes as less than 1% (- 1988), (World Health Organization 2023).

The requirements for using this method as an NFP are: the woman must remain in amenorrhea from birth, breastfeed exclusively, and it can only be used during the first six months postpartum. After six months, the effectiveness of this method decreases when the baby is started on complementary foods, something women should be aware of if this is their only method of contraception.

This method is based on the inhibition of ovulation that occurs during exclusive breastfeeding. Frequent sucking of the nipple by the baby stimulates the release of oxytocin and prolactin by the mother. The latter hormone suppresses pituitary secretion of gonadotropin-releasing hormone (GnRH), reducing the release of hypothalamic luteinizing hormone (LH) and follicle-stimulating hormone (FSH); ultimately, ovulation is inhibited. For this inhibition stimulus to be effective, the baby must be at the breast suckling as much as possible, and feeding frequency must be high, including nighttime feedings. No intervals longer than 4 to 6 hours should pass without breastfeeding (Chowdhury et al. 2015).

The LAM method has an effectiveness rate of up to 98% in amenorrheic women who exclusively breastfeed during the first 6 months after delivery. Pregnancy rates vary, ranging from 0.45% to 7.5%, depending on the patient's eligibility (Van der Wijden C, Kleijnen J, and Van den Berk T 2022).

Among the advantages of this method are: it is cost-effective and free, natural, non-invasive, and accessible to most women. It promotes breastfeeding, providing the world-renowned benefits of exclusive breastfeeding for the first six months to infants; and to maternal benefits such as breastfeeding protection against breast and ovarian cancer and a reduced risk of type 2 diabetes (Chowdhury et al. 2015).

Regarding the method's drawbacks, particularly for mothers, we can highlight its limited duration, the requirement for exclusive breastfeeding, and the potential for method failure, since ovulation can precede menstruation. And, like other NFP methods, it also offers no protection against STIs (Van der Wijden and Manion 2015).

Conclusion

All NFP methods are based on a deep understanding of the menstrual cycle and require a high level of commitment and daily observation to achieve effectiveness in preventing pregnancy.

There are a variety of natural methods within NFP, each with its own particular characteristics, allowing each to be tailored to the needs, preferences, and physiological conditions of each woman and couple.

The effectiveness of these techniques varies depending on the method used and its application. Symptothermal and cervical mucus methods, when used correctly and with adequate training, offer levels of effectiveness comparable to barrier contraceptive methods; while methods such as the rhythm method have higher failure rates under typical use conditions. It should be noted that none of these methods protect against sexually transmitted infections (STIs), and all require consistency, education, and follow-up. Certain factors such as menstrual irregularities, medical conditions, or stress can reduce their effectiveness.

A fundamental advantage of NFP is its high educational and empowering potential, as it promotes sexual and reproductive education, fosters self-awareness, and can strengthen communication and commitment within couples regarding fertility, becoming a comprehensive health tool beyond its contraceptive function.

References

-. 1988. "Breastfeeding as a Family Planning Method." *Lancet* (London, England) 2 (8621): 1204–5.

Arévalo, Marcos, Victoria Jennings, Minna Nikula, and Irit Sinai. 2004a. "Efficacy of the New Two-Day Method of Family Planning." *Fertility and Sterility* 82 (4): 885–92. https://doi.org/10.1016/j.fertnstert.2004.03.040.

———. 2004b. "Efficacy of the New Two-Day Method of Family Planning." *Fertility and Sterility* 82 (4): 885–92. https://doi.org/10.1016/j.fertnstert.2004.03.040.

Arévalo, Marcos, Victoria Jennings, and Irit Sinai. 2002. "Efficacy of a New Method of Family Planning: The Standard Days Method." *Contraception* 65 (5): 333–38. https://doi.org/10.1016/S0010-7824(02)00288-3.

Ashley Jensen, and Jane Wrede. 2020. "Fertility Awareness-Based Methods for Family Planning: A Literature Review." *Journal of Christian Nursing: A Quiarterly Publication of Nurses Christian Fellowship* 37 (4): 212–20.

Bettina Böttcher, Maria J. Beckermann, Barbara Berger, Jann Frederik Cremers, Elisabeth D'Costa, Petra Frank-Herrmann, Tanja Freundl-Schütt, et al. 2024. "*S2k-Guideline Non-Hormonal Contraception, Part 1: Natural Family Planning, Lactational Amenorrhea, Barrier Methods, Coitus Interruptus*." Thieme 84 (No. 015-095): 697–714.

Chowdhury, Ranadip, Bireshwar Sinha, Mari Jeeva Sankar, Sunita Taneja, Nita Bhandari, Nigel Rollins, Rajiv Bahl, and Jose Martines. 2015. "Breastfeeding and Maternal Health Outcomes: A Systematic Review and Meta-analysis." *Acta Paediatrica* 104 (S467): 96–113. https://doi.org/10.1111/apa.13102.

Colombo, B, and G Masarotto. 2000. "Daily Fecundability: First Results from a New Data Base." *Demographic Research* 3 (September):[39] p.

Ecochard, Rene, Olivia Duterque, Rene Leiva, Thomas Bouchard, and Pilar Vigil. 2015. "Self-Identification of the Clinical Fertile Window and the Ovulation Period." *Fertility and Sterility* 103 (5): 1319-1325.e3. https://doi.org/10.1016/j.fertnstert.2015.01.031.

Fehring RJ, Schneider M, and Raviele K. 2012. "Efficacy of Cervical Mucus Observations plus Electronic Hormonal Fertility Monitoring as a Method of Natural Family Planning." *Journal of Obstetric, Gynecologic & Neonatal Nursing* 41 (5): 583–91.

Fletcher, RH, SW Fletcher, and GS Fletcher. 2014. *Clinical Epidemiology: The Essentials*. Edited by Lippincott Williams & Wilkins. 5th ed.

Frank-Herrmann, P., J. Heil, C. Gnoth, E. Toledo, S. Baur, C. Pyper, E. Jenetzky, T. Strowitzki, and G. Freundl. 2007. "The Effectiveness of a Fertility Awareness Based Method to Avoid Pregnancy in Relation to a Couple's Sexual Behavior during the Fertile Time: A Prospective Longitudinal Study." *Human Reproduction* 22 (5): 1310–19. https://doi.org/10.1093/humrep/dem003.

Frank-Herrmann, Petra, C Gnoth, S Baur, T Strowitzki, and G Freundl. 2005. "Determination of the Fertile Window: Reproductive Competence of Women – European Cycle Databases." *Gynecological Endocrinology* 20 (6): 305–12. https://doi.org/10.1080/09513590500097507.

Fritz, M. A., and L. Speroff. 2011a. *Clinical Gynecologic Endocrinology and Infertility*. 8th ed. Vol. Chapter 1.

———. 2011b. *Clinical Gynecologic Endocrinology and Infertility*. 8th ed.

Grimes, David A, Maria F Gallo, Vera Halpern, Kavita Nanda, Kenneth F Schulz, and Laureen M Lopez. 2004. "Fertility Awareness-Based Methods for Contraception." *Cochrane Database of Systematic Reviews* 4 (October). https://doi.org/10.1002/14651858.CD004860.pub2.

Manhart, Michael D., Marguerite Duane, April Lind, Irit Sinai, and Jean Golden-Tevald. 2013. "Fertility Awareness-Based Methods of Family Planning: A Review of Effectiveness for Avoiding Pregnancy Using SORT." *Osteopathic Family Physician* 5 (1): 2–8. https://doi.org/10.1016/j.osfp.2012.09.002.

World Health Organization. 2023. "*Family Planning/Contraceptive Methods*." September 5, 2023.

Padilha, Tarcisio, and Edson Adolfo Deretti. 2021. "Billings Ovulação Method: Between Efficiency and Deconhecimento." *Bioethics Magazine* 29 (1): 208–19. https://doi.org/10.1590/1983-80422021291460.

Pallone, SR, and GR Bergus. 2009. "Fertility Awareness-Based Methods: Another Option for Family Planning." *The Journal of the American Board of Family Medicine* 22 (2): 147–57. https://doi.org/10.3122/jabfm.2009.02.080038.

Porta, M. 2014. *A Dictionary of Epidemiology*. Edited by Oxford University Press. 6th ed.

Rachel Peragallo Urrutia, Chelsea B Polis, Elizabeth T Jensen, Margaret E Greene, Emily Kennedy, and Joseph B Stanford. 2018. "Effectiveness of Fertility Awareness-Based Methods for Pregnancy Prevention: A Systematic Review." *Obstetrics and Gynecology* 132 (3): 591–604.

Riddle, J. M. 1992. *Contraception and Abortion from the Ancient World to the Renaissance*. Cambridge, MA: Harvard University Press.

Shacter, Hannah E., Rebekah E. Gee, and Judith A. Long. 2007. "Variation in Availability of Emergency Contraception in Pharmacies." *Contraception* 75 (3): 214–17. https://doi.org/10.1016/j.contraception.2006.11.005.

Trussell, James. 2011. "Contraceptive Failure in the United States." *Contraception* 83 (5): 397–404. https://doi.org/10.1016/j.contraception.2011.01.021.

Urrutia, Rachel Peragallo, and Chelsea B Polis. 2019. "Fertility Awareness Based Methods for Pregnancy Prevention." *BMJ*, July. https://doi.org/10.1136/bmj.l4245.

Wijden C, Van der, Kleijnen J, and Van den Berk T. 2022. "Lactational amenorrhea for family planning (Cochrane Review)." *The Cochrane Library Plus*, October.

Wijden, Carla Van der, and Carol Manion. 2015. "Lactational Amenorrhea Method for Family Planning." *Cochrane Database of Systematic Reviews 2015* (10). https://doi.org/10.1002/14651858.CD001329.pub2.

Wilcox, A. J, D Dunson, and DD Baird. 2000. "The Timing of the 'Fertile Window' in the Menstrual Cycle: Day Specific Estimates from a Prospective Study." *BMJ* 321(7271): 1259–62. https://doi.org/10.1136/bmj.321.7271.1259.

World Health Organization. 2018. *Family Planning: A Global Handbook for Providers: Evidence-Based Guidance Developed through Worldwide Collaboration*, 3rd Ed. 3rd ed.

World Health Organization, and Johns Hopkins. 2022. *Family planning a global handbook for providers*. Edited by United States Agency for International Development Bureau for Global Health Office of Population and Reproductive Health. 4th ed.

Chapter 5

Barrier Contraceptive Methods

M. Cebrián Marcilla[1,*], MD
M. Moreno Palmero[1], MD
M. M. Castillo García[1], MD
Ll. Belmonte Andújar[2], PhD
and A. M. Fuentes Rozalén[3], MD
[1]Obstetrics and Gynecology Department, University and Hospital of Albacete, Albacete, Spain
[2]Medical Science Department, School of Medicine of Albacete, Universidad de Castilla-La Mancha, Spain
[3]Instituto Bernabeu of Alicante, Spain

Abstract

The main ones include the male and female condom, diaphragm, cervical cap, contraceptive sponge, spermicides and vaginal pH-regulating gels. The condom is the most accessible method and the only one that, when used correctly, effectively protects against sexually transmitted infections, including the human immunodeficiency virus. Other devices, such as the diaphragm and cervical cap, require precise placement and concomitant use of spermicides to optimise their efficacy, which decreases after vaginal delivery. The contraceptive sponge combines barrier and spermicide, allowing multiple intercourse without removal, although it presents a risk of irritation and toxic shock syndrome if used for prolonged periods. Spermicides used alone have low efficacy and may increase vulnerability to sexually transmitted infections. PH-regulating gels represent a non-hormonal alternative in development, with potential for future innovations based on topical monoclonal antibodies. The general advantages of these methods include immediate reversibility, low cost, user autonomy and absence of systemic hormonal effects. However, their variable efficacy and the need for adequate education limit their exclusive use. Combination with hormonal methods can enhance contraceptive and STI protection, optimising reproductive health.

Keywords: contraception, barrier, condom, diaphragm, sponge, spermicides, autonomy

---

* Corresponding Author's Email: marta.ceb.mar@gmail.com

In: Advances in Reproductive Health
Editors: Llanos Belmonte Andujar and Ana Fuentes Rozalen
ISBN: 979-8-90134-038-7

Introduction

Barrier methods are a type of contraceptive that prevent sperm from reaching the egg by blocking their passage into the female reproductive system. They work by creating a physical or chemical barrier that stops fertilization. This group includes the male and female condom, the diaphragm, the cervical cap, and the vaginal sponge. Although spermicides and vaginal pH regulators are not physical barriers, they are sometimes included in this category because they are used in combination with these methods and help prevent pregnancy.

The contraceptive effectiveness varies depending on the type of method, correct use, and user adherence, with failure rates ranging from 2% to 28% according to data on typical use (WHO 2022; Trussell 2011).

History and Development of Barrier Methods

The use of barrier methods to prevent pregnancy is very old. It is known that in civilizations such as Egypt and Rome, linen wrappings or animal bladders were used as protection (Service 2023). As early as the 19th century, thanks to the vulcanization of rubber, reusable condoms began to be manufactured, which made these methods more durable and accessible. Later, in 1920, the use of latex made it possible to produce condoms on a large scale and with better quality. Other methods such as the diaphragm and the cervical cap, designed to cover the cervix, became especially popular in Europe and the United States at the beginning of the 20th century (Dittrick Medical History Center, accessed 2025). During the first decades of the 20th century, these methods were practically the only option available to many women. However, their use has declined over time. According to the 1995 National Survey of Family Growth, the use of female-controlled barrier methods reached one of its lowest recorded levels (Gilliam and Derman 2000).

The contraceptive sponge is a method that combines a physical barrier with chemical spermicides. Its origins go back to ancient times in civilizations such as Egypt and Greece, where natural sea sponges soaked in substances like vinegar or boric acid were used to prevent pregnancy, while more recent versions are made of synthetic materials impregnated with spermicides (Dittrick Medical History Center, accessed 2025).

Importance in Reproductive Health

Barrier methods are very important for reproductive health for several reasons. First, they are non-hormonal contraceptive methods, which makes them ideal for people who do not want to use hormonal contraception or who have health conditions that prevent its use. Second, they are the only contraceptive methods that offer dual protection: they help prevent pregnancy and also reduce the risk of sexually transmitted infections (STIs), including HIV.

However, it is important to keep in mind that, in general terms, barrier methods tend to be less effective than hormonal methods. For this reason, it is essential to use them correctly and consistently to ensure their effectiveness (CDC 2025; Chappell, Griffin and Howard 2022; Dittrick Medical History Center, accessed 2025).

From a public health perspective, they are a key tool because they are easy to obtain, affordable, and do not require a prescription. All of this makes them essential in family planning and disease prevention programs. In addition, they allow each person to have more control over their sexual and reproductive life, which is closely linked to the respect for their sexual and reproductive rights (Nabhan et al. 2023).

Main Barrier Methods

Male Condom

The male condom (Figure 1) is a barrier contraceptive method that is placed over the erect penis and acts as a physical barrier that blocks sperm from entering the uterus, preventing them from reaching the egg.

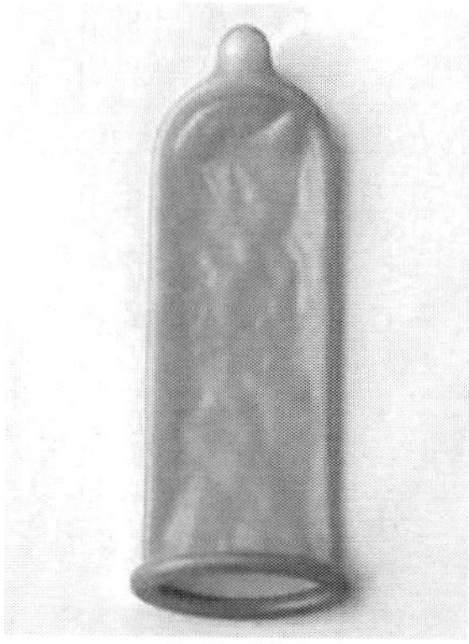

Figure 1. Male condom.

Types of Condoms and Advances in Materials

There are multiple types of male condoms, primarily distinguished by the material they are made from. Latex remains the most widely used material globally, thanks to its excellent elasticity, durability, and low cost. However, its use can trigger allergic reactions in approximately 4% of the population, which justifies the need to offer safe alternatives for people with sensitivity to this material (Trussell 2011; WHO 2023).

In such cases, latex-free condoms are recommended. Among them, those made of polyurethane—a synthetic plastic that is thinner and allows better heat transmission—stand out as they can enhance the sensation of natural intimacy during sex. However, its lower elasticity can result in a looser fit and a slightly higher risk of slippage (Workowski et al. 2021; CDC 2025a). On the other hand, polyisoprene, a synthetic rubber derivative, offers properties similar to latex in terms of comfort and strength, but without the proteins that cause allergic reactions, making it a safe and effective option (Tsikouras et al. 2024; Kopa et al. 2024a; Frezieres et al. 1999; Crosby et al. 2013).

Another less common alternative is the condom made from natural membranes, such as sheep cecum (commonly known as "lambskin"). While it offers a more natural-feeling experience due to its texture and porosity, it does not provide protection against STIs (Trussell 2011; WHO 2023).

Condoms are available in lubricated, flavored, or textured versions, adapting to different individual preferences. It is essential to remember that oil-based lubricants should be avoided with latex and polyisoprene condoms, as they can weaken the material and increase the risk of breakage. Instead, compatible lubricants such as water- or silicone-based options should be used (Workowski et al. 2021; CDC 2025a).

In the field of innovation, the industry has developed condoms made with graphene, an ultra-strong and flexible material that improves heat transfer and sensitivity, offering an experience closer to skin-to-skin contact (Tsikouras et al. 2024; Kopa et al. 2024a; Frezieres et al. 1999; Crosby et al. 2013). Likewise, hydrogel condoms are currently being studied as a self-lubricating, latex-free option, ideal for people with allergies and promising better comfort and tolerance (Beksinska et al. 2020).

Among the latest innovations is the Lelo Hex condom, made from natural latex with a hexagonal structure composed of 350 interconnected cells. This design allows it to adapt better to the anatomy, provides greater strength, and reduces the risk of breakage without sacrificing sensitivity (Woo 2016).

A new type of pre-erection condom has also been developed and is already being marketed in the United Kingdom and Germany. It is applied while the penis is still flaccid and stays in place with a base ring. Its goal is to reduce the interruption of the intimate moment and provide a helpful alternative for men with anxiety-induced erectile dysfunction when using condoms (Godoy 2024).

Furthermore, in response to growing environmental awareness and the demands of consumers who follow a vegan lifestyle, condoms made from biodegradable materials and recyclable packaging are being developed. These products not only reduce environmental impact, but are also made without animal-derived ingredients and are not tested on animals, while maintaining the same contraceptive effectiveness as traditional condoms (Euronews 2019).

Correct Way of Use

The correct use of the male condom is essential to ensure both its contraceptive effectiveness and its ability to prevent sexually transmitted infections. It should be put on before any genital contact, as pre-ejaculate fluid can also contain sperm (WHO 2023). In addition to its primary role as a contraceptive method, the condom also serves as a backup in case of failure of other methods, such as missed doses of hormonal contraceptives (Kopa et al. 2024a).

To use a condom correctly, it should be applied to the erect penis, leaving a small space at the tip (the reservoir) to collect semen. It is important to squeeze the air out of the tip before unrolling it completely to the base of the penis. After intercourse, it should be removed while the penis is still erect, holding the base firmly to prevent leakage. Condoms should not be reused, should not be opened with sharp objects, and must be stored properly to ensure their effectiveness (Trussell 2011; ACOG 2025).

Mistakes such as not leaving space at the tip, not unrolling the condom fully, or using incompatible lubricants can compromise its effectiveness. These errors, though common, are easily prevented with proper sexual education (Workowski et al. 2021).

Effectiveness and Prevention of STIs

With correct and consistent use, the failure rate according to the Pearl Index is only about 2% per year, although with typical use it can rise to 13% (Trussell 2011; Kopa et al. 2024a; Majra 2010). Combining condoms with another method, such as the use of spermicides, represents a more effective strategy to prevent both pregnancy and sexually transmitted infections (ACOG 2025).

The male condom is the only contraceptive method that effectively protects against most STIs, including HIV, chlamydia, gonorrhea, syphilis, and herpes simplex (American College of Obstetricians and Gynecologists 2025). Various studies indicate that it reduces the risk of acquiring HIV by between 80% and 90%, a figure that improves with correct and systematic use. For STIs such as HPV (Human Papillomavirus) or herpes, which can be transmitted through skin-to-skin contact, protection is partial (WHO 2023).

The increase in STIs, especially among young people, has been linked to the use of social networks and dating apps, reinforcing the need to promote condom use through comprehensive and evidence-based sexual education (Beksinska et al. 2020).

Education and Counselling

Good professional counseling improves the acceptance and correct use of condoms. Social or cultural stigma must also be addressed through education, ideally starting at an early age and reinforced in healthcare, school, and community settings (WHO 2023).

Having clear and contextualized information allows people to make informed decisions, improve sexual autonomy, reduce unplanned pregnancies, and effectively and empathetically prevent STIs.

Condoms and Sexual Dysfunction

The condom can have both positive and negative impacts on sexual function. Some models are designed to delay ejaculation, helping those seeking greater ejaculatory control. In other cases, condoms may be associated with psychogenic erectile dysfunction, especially due to reduced sensitivity or their effect on arousal. Ultrathin condoms represent an effective alternative in these cases (Tsikouras et al. 2024; Kopa et al. 2024a; Randolph et al. 2007; Service et al. 2023), as does the development of the new pre-erection condoms mentioned earlier (Godoy 2024).

Female Condom

Characteristics and Materials

The female condom, also known as the internal condom (Figure 2), provides protection against both unplanned pregnancies and sexually transmitted infections. Unlike the male condom, it is inserted inside the vagina before sexual intercourse, giving the user greater control over her sexual health (Tsikouras et al. 2024; Harris et al. 2022).

It consists of a sheath with two flexible rings: one closed ring that is inserted and remains at the end of the vagina, and an external ring that stays outside the body covering part of the vulva. This design allows for greater coverage of the external genitalia, thereby reducing the risk of transmission of sexually transmitted infections, especially those spread by skin-to-skin contact (Workowski et al. 2021).

Currently, there are different versions made from materials such as nitrile, polyurethane, or latex. The most widely used model is the FC2 (Female Condom), approved by the FDA (Food and Drug Administration), made of nitrile and pre-lubricated with silicone. Other versions, such as Cupid FC or VA w.o.w ("Added Value Week after Week"), include a medical sponge to facilitate insertion (Tsikouras et al. 2024).

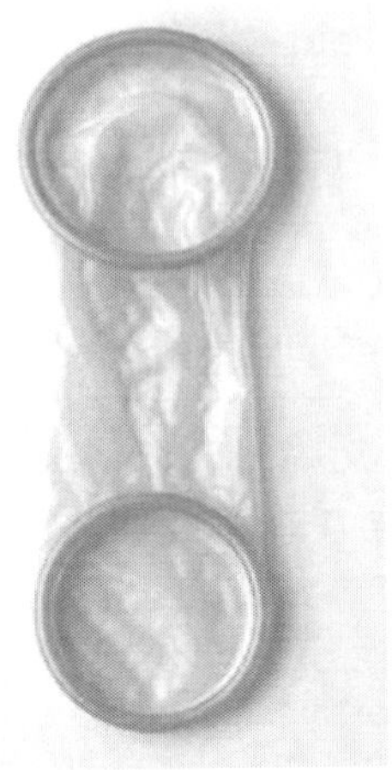

Figure 2. Female condom.

Instructions for Use

Proper use of the female condom is essential to ensure its effectiveness. Although it may seem more complex at first, once the procedure is learned, insertion is simple (Harris et al. 2022).

- It is recommended to use a new condom for each sexual encounter.
- Before opening the package, check the expiration date and the condition of the wrapper.
- With clean hands, squeeze the inner ring and insert it into the vagina, pushing it with a finger as deep as possible.
- The outer ring should remain outside, covering the labia.
- During penetration, the penis must enter the sheath. If it enters outside, stop and reposition.
- After intercourse, twist the outer ring to prevent spillage and gently remove it.
- The condom should be disposed of in a trash bin (never in the toilet).

An important warning is not to use it simultaneously with a male condom, as friction between the two can cause tearing or displacement (Tsikouras et al. 2024). Additionally, condoms should not be carried in the back pocket or wallet, as heat and friction can damage them (ACOG 2025).

Advantages and Disadvantages

The female condom offers significant advantages. Being a non-hormonal method, it does not interfere with medical treatments or breastfeeding, and it is suitable for people with latex allergies (depending on the model). Additionally, it can be inserted up to 8 hours before intercourse, reducing the need to interrupt the intimate moment (WHO, accessed 2025; ACOG 2025; Harris et al. 2022).

Some models even provide additional clitoral stimulation thanks to the external ring, which can be perceived as an extra benefit by some users (Fasehun et al. 2022).

However, its use requires practice, it may be uncomfortable at first, and in some countries, availability is limited and the price is high. Furthermore, studies show it has a typical-use failure rate close to 21%, compared to 13% for the male condom (Trussell 2011; Service et al. 2023; Tsikouras et al. 2024).

Diaphragm

Operation and Placement

The diaphragm (Figure 3) is a barrier contraceptive method consisting of a flexible silicone or latex dome that is inserted into the vagina before sexual intercourse, covering the cervix to prevent sperm from entering the uterus (Harris et al. 2022; Kilbourne Brook and Coffey 2024).

Its effectiveness largely depends on correct placement and the complementary use of a spermicide (Trussell 2011).

For insertion, it is recommended to adopt a comfortable position, such as standing with one leg raised, squatting, or lying down. Using the fingers, the diaphragm is folded and inserted deeply into the vagina, ensuring it completely covers the cervix. Once in place, it should remain for at least six hours after intercourse to ensure all sperm have been immobilized, but it should not be kept in for more than 24 consecutive hours to avoid the risk of infection (ACOG 2025; Tsikouras et al. 2024; Harris et al. 2022; WHO 2022; Johns Hopkins Center for Communication Programs 2022).

It is important to highlight that the diaphragm requires a prior gynecological evaluation, as there are different sizes, and an improper fit can significantly reduce its effectiveness. Therefore, it can only be obtained with a prescription. After events such as childbirth, abortion, or significant changes in body weight, the appropriate size may need to be reassessed (ACOG 2025; CDC 2025b).

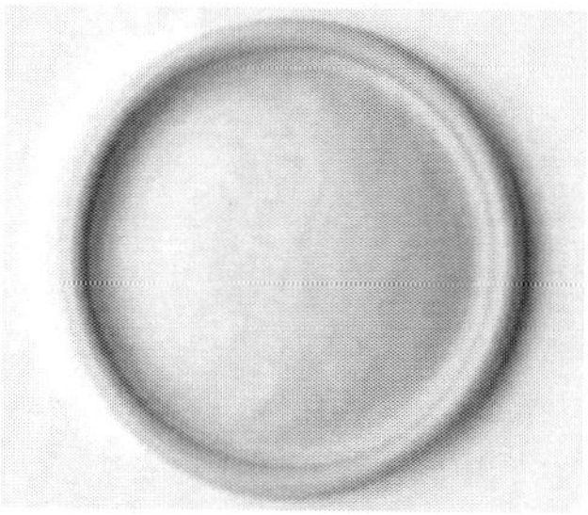

Figure 3. Diaphragm.

Use with Spermicides

The use of the diaphragm should always be accompanied by a spermicide, typically based on nonoxynol-9, thereby increasing the method's effectiveness. The spermicide is applied inside the diaphragm before insertion, and if multiple sexual acts occur, additional spermicide must be applied without removing the device (Tsikouras et al. 2024).

Although spermicides are essential for the diaphragm's proper functioning, frequent use may cause vaginal irritation or increase the risk of urinary tract infections in some women. Therefore, it is advisable to alternate its use or consider other options if recurrent discomfort occurs (Harris et al. 2022; Roddy et al. 1998).

Advantages:

- It is a hormone-free contraceptive method; therefore, it does not interfere with the endocrine balance nor does it have systemic side effects (Fasehun et al. 2022).
- It can be inserted hours before sexual intercourse, allowing for greater freedom and intimacy at the moment (Kilbourne Brook and Coffey 2024).
- It is reusable and, with proper care, can last up to two years, making it an economical long-term option (ACOG 2025; Kilbourne Brook and Coffey 2024).
- It is compatible with breastfeeding and most medications.

Disadvantages:

- It requires a medical prescription, prior planning, and some practice to insert it correctly, which may hinder its acceptance or continued use.
- Its effectiveness is lower than that of other methods, with a pregnancy rate of approximately 6% with perfect use and up to 16% with typical use (Trussell 2011).
- It does not protect against sexually transmitted infections. The spermicide used with the diaphragm may increase the risk of contracting HIV from an infected partner, so its use alongside condoms is recommended in sexual encounters with exposure risk (ACOG 2025).
- It may increase the risk of urinary tract infections, especially if used for prolonged periods, combined with spermicide, or if good hygiene is not maintained (ACOG 2025; CDC 2025b).
- The spermicide can cause burning and vaginal irritation. Some people may be allergic to the spermicide or latex and experience a reaction (ACOG 2025).

Cervical Cup

Definition and General Characteristics

The cervical cap (Figure 4) is a reusable barrier contraceptive method made of silicone that is inserted into the vagina and fits directly over the cervix, preventing sperm from entering the uterus. Unlike other barrier methods, the cervical cap stays in place by suction on the cervix, without needing support from the vaginal walls. It is a hormone-free option and designed for autonomous use, especially recommended for women seeking female-controlled contraception (WHO 2022; Johns Hopkins Center for Communication Programs 2022).

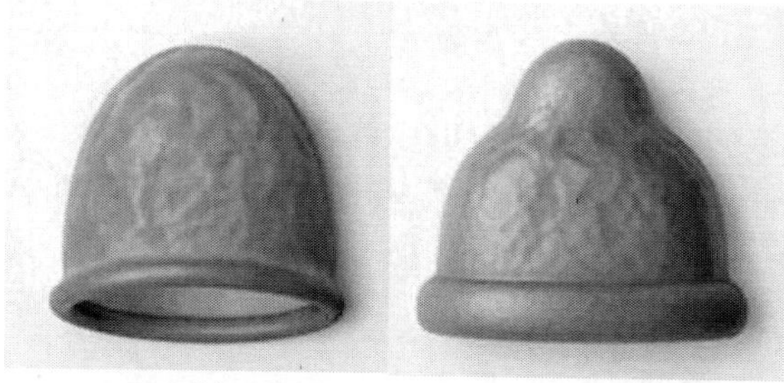

(a) (b)

Figure 4a-4b. Cervical cap.

Currently, the most commonly available model is the FemCap, offered in different sizes depending on whether the woman has had vaginal births, which affects cervical anatomy. The device is discreet, not noticeable during sexual intercourse, and its mechanism of action depends both on its sealing ability and its use together with spermicide (Trussell, 2011; ACOG 2025; CDC 2025b).

The cervical cap does not protect against sexually transmitted infections, including HIV. For additional protection, it is recommended to use it together with an internal or external condom (ACOG 2025).

Instructions for Insertion and Removal

Proper use of the cervical cap requires some familiarity. It can be inserted several hours before intercourse (up to six hours) (CDC 2025b), allowing for flexible planning. To insert it correctly, the following steps should be followed:

- Apply spermicide inside the cervical cap.
- Slightly fold it to facilitate insertion into the vagina.
- Guide it up to the cervix, where it should fit firmly, creating a seal.
- Check that the cervix is completely covered.

After intercourse, the cervical cap should remain in place for at least six hours but must not be worn for more than 48 continuous hours to avoid irritation, changes in vaginal pH, or infections (ACOG 2025; WHO 2022; Johns Hopkins Center for Communication Programs 2022).

Contraceptive Effectiveness

The effectiveness of the cervical cap varies depending on the user's profile and consistency of use. In women who have not had vaginal births, the typical-use failure rate is approximately 14% per year. However, in those who have had vaginal deliveries, this rate rises to around 29% (Trussell 2011). This difference is due to changes in the shape and size of the cervix after childbirth, which make it harder to achieve a tight seal. Therefore, effectiveness improves significantly when combined with the proper use of spermicides and thorough instruction on correct placement (Trussell 2011; ACOG 2025; CDC 2025b).

Benefits and Limitations

Among the main advantages of the cervical cap are the following:

- It contains no hormones.
- It can be inserted in advance, which favors spontaneity.
- It is reusable, making it economically accessible in the long term.
- It is compatible with breastfeeding and does not interfere with sexual desire.

However, it also has some drawbacks:

- Its effectiveness is considerably lower in women with a history of vaginal births.
- Its insertion can be challenging at first and requires practice.
- It does not provide protection against sexually transmitted infections.
- It may cause discomfort, irritation, or increase the risk of infections if kept in place for more than 48 hours.

Fundamental Differences Between Cervical Cap and Diaphragm

Although both methods belong to the barrier contraceptive category and are used with spermicides, they have important differences. The cervical cap is smaller and fits directly onto the cervix by suction, while the diaphragm is larger and rests on the vaginal dome, covering the cervix. The cervical cap can remain in place for up to 48 hours, whereas the diaphragm's maximum recommended time is 24 hours.

Regarding effectiveness, the cervical cap is less effective in women who have had vaginal deliveries, unlike the diaphragm, whose effectiveness remains more consistent across different groups. Both methods require a prior medical evaluation to select the appropriate size. However, inserting the cervical cap may be more complex due to its smaller size and the need for an exact fit. Neither method provides protection against sexually transmitted infections.

Contraceptive Sponge

Definition and Characteristics

The contraceptive sponge (Figure 5) is a barrier method that works in two ways: first, it forms a physical barrier between sperm and the cervix; second, it releases spermicide (usually nonoxynol-9) that immobilizes or destroys sperm upon contact (Xu et al. 2022; Harris et al. 2022; ACOG 2025; Kuyoh et al 2003). Its anatomical design includes a slight concavity that fits the cervix, and a removal loop to facilitate extraction (ACOG 2025; WHO 2022; Johns Hopkins Center for Communication Programs 2022; Global Library of Women's Medicine, accessed 2025).

The most widely available commercial product is the Today Sponge, a polyurethane sponge approximately 5 cm in diameter and 1.9 cm thick, containing 1 gram of nonoxynol-9. Its anatomical design includes a slight concavity that fits the cervix and a nylon loop to facilitate removal (Xu et al. 2022; Kuyoh et al 2003). The sponge comes pre-moistened, and its activation occurs by wetting it with at least 30 mL of water, allowing gradual release of the spermicide through the porous material (ACOG 2025). It is available over the counter, which makes it easily accessible.

It should be inserted before sexual intercourse, preferably a few minutes in advance to allow activation of the spermicide and can be placed up to 24 hours beforehand. Removal is not required between sexual acts, but it must be left in place for at least 6 hours after the last intercourse (ACOG 2025).

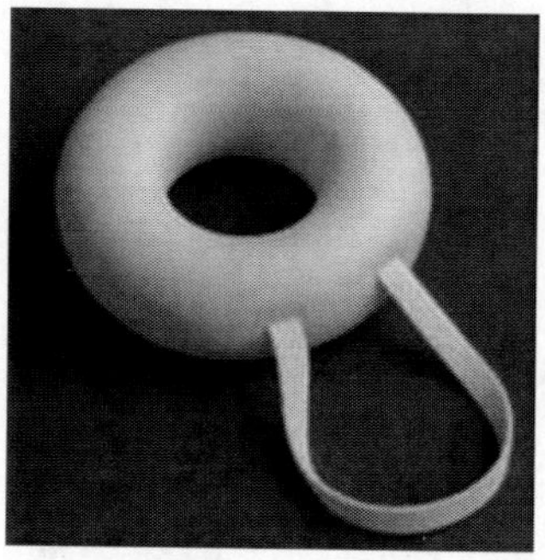

Figure 5. Contraceptive sponge.

The sponge does not protect against sexually transmitted infections (STIs), including HIV. A condom should be used in addition to the sponge to protect against STIs (ACOG 2025).

Insertion and Removal Instructions

- *Activation*: Completely moisten the sponge with clean water to activate the spermicide.
- *Preparation*: Gently fold the sponge between your fingers to facilitate insertion.
- *Placement:* Insert it deeply into the vagina, ensuring the concavity covers the cervix. Confirm proper positioning by touch.
- *Duration:* It can be placed up to 24 hours before intercourse. No removal is needed between sexual acts within this period, but it must remain in place for at least 6 hours after the last sexual act.
- *Removal:* Remove by gently pulling the ribbon. It should not be left in place for more than 30 hours total to avoid risks such as toxic shock syndrome (Tsikouras et al. 2024; Xu et al. 2022; ACOG 2025).

Contraceptive Effectiveness

The effectiveness of the contraceptive sponge varies depending on whether a woman has had vaginal deliveries. In nulliparous women, the typical-use failure rate is approximately 12% per year; in multiparous women, it rises to around 24% (Trussell 2011; Xu et al. 2022). These differences are related to changes in cervical anatomy and the difficulty in achieving a complete seal.

Clinical studies have shown that the sponge has lower contraceptive efficacy and a higher discontinuation rate compared to other methods like the diaphragm (Kuyoh et al. 2003). Therefore, it is not recommended as a primary method for multiparous women who require high effectiveness.

If you wish to use the sponge after childbirth, you should wait 6 weeks until the uterus and cervix have returned to their normal size (ACOG 2025).

Effectiveness improves with correct and consistent use, as well as when combined with other barrier methods.

Advantages:

- Does not contain hormones, thus avoiding systemic side effects.
- Can be used spontaneously up to 24 hours before sexual intercourse.
- Allows for multiple acts of intercourse within the same usage period.
- Does not require medical intervention for acquisition or use.

Disadvantages:

- Lower effectiveness in women who have had vaginal births.
- Possible local adverse effects, such as vaginal irritation or dysbiosis, due to the non-selective effect of nonoxynol-9 on epithelial cells and the microbiota (Xu et al. 2022).
- Does not protect against sexually transmitted infections, including HIV; simultaneous use of condoms is recommended for dual protection (Kuyoh et al. 2003; ACOG 2025).
- Rare but serious risk of toxic shock syndrome if the recommended usage time is exceeded (Tsikouras et al. 2024).

Clinical and Educational Considerations

The contraceptive sponge represents a valid option for women seeking autonomous, hormone-free methods, especially in contexts where access to healthcare services is limited (Kuyoh et al. 2003; ACOG 2025). However, it is essential to provide clear information about correct use, time limits, and the need to monitor for signs of infections or adverse reactions.

This method can be a good temporary or complementary alternative but should not be recommended as the primary option for multiparous women who require high contraceptive efficacy (Kuyoh et al. 2003).

PH Regulating Contraceptive Gel

In recent years, there has been a growing interest in non-hormonal methods of contraception that allow greater autonomy and control for women. Among these options is the pH-regulating contraceptive gel, a product that offers a safe, effective and hormone-free alternative for pregnancy prevention.

How Does It Work?

This gel works by changing the pH of the vagina to a more acidic environment (around 3.5), which hinders sperm motility. Under normal physiological conditions, semen has an alkaline pH which neutralises vaginal acidity to allow sperm to survive. The gel counteracts this effect, maintaining a low pH that interferes with their viability and motility (Coppola 2021).

The most representative example is the product Phexxi®, approved by the FDA (Food and Drugs Administration) in 2020. Its formulation includes lactic acid, citric acid and tartaric acid, ingredients that, in addition to modifying the pH, respect the vaginal flora and do not alter the natural microbiota when used correctly (FDA 2020).

Application and Use

The gel should be applied to the vagina immediately before sexual intercourse (up to one hour before). It comes in pre-filled doses in single-use applicators, similar to some vaginal treatments. It does not need to be withdrawn after intercourse, as it is eliminated by normal physiological mechanisms.

A new dose should be applied before each new sexual intercourse. It is not recommended for use more than once in 24 hours if the person has vaginal irritation or sensitivity.

Effectiveness

Its efficacy with typical use is approximately 86%, while with perfect use it can reach up to 93% (Thomas et al. 2020), which puts it within the efficacy range of other non-hormonal methods, such as the male condom or diaphragm (Thomas et al. 2020).

It does not protect against sexually transmitted infections (STIs), so its use in combination with barrier methods is recommended if dual protection is desired.

Safety and Tolerability

One of the strengths of the contraceptive gel is that it does not interfere with hormones, making it suitable for women who cannot tolerate hormonal contraceptives or have medical contraindications. Mild side effects have been reported, such as a burning sensation or transient vaginal itching, but it is generally considered well tolerated (Coppola 2021).

In addition, the gel can be used on an ad hoc basis, for example for occasional intercourse, making it a flexible option.

Advantages:

- It does not contain hormones, so it does not interfere with endocrine balance.
- It is locally acting and does not require medical procedures or prescription in some countries.
- It offers a contraceptive option controlled by the woman, without the need for coordination with the partner.
- It can be used on an ad hoc basis, making it ideal for those who do not have frequent sexual intercourse.

Disadvantages:

- Lower efficacy compared to hormonal methods or long-acting devices.
- Possible local side effects such as vaginal burning, itching or discomfort (Chappell, Griffin and Howard 2022).
- Requires reapplication before each intercourse, which may be uncomfortable or interfere with spontaneity.
- Does not protect against STIs.

Clinical and Educational Considerations

PH-regulating gel represents an important innovation in the field of non-hormonal contraception, especially for those who cannot or do not wish to use hormonal methods. Its ease of use, autonomy and tolerance make it a viable alternative, particularly in transitional stages (such as postpartum or perimenopause) or in combination with other methods.

However, proper education in its correct use and clinical follow-up is required if adverse reactions are observed. It is also essential to report that it is not a substitute for STI protection.

Emerging Innovations: Monoclonal Antibodies as Topical Contraceptives

The field of topical contraception is undergoing a major evolution with the development of sperm-targeted monoclonal antibodies. A recent study has identified the human contraceptive antibody HCA (Human Contraceptive Antibody), designed to specifically bind to the CD52g glycoprotein present on human spermatozoa, causing their agglutination and immobilisation (Baldeon-Vaca et al. 2021).

This antibody was produced in plants of the genus Nicotiana and demonstrated efficacy in vaginal physiological conditions, including an acidic environment and the presence of diverse microbiota. Furthermore, it did not produce inflammatory effects in human vaginal tissue models, positioning it as a promising non-hormonal topical alternative for on-demand use (Baldeon-Vaca et al. 2021).

Although still in the research phase, its future integration into formulations such as vaginal gels or films could represent a significant advance, especially if combined with other agents such as pH regulators or microbicides, offering dual protection against pregnancy and STIs (Baldeon-Vaca et al. 2021).

Spermicides

This method of contraception will be discussed in detail in the next chapter of this book.

Benefits and Limitations of Barrier Methods

Protection from Sexually Transmitted Infections (STIs)

One of the greatest benefits of barrier methods, especially male and female condoms, is their *dual function:* in addition to preventing unintended pregnancy, they reduce the risk of STI transmission. This is a unique feature compared to hormonal, surgical or natural methods, which do not offer this type of protection (WHO 2022; Johns Hopkins Center for Communication Programs, 2022).

Studies have shown that correct and consistent use of male condoms can reduce the risk of HIV transmission by more than 80% (CDC 2021), as well as significantly reduce the incidence of other STIs such as gonorrhoea, chlamydia and syphilis. They also offer some protection against skin-to-skin infections, such as genital herpes and human papillomavirus (HPV), although this protection is partial, as they do not cover the entire genital area.

In contrast, methods such as spermicides, especially those containing nonoxynol-9, do not protect against STIs and their frequent use may even increase the risk of HIV transmission by damaging the vaginal mucosa (Roddy et al. 1998).

Accessibility and Cost

Barrier methods are, for the most part, accessible and affordable, available without a prescription and widely distributed in pharmacies, health centres, public campaigns and vending machines. Their non-hormonal nature and easy reversibility make them a popular choice among young people or those who want a method without systemic effects.

Cost varies: condoms are inexpensive and often free, while other methods such as the diaphragm or cervical cap require a somewhat higher initial investment, but are reusable. The sponge, pH gel or spermicides, on the other hand, are a recurrent expense.

Compared to hormonal methods, which may require doctor visits and prescription, or surgical methods, which involve invasive procedures, barrier methods represent a more flexible and affordable option.

Health Impact and Side Effects

One of the most notable advantages of barrier methods is their low systemic impact. As they do not interfere with the endocrine system, they are ideal for people with medical contraindications to the use of hormonal contraceptives or who prefer to avoid alterations in their menstrual cycle.

In terms of adverse effects, the most common include:

- Genital irritation or allergic reactions, particularly from latex or nonoxynol-9.
- Possible interference with sexual spontaneity due to the need for prior insertion.
- In some cases, such as condom use, changes in sexual sensitivity may be experienced (Kopa et al. 2024b).

However, as non-invasive methods with immediate reversible effect, they do not affect long-term fertility and do not require recovery periods after discontinuation.

Combined Use with Other Contraceptive Methods

Barrier Methods and Hormonal Contraceptives

Combining barrier methods with hormonal contraceptives (such as the pill, the vaginal ring, the patch, the implant or the hormonal IUD (intrauterine device) offers dual protection: the hormonal component ensures high contraceptive efficacy (with failure rates of less than 1% in perfect use), while the barrier method protects against STIs, which the hormonal method does not (WHO 2022; Johns Hopkins Center for Communication Programs 2022).

This combination is especially recommended for:

- New or non-monogamous couples.
- Young people with an active sex life.
- Users of hormonal contraception who want more peace of mind.

- Women who have started a new contraceptive and are going through the adaptation or waiting period until it is fully effective.

In addition, using a condom in conjunction with a hormonal method enhances contraceptive security in case of forgetfulness, vomiting, drug interactions or errors in hormonal use.

Barrier Methods in Family Planning

Barrier methods also play an important role in modern family planning, whether as a primary, supplementary or backup method.

Their use is particularly valuable in the following situations:

- During postpartum and breastfeeding, when some hormonal methods are contraindicated or temporarily inadvisable.
- In combination with natural methods, as a back-up on fertile days detected by the rhythm method or cervical mucus monitoring.
- During transition between contraceptive methods, e.g., while awaiting insertion of an IUD or effectiveness of an implant.
- In sporadic sexual intercourse, where a method of continuous use is not required, barrier methods allow for timely protection.

Versatility, low cost, ease of acquisition and lack of systemic effects make barrier methods easily integrated into combination strategies, allowing for greater personalisation of sexual and reproductive health care.

Conclusion

Barrier methods of contraception remain a key option in the range of family planning strategies. Despite the rise of newer methods, these devices offer unique advantages that make them especially relevant today.

First, they are the only methods that combine contraceptive protection and prevention of sexually transmitted infections (STIs), which is essential for many people, especially in high-risk settings. Moreover, because they do not contain hormones, they represent a safe alternative for those who cannot or do not wish to use hormonal contraceptives.

However, it is important to remember that, in general, they can be somewhat less effective than other methods if they are not used correctly and consistently. Therefore, education on their proper use and knowledge of the different options available - such as condoms, diaphragms, cervical caps, spermicides and pH-regulating gels - is key to informed decision-making.

In addition, recent advances in materials and design, such as vegan condoms, pre-erection models or condoms made with improved latex, show that these methods continue to evolve to meet today's needs, both functionally, ethically and environmentally.

Choosing an appropriate barrier method requires consideration of personal, medical and relational factors, so professional counselling is essential. Overall, barrier methods are a versatile, accessible and respectful tool for sexual and reproductive health.

References

American Academy of Family Physicians. 2021. *Sexually transmitted infections treatment guidelines, 2021.* American Academy of Family Physicians. https://www.aafp.org/dam/AAFP/documents/patient_care/public_health/STI-Updates-2021.pdf.

American College of Obstetricians and Gynecologists. n.d. *Barrier methods of birth control: Spermicide, condom, sponge, diaphragm, and cervical cap.* https://www.acog.org/womens-health/faqs/barrier-methods-of-birth-control. *Accessed 27 June 2025.*

American College of Obstetricians and Gynecologists. n.d. *Eficacia de los métodos anticonceptivos* [Effectiveness of contraceptive methods]. https://www.acog.org/es/recursos-para-pacientes/preguntas-frecuentes/eficacia-de-los-metodos-anticonceptivos. *Accessed 27 June 2025.*

BaldeonVaca, Galo, Marathe, Jay G., Politch, John A., Mausser, Eric, Pudney, John, Doud, James, Nador, Estela, Fichorova, Raina N., Anderson, David J., and CuUvin, Susan. 2021. "Production and characterization of a human antisperm monoclonal antibody against CD52g for topical contraception in women." *eBioMedicine* 69. https://doi.org/10.1016/j.ebiom.2021.103470.

Beksinska, Mags, Nkosi, Palesa, Mabude, Zukiswa, Mantell, Jennifer E., Zulu, Buyiswa, Milford, Clare, and Smit, Jannie A. 2020. "Lessons from the evaluation of the South African national female condom programme." *PLOS ONE* 15 (8): e0236984. https://doi.org/10.1371/journal.pone.0236984.

Centers for Disease Control and Prevention. 2025a. *Condom use: An overview.* Centers for Disease Control and Prevention. https://www.cdc.gov/condom-use.

Centers for Disease Control and Prevention. 2025b. *Contraception and birth control methods.* Centers for Disease Control and Prevention. https://www.cdc.gov/reproductivehealth/contraception/index.htm.

Chappell, Benjamin T., Griffin, Bryan L., and Howard, Brandon. 2022. "Mechanisms of action of currently available womancontrolled, vaginally administered, nonhormonal contraceptive products." *Therapeutic Advances in Reproductive Health* 16. https://doi.org/10.1177/26334941221120465.

Coppola, John S. 2021. "A new vaginal pH regulator for hormonefree, ondemand contraception." *Nursing for Women's Health* 25 (2): 152–155. https://doi.org/10.1016/j.nwh.2021.02.002.

Crosby, Richard A., Milhausen, Robin R., Mark, Karen P., Yarber, William L., Sanders, Scott A., and Graham, Charles A. 2013. "Understanding problems with condom fit and feel: An important opportunity for improving clinicbased safer sex programs." *The Journal of Primary Prevention* 34 (1–2): 109–115.

Dittrick Medical History Center. n.d. *Condoms and sponges.* https://artsci.case.edu/dittrick/online-exhibits/condoms-and-sponges. *Accessed 27 June 2025.*

European Pharmaceutical Review. n.d. *FDA approves Phexxi™ vaginal gel for prevention of pregnancy.* https://www.europeanpharmaceuticalreview.com/news/122035/fda-approves-phexxi-vaginal-gel. *Accessed 27 June 2025.*

Euronews. 2019. "Ecofriendly sex life: Are condoms good for the environment?" *ONE Only Natural Energy*, August 8. https://www.euronews.com/green/2019/08/08/eco-friendly-sex-life-are-condoms-good-for-the-environment.

Fasehun, Linda, Lewinger, Susan, Fasehun, Olufunmilayo, and Brooks, Merle. 2022. "Barriers and facilitators to acceptability of the female condom in low and middleincome countries: A systematic review." *Annals of Global Health* 88 (1). https://doi.org/10.5334/aogh.3830.

Frezieres, Roberto G., Walsh, Terri L., Nelson, Ana L., Clark, Vickie A., and Coulson, Alan H. 1999. "Evaluation of the efficacy of a polyurethane condom: Results from a randomized, controlled clinical trial." *Family Planning Perspectives* 31 (2): 81–87.

Gilliam, Michele L. and Derman, Rita J. 2000. "Barrier methods of contraception." *Obstetrics and Gynecology Clinics of North America* 27 (4): 841–858.

Godoy, Juan M. 2024. "Cómo funciona el preservativo preerección que se coloca dos horas antes de tener relaciones sexuales" [How the preerection condom works]. *Infobae*, April 26. https://www.infobae.com/salud/2024/04/26/preservativo-pre-ereccion-nueva-tecnologia.

Harris, Deborah M., Dam, Anna, Morrison, Kim, Mann, Christine, Jackson, Amanda, Bledsoe, Stephanie M., Rowan, Amy, and Longfield, Katherine. 2022. "Barriers and enablers influencing women's adoption and continuation of vaginally inserted contraceptive methods: A literature review." *Studies in Family Planning* 53 (3): 455–490.

KilbourneBrook, Marion and Coffey, Patricia S. 2024. "Learnings from an innovative model to expand access to a new and underutilized nonhormonal contraceptive diaphragm." *Global Health: Science and Practice* 12 (5). https://doi.org/10.9745/GHSP-D-23-00315.

Kopa, Zorica, Scafa, Raffaela, Graziani, Andrea, Goulis, Dimitrios G., and Ferlin, Angelo. 2024. "Male contraception: Focus on behavioral and barrier methods." *Andrology* 12 (7): 1535–1540.

Kuyoh, M. A., C. Toroitich-Ruto, D. A. Grimes, K. F. Schulz, and M. F. Gallo. 2003. "Sponge versus Diaphragm for Contraception: A Cochrane Review." *Contraception* 67, no. 1 (January): 15–18. https://doi.org/10.1016/s0010-7824(02)00434-1.

Majra, Jay P. 2010. "Use of condoms: Clarifying the message." *Indian Journal of Community Medicine* 35 (2): 362.

Nabhan, Anu, Kabra, Renu, Ashraf, Asim, Elghamry, Farah, Kiarie, James, Atwa, Eman, Bahnasy, Samah, Salem, Rania, and Abdulkarim, Amal. 2023. "Implementation strategies, facilitators, and barriers to scaling up and sustaining demand generation in family planning: A mixedmethods systematic review." *BMC Women's Health* 23 (1): 574. https://doi.org/10.1186/s12905-023-02520-4.

Randolph, Michael E., Pinkerton, Scott D., Bogart, Laura M., Cecil, Heather, and Abramson, Paul R. 2007. "Sexual pleasure and condom use." *Archives of Sexual Behavior* 36 (6): 844–848.

Roddy, Robert E., Zekeng, Libii, Ryan, Kelly A., Tamoufé, Umberto, Weir, Stephanie S., and Wong, Eric L. 1998. "A controlled trial of nonoxynol 9 film to reduce maletofemale transmission of sexually transmitted diseases." *The New England Journal of Medicine* 339 (8): 504–510.

Service, Christopher A., Puri, Deepak, Hsieh, TerryCheng, and Patel, Devesh P. 2023. "Emerging concepts in male contraception: A narrative review of novel, hormonal and nonhormonal options." *Therapeutic Advances in Reproductive Health* 17. https://doi.org/10.1177/26334941231203426.

Thomas, Michael A., Chappell, Benjamin T., Maximos, Brittany, Culwell, Kelly R., Dart, Corinne, and Howard, Brandon. 2020. "A novel vaginal pH regulator: Results from the phase 3 AMPOWER contraception clinical trial." *Contraception: X* 2. https://doi.org/10.1016/j.conx.2020.100020.

Trussell, James. 2011. "Contraceptive failure in the United States." *Contraception* 83 (5): 397–404.

Tsikouras, Panagiotis, Nikolettos, Nikolaos, Rath, Wolfgang, and Von Tempelhoff, Friedrich, eds. 2024. *Conception and family planning – New aspects*. Vol. 2. London: IntechOpen. https://doi.org/10.5772/intechopen.102930.

Woo, Eugenio. 2016. "Empresa consigue crear un condón irrompible: 'No era el látex, era la estructura'" [Company creates unbreakable condom: "It wasn't the latex, it was the structure"]. *BioBioChile*, June 17. https://www.biobiochile.cl/noticias/salud-y-bienestar.

Workowski, Kimberly A., Linda H. Bachmann, Patricia A. Chan, Christine M. Johnston, Christine A. Muzny, Ian Park, Holly Reno, Jeanne M. Zenilman, and Gail A. Bolan. 2021. *Sexually Transmitted Infections Treatment Guidelines, 2021*. Centers for Disease Control and Prevention. https://www.cdc.gov/std/treatment-guidelines/default.htm.

World Health Organization. 2022. *Family planning: A global handbook for providers*. Geneva: World Health Organization. https://www.who.int/publications/i/item/9789243565400.

World Health Organization. n.d. *WHO_RHR_07.18_eng.pdf*. https://apps.who.int/iris/handle/10665/69729. *Accessed 27 June 2025.*

World Health Organization. 2023. *Integrating the prevention and control of noncommunicable diseases in HIV/AIDS, tuberculosis, and sexual and reproductive health programmes: Implementation guidance*. Geneva: World Health Organization. https://www.who.int/publications/i/item/9789240072130.

Xu, Murong, Mingpeng Zhao, Raymond Hang Wun Li, Zhixiu Lin, Jacqueline Pui Wah Chung, Tin Chiu Li, Tin-Lap Lee, and David Yiu Leung Chan. 2022. "Effects of Nonoxynol-9 (N-9) on Sperm Functions: Systematic Review and Meta-Analysis." *Reproduction & Fertility* 3 (1): R19–R33. https://doi.org/10.1530/RAF-21-0024.

Chapter 6

Spermicides

M. M. Castillo García[1,*], MD
A. Serrano Sánchez[1], MD
P. Mora Ábalos[1], MD
M. Cebrián Marcilla[1], MD
and Ll. Belmonte Andújar[1,2], MD
[1]Obstetrics and Gynecology Department, University and Hospital of Albacete, Albacete, Spain
[2]Medical Science Department, School of Medicine of Albacete, Universidad de Castilla-La Mancha, Spain

Abstract

Spermicides are non-hormonal, local contraceptive methods that act by inactivating spermatozoa through various mechanisms, such as altering vaginal pH or disrupting their cell membranes. Although their effectiveness as a stand-alone method is limited, they still represent a valid option for those seeking timely, hormone-free contraception with user autonomy. This chapter reviews their historical development, the principal compounds used – such as nonoxynol-9, benzalkonium chloride, and the more recently approved acidifying gels – as well as their clinical efficacy, safety profile, and possible effects on the vaginal microbiota. Combinations with barrier methods and current research into spermicides with antimicrobial potential are also explored. Far from being obsolete, spermicides are being re-engineered into safer and more versatile forms that better respond to the needs of many women. Their development remains essential in the pursuit of more accessible, autonomous, and physiology-friendly contraceptive methods.

Keywords: spermatocidal agents, spermicide, nonoxynol, vaginal pH modulator gel, phexxi, non hormonal contraception, microbicide

[*] Corresponding Author's Email: mm.castillogarcia13@gmail.com

In: Advances in Reproductive Health
Editors: Llanos Belmonte Andujar and Ana Fuentes Rozalen
ISBN: 979-8-90134-038-7

Introduction

Among the wide range of contraceptive methods currently available, spermicides represent a category of chemical-based contraception designed to locally inhibit the fertilising capacity of spermatozoa by altering their motility, viability, or structural integrity within the female genital tract (Grimes et al., 2013).

Although their efficacy as a stand-alone method has long been debated—due to relatively high failure rates and unplanned pregnancies—spermicides continue to undergo research and reformulation, particularly in combination with emerging pharmaceutical forms such as pH-modulating vaginal gels and microbicidal agents (Grimes et al., 2013; Marinaro and Goldstein, 2025).

Spermicides have been used for several decades. Despite having lower efficacy than many other contraceptive methods, they remain a valid non-hormonal alternative for those wishing to avoid the side effects of hormonal contraceptives or who are unable to use them for medical or personal reasons. This method also offers other benefits, including accessibility, ease of use, and the possibility of combining them with other methods such as the male or female condom or diaphragm. Moreover, they are particularly useful in situations where immediate contraceptive control is desired without medical intervention or long-term commitment (Encyclopedia of Reproduction, 2018; Hassoun, 2018).

History and Evolution of Spermicides

The history of spermicides as a chemical contraceptive method can be traced back to ancient civilisations such as the Egyptians, Greeks, and Romans, where various natural substances and plant extracts with potential spermicidal properties were used. Ancient Egyptian texts like the Ebers Papyrus mention mixtures of natural ingredients aimed at achieving contraceptive effects—e.g., honey with sodium bicarbonate, crocodile dung with herbal paste, or acacia (which ferments to lactic acid, a compound with spermicidal action). These mixtures, often inserted into the vagina, may have worked as much through their barrier properties as their chemical effects (Riddle, 1997).

Another traditional and well-known method in Mediterranean cultures was the use of lemon juice as a spermicide. "Primitive vaginal sponges" soaked in lemon juice were reportedly used for centuries, particularly in historic Constantinople. Even today, in some regions where access to modern contraception is limited, lemon juice douching is still used as a folk method to prevent pregnancy (Clarke, McCoombe, and Short, 2006).

Scientific progress over time introduced experimentation with botanical extracts (e.g., cedarwood, olive, and frankincense oils), mineral oxides, and various acidic or soapy substances. Some early spermicides contained metallic salts—effective but often toxic (Evolutionary History of Contraception – Annals RANM, 2018).

The first commercially available spermicides appeared in the late 19th and early 20th centuries. Often used alongside barrier methods like diaphragms and cervical caps, their popularity declined in the latter half of the 20th century due to rising awareness and incidence of sexually transmitted infections (STIs) (Uribe-Clavijo et al., 2012).

The modern era of spermicides began in the mid-20th century with the introduction of surfactants such as benzalkonium chloride and especially nonoxynol-9 (N-9)—a non-ionic surfactant with proven sperm-immobilising and lytic properties. N-9 became the gold standard spermicide for years (Iyer & Poddar, 2008a; Batár, 2010).

However, by the late 1990s and early 2000s, concerns arose regarding its safety—especially with frequent or prolonged use. Studies by the WHO revealed that repeated exposure to N-9 could damage the vaginal and cervical epithelium, increasing susceptibility to STIs, including HIV. As a result, some jurisdictions began withdrawing products with high concentrations of N-9 (Wilkinson et al., 2002).

This led to the development of safer alternatives that modify the vaginal environment without damaging the mucosa. In this context, products such as *Phexxi®*—a non-hormonal gel containing lactic acid, citric acid, and tartaric acid—have emerged. Approved by the FDA in 2020, Phexxi® acidifies the vaginal environment to inhibit sperm motility without harming vaginal tissues (Su and Vincent, 2022).

Vaginal Microbiota, Vaginal pH and Their Interaction with Sperm: Biological Basics for Acidifying Spermicides

The vaginal microbiota constitutes the first line of defence in the female genital tract, and its composition is strongly influenced by hormonal factors, particularly oestrogens. Under the influence of these hormones, the vaginal epithelium promotes the accumulation of glycogen, which is subsequently fermented by bacteria of the *Lactobacillus* genus. This fermentation produces lactic acid, which maintains an acidic vaginal pH (ranging from 3.5 to 4.5). Such an acidic environment is essential for preserving a protective barrier against pathogens and simultaneously represents a natural defence against fertilisation by influencing sperm motility and viability (Pendharkar et al. 2023).

The acidic environment generated by *Lactobacillus* not only reduces the risk of infections but also negatively affects sperm motility and viability. Several *in vitro* studies have demonstrated that a pH below 6.0 significantly reduces progressive sperm motility by causing mitochondrial disruption and damaging the plasma membrane, thereby compromising the sperm's ability to reach and fertilise the ovum (Zhou et al. 2015). Furthermore, *Lactobacillus* strains that produce hydrogen peroxide enhance the antimicrobial effect of the environment, acting synergistically with lactic acid to inhibit pathogens responsible for sexually transmitted infections, such as *Neisseria gonorrhoeae*, *Chlamydia trachomatis*, herpes simplex virus, and HIV (Pendharkar et al. 2023).

Human semen is alkaline (pH between 7.2 and 8.0), which temporarily neutralises vaginal acidity following ejaculation. This transient increase in pH creates a favourable environment for sperm motility but concurrently reduces the effectiveness of the vagina's natural antimicrobial barrier. Studies indicate that when vaginal pH exceeds a threshold of 5.0, the likelihood of vaginal and sexually transmitted infections increases, particularly during microbial imbalances such as bacterial vaginosis (Bayer and Jensen 2014).

Based on these physiological interactions, spermicidal formulations have been developed to maintain vaginal acidity even in the presence of semen. Unlike classical surfactants such as nonoxynol-9—which function by physically disrupting the sperm membrane and may cause mucosal irritation—acidifying spermicides reduce sperm motility by maintaining a vaginal pH that is unfavourable for sperm activity (Xu et al. 2022; Nelson 2018).

Several compounds have been studied for this purpose, including lactic acid, citric acid, and potassium bitartrate. For instance, citric acid at concentrations as low as 0.01% has been shown to significantly hinder sperm penetration into cervical mucus, with 0.1% concentrations capable of completely inhibiting it (Su and Vincent 2022). Similarly, lemon juice (rich in citric acid) has demonstrated immediate *in vitro* spermicidal effects by completely immobilising spermatozoa (Suthutvoravut and Kamyarat 2016).

Modern formulations, such as BufferGel, utilise buffering agents to preserve vaginal acidity post-ejaculation. These preparations not only serve contraceptive purposes but have also shown efficacy comparable to pharmacological treatments in managing infections like bacterial vaginosis by rapidly restoring the acidic balance of the vaginal ecosystem (Bayer and Jensen 2014; Williams et al. 2007).

Classification and Mechanisms of Action of Different Spermicides

Surfactant Agents

Nonoxynol-9 (N-9)

Nonoxynol-9 (N-9) is a widely used non-ionic surfactant present in topical contraceptive formulations intended for vaginal use. Its spermicidal action is based on the irreversible disruption of the sperm plasma membrane, leading to cell lysis and loss of function. This compound acts rapidly upon contact, directly interfering with multiple sperm functions, affecting both membrane integrity as well as sperm motility and fertilising capacity (Iyer & Poddar, 2008b; Xu et al., 2022).

Mechanism of Action

Nonoxynol-9 has non-ionic surfactant properties, enabling it to integrate into the lipid bilayers of biological membranes. In sperm cells, this action disrupts the phospholipid architecture of the plasma membrane, promoting pore formation, increased cellular permeability, and loss of essential intracellular contents (Ingram et al., 2006).

This process entails:

- Mitochondrial membrane depolarisation, impairing ATP production in the midpiece.
- Alterations in the acrosome, essential for the acrosomal reaction prior to fertilisation.
- Decondensation of nuclear chromatin, which prevents fusion with the oocyte.
- A significant reduction in rapid progressive motility within cervical mucus, as demonstrated by multiple in vivo postcoital studies.

This spermicidal effect occurs within an extremely short contact time, with the ability to immobilise and lyse sperm within minutes of application. Additionally, N-9 interferes with other physiological functions such as the generation of reactive oxygen species (ROS), acrosin activity, tyrosine phosphorylation, and hemizona binding – all crucial to sperm activation and fertilising potential (Xu et al., 2022).

Although N-9 initially demonstrated some microbicidal and antiviral activity, later studies revealed that its effect on the cervicovaginal epithelium may damage the mucosa and cause vaginal dysbiosis, thereby facilitating the entry of sexually transmitted pathogens, including the human immunodeficiency virus (HIV) (Alfaiate et al., 2021).

Method of Use and Duration of Effect

The use of N-9 depends on the specific pharmaceutical formulation and is intended for immediate application or use within minutes prior to intercourse. It can be used at any time during the menstrual cycle. Instructions for use vary:

- Vaginal suppositories and films: require a waiting period of 10–15 minutes before intercourse to ensure proper dissolution and distribution of the active ingredient.
- Creams, foams, and gels: may be applied directly into the vaginal canal immediately before sexual activity (from 0 to 59 minutes), as their formulation allows for rapid dispersion within the vaginal environment. (Xu et al., 2022)

In all cases, a new dose is required for each act of intercourse, as the spermicidal effect does not persist beyond a single application.

The window of efficacy is limited to one sexual encounter, and its effectiveness diminishes significantly if the minimum waiting time is not observed (in the case of films/suppositories) or if repeated ejaculation occurs without reapplication. The typical-use failure rate ranges from 18% to 28% per year, though this may be reduced when combined with barrier methods (such as the diaphragm or condom). When using N-9 with a diaphragm or cervical cap, it is essential to ensure compatibility with these devices ("Contraception and Abortion - ClinicalKey," n.d.).

Additionally, despite its ease of use, current formulations present notable limitations in terms of intravaginal retention. Pharmacokinetic studies have shown that within two hours of application, 60% to 93% of the active compound may be lost due to vaginal discharge. For example:

- Contraceptive Vaginal Film (VCF): 77% Loss
- Creams such as Delfen®, Conceptrol®, Advantage S®, Semicid®: Losses between 81% and 93%

These losses directly compromise the efficacy of N-9, particularly during prolonged or delayed intercourse, highlighting the need for improved bioadhesive and viscosity properties in these spermicides (Garg et al., 2001).

Contraceptive Efficacy

In terms of contraceptive effectiveness, relatively high pregnancy rates have been observed when N-9 is used as the sole method of contraception. Various studies have reported a Pearl Index of approximately 18% with perfect use and 28% with typical use (Serfaty, 2017).

While these figures reflect a reduction in risk compared to no contraception, they indicate limited effectiveness, particularly in comparison with hormonal methods or intrauterine devices. The World Health Organization (WHO) has acknowledged these limitations, advising against its use as a sole method, especially in populations at risk of sexually transmitted infections (STIs) (Xu et al., 2022; "Contraceptive Efficacy | GLOWM," n.d.).

A Cochrane review found that the probability of pregnancy after six months of N-9 use ranged between 14% and 22%, depending on the administered dose (52.5 mg, 100 mg, or 150 mg). However, these results are limited by high dropout rates (up to 39%), which hindered a robust meta-analysis (Grimes et al., 2013).

Safety and Tolerability

Despite its widespread availability and long-standing use, the safety profile of nonoxynol-9 has been the subject of considerable concern. Frequent or repeated use has been associated with several local side effects, primarily irritation, epithelial damage, mucosal inflammation, and ulceration of the vaginal and cervical epithelium. This toxicity has been documented in both animal and human models, with prolonged use linked to epithelial atrophy, leukocyte infiltration, and increased expression of inflammatory cytokines such as IL-1 and IL-6 (Alfaiate et al., 2021; Serfaty, 2017).

Significant alterations in the vaginal microbiota have also been reported following continued use, including increased colonisation by species associated with bacterial vaginosis, such as *Gardnerella vaginalis*. Although the increase observed was mild, it is associated with an imbalance in the protective microbiota, potentially heightening the risk of vaginal infections (Wilkinson et al., 2002).

The most commonly reported adverse effects include vaginal irritation, itching, stinging, burning sensations, and dysuria, experienced by both users and their partners. These symptoms are typically transient but may occasionally require a change of formulation or discontinuation (*Amaral et al., 2004;* "Contraception and Abortion - ClinicalKey," n.d.).

One of the most pressing safety concerns regarding N-9 is its potential to increase the risk of STI transmission. Although it was initially believed to offer microbicidal protection against pathogens such as HIV, chlamydia, or gonorrhoea, clinical evidence suggests the contrary. Frequent use of N-9 has been linked to an increased risk of HIV acquisition, attributed to epithelial microlesions and disruption of the mucosal barrier, facilitating viral entry (Roddy et al., 2002; Serfaty, 2017).

Its use has also been associated with a higher frequency of genital epithelial lesions, particularly among women using the product frequently. These lesions are often observed on the vulva, away from the highest concentrations of N-9, suggesting aetiological links with both microbiota imbalances and irritative or hypersensitivity reactions. Some evidence even suggests that certain STIs, such as reactivated genital herpes, may play a role (Wilkinson et al., 2002).

A clinical trial conducted in Africa demonstrated a significant increase in HIV infection risk in women who used N-9 repeatedly, prompting public health agencies such as the CDC and WHO to advise against its use among individuals at high risk of STI exposure (Alfaiate et al., 2021).

Considerations During Pregnancy and Lactation

No association has been found between N-9 use and congenital malformations or adverse foetal outcomes (Gallaway et al., 2009). A meta-analysis and follow-up studies did not indicate significant teratogenicity, except for a statistically weak association with perimembranous ventricular septal defects, likely to be incidental (Einarson et al., 1990).

However, animal studies have shown that N-9 can cross the vaginal mucosa and enter the systemic circulation and breast milk, and it is therefore contraindicated during breastfeeding (Serfaty, 2017).

Benzalkonium Chloride

Benzalkonium chloride (BZK) is a cationic compound belonging to the quaternary ammonium salt family, widely used as an antiseptic, bactericide, and, in particular, as a spermicide (Alfaiate et al., 2021).

Mechanism of Action

BZK's spermicidal effect stems primarily from its cationic surfactant activity: this property allows it to interact with the sperm cell membrane (composed of a negatively charged lipid bilayer), facilitating electrostatic binding and subsequent structural disruption of the membrane.

BZK acts via multiple synergistic mechanisms, similar to those of nonoxynol-9:

- Destabilisation of the sperm membrane: It interacts with the phospholipids of the sperm plasma membrane, causing pore formation and increased cellular permeability, leading to rapid cell death due to osmotic imbalance.
- Enzymatic inactivation: It inhibits key enzymes required for sperm survival and motility, including those involved in cellular respiration and glycolysis.
- Acrosome alteration: It partially denatures acrosin, an enzyme essential for oocyte penetration, thereby preventing fertilisation.
- Modification of cervical mucus: It significantly alters the mesh-like structure of cervical mucus by disrupting glycoprotein networks, increasing viscosity and impairing sperm migration towards the uterus (Serfaty, 2017).

Method of Use and Duration of Effect

BZK is available in a wide variety of pharmaceutical forms, allowing adaptation to the preferences and needs of individual users. Pharmatex® formulations include: vaginal creams with applicator, suppositories and mini-suppositories, pessaries and mini-pessaries, effervescent vaginal tablets, and soft vaginal capsules (Alfaiate et al., 2021).

Each formulation has specific features regarding onset of action, ease of use, and tolerability. For example, effervescent tablets require prior dissolution, while soft capsules may be more comfortable for women with vaginal dryness.

BZK should be applied intravaginally at least 5–15 minutes before each act of intercourse. Its spermicidal effect lasts between 4 and 6 hours, provided no further intercourse occurs; in such cases, a new dose must be applied. Vaginal douching should be avoided before and after use—especially with anionic soaps—as these may form insoluble compounds with BZK, neutralising its action.

It is essential that users understand that BZK's contraceptive effectiveness strictly depends on correct application, full vaginal coverage, and consistent use before every act of intercourse. Failure to adhere to these instructions may significantly reduce its efficacy (Serfaty, 2017).

Contraceptive Effectiveness

In several controlled clinical studies, BZK has demonstrated moderate contraceptive effectiveness when used correctly:

- Pearl Index: between 1.1 and 1.4 in prospective multicentre studies.

These values suggest that it is less effective than hormonal methods or intrauterine devices, but it remains a suitable option for women seeking non-hormonal, locally acting contraceptives.

It is important to note that effectiveness depends heavily on strict adherence to instructions, adequate vaginal coverage, and accurate user education, as application errors or inconsistent use markedly reduce effectiveness (Alfaiate et al., 2021; Su & Vincent, 2022).

Safety and Tolerability

BZK has shown good overall tolerability in humans. In clinical studies, only 22.6% of users reported adverse effects, with a treatment discontinuation rate of just 2.4% (Su & Vincent, 2022).

The most frequently reported side effects include: sensations of warmth, stinging, burning, or vaginal/penile irritation after intercourse. These reactions are usually mild and transient, rarely requiring treatment suspension.

Although *in vitro* cytotoxicity has been observed in HeLa cell cultures, clinical effects on the human vaginal mucosa have been minimal, with no significant changes in vaginal pH or commensal flora. Compared with nonoxynol-9 (N-9), BZK is less toxic and less likely to induce severe epithelial damage, making it a safer option at the mucosal level (Alfaiate et al., 2021).

Nonetheless, frequent or incorrect use of spermicides, including BZK, may potentially increase the risk of sexually transmitted infection (STI) transmission due to microlesions of the epithelium. Although BZK has demonstrated some in vitro antimicrobial and antiviral activity, it should not be considered protective against STIs (Su & Vincent, 2022).

Considerations During Pregnancy and Lactation

Regarding systemic exposure, BZK is not significantly absorbed via the vaginal route, which rules out major teratogenic or systemic effects. Animal and human studies have not demonstrated passage into the bloodstream or breast milk; therefore, it is not contraindicated during breastfeeding nor in the event of accidental use in early pregnancy (Serfaty, 2017).

Vaginal pH Regulating Gels

Vaginal pH-regulating gels represent an innovation in the field of non-hormonal contraception, offering a pericoital, topical option that functions by maintaining an acidic vaginal environment to immobilise sperm and potentially reduce the risk of sexually transmitted infections (STIs). Unlike traditional spermicides, these gels do not contain cytotoxic agents, but instead use a combination of organic acids that exert their effect by modifying the vaginal microenvironment (Garg et al., 2001).

Mechanism of Action

Products marketed under the names *Amphora™*, *ACIDFORM*, and its current approved form *Phexxi®* consist of a viscous, whitish, bioadhesive gel composed of three main active ingredients: lactic acid (90 mg), citric acid (50 mg), and potassium bitartrate (20 mg).

These are combined with excipients such as benzoic acid (preservative), alginic acid and xanthan gum (gelling agents), glycerin (humectant), sodium hydroxide, and purified water. The formulation has an initial pH of approximately 3.55 and is designed to maintain vaginal acidity even after exposure to semen, which is alkaline and tends to neutralise the physiological vaginal pH. (Su & Vincent, 2022)

The mechanism of action is based on the gel's ability to resist the buffering effect of semen, preserving an acidic pH that is incompatible with sperm motility. At pH levels below 5, sperm motility is significantly reduced, and the acrosome reaction is inhibited, thereby blocking fertilisation. Unlike classical spermicides such as nonoxynol-9, which act through direct disruption of the sperm membrane, acidifying gels act indirectly, reducing viability through a hostile pH environment while preserving the integrity of the vaginal epithelium. (Nelson, 2018)

Method of Use and Duration of Effect

The formulation is provided in single-use, pre-filled vaginal applicators (5g of gel). It is administered intravaginally up to one hour before intercourse, with no waiting time required after insertion. A new dose must be applied before each act of intercourse. However, it is not recommended to use it more than once within 24 hours if vaginal irritation symptoms are present.

Notably, the product was approved by the FDA in 2020 as a prescription-based, non-hormonal contraceptive method in certain countries (e.g., the United States). This gel may be used in combination with other barrier methods such as male condoms, diaphragms, or cervical caps. However, simultaneous use with vaginal contraceptive rings is not recommended (Su & Vincent, 2022).

Clinical studies have shown that the gel possesses superior bioadhesive and viscosity-retention properties compared to other vaginal formulations, allowing:

- The gel to remain in the vagina for up to 10–12 hours after application.
- Peak spermicidal effect to persist for at least 8 hours post-insertion (Garg et al., 2001).

Colposcopic observations confirmed the continuous presence of the gel on the vaginal mucosa for up to 12 hours post-application. This persistence, along with resistance to dilution by vaginal fluids and semen, ensures sustained activity within that timeframe, provided no further intercourse occurs.

Nonetheless, the product is exclusively preventive and pericoital; it has no postcoital effect and offers no prolonged contraceptive protection. It is not a substitute for continuous-use methods such as IUDs or long-acting hormonal contraceptives (Bayer & Jensen, 2014).

Contraceptive Efficacy

Vaginal pH-regulating gels such as ACIDFORM (commercially Amphora™, now Phexxi®) exert their contraceptive effect by acidifying the vaginal environment, counteracting the alkaline pH of semen.

In several laboratory studies, ACIDFORM demonstrated strong buffering capacity—up to four times greater than comparable products—effectively acidifying even large volumes of ejaculate. Postcoital tests revealed that the number of progressively motile sperm in cervical mucus was nearly zero following ACIDFORM application, suggesting rapid and effective immobilisation (Bayer & Jensen, 2014; Garg et al., 2001).

Moreover, the spermicidal efficacy of ACIDFORM was shown to depend on its concentration relative to semen volume: a gel/semen ratio of **1:3.4** reduced the pH of the ejaculate to 5—sufficient to completely inhibit sperm motility. This finding supports the recommendation to apply at least 5g of the product vaginally before intercourse (Bayer & Jensen, 2014).

Phexxi®, the currently marketed formulation, has undergone evaluation in controlled clinical trials to determine its real-world efficacy. In a multicentre phase III trial in the United States involving over 1,100 women of reproductive age, a cumulative pregnancy rate of 13.7% was observed over seven cycles of use (Pearl Index: 27.5 per 100 woman-years), indicating moderate effectiveness under typical use.

Importantly, under perfect use conditions—correct application before every act of intercourse without omissions—the Pearl Index dropped to 6.7, placing the product in a range comparable to the diaphragm and traditional barrier methods. This difference between typical and perfect use highlights the significant impact of adherence, a common issue with pericoital contraceptive methods (Su & Vincent, 2022).

Safety and Tolerability

Phase I and II studies with ACIDFORM reported good tolerability when applied daily over several consecutive days. In a controlled clinical trial, daily use for six days did not produce clinical signs of vulvovaginal irritation or lesions detectable by colposcopy. No alterations in vaginal pH or microbiota were observed in healthy women (Garg et al., 2001).

With the commercial release of Phexxi®, large-scale phase III studies confirmed these findings. In a multicentre trial, adverse effects reported by women included mild genital irritation (burning, stinging, itching) in approximately 20% of users, urinary tract infections in 6%, candidiasis in 3%, and bacterial vaginosis in another 3%. Fewer than 2.4% of participants discontinued use due to adverse effects, indicating high clinical acceptability (Su & Vincent, 2022).

Nonetheless, a minority of women (~3%) developed episodes of bacterial vaginosis during Phexxi use. This suggests that, although the risk of dysbiosis is low, certain gel components—such as benzoic acid or specific excipients—may transiently alter microbial balance in predisposed individuals.

A key consideration in evaluating vaginal products is their effect on STI susceptibility, particularly HIV. The development of these gels was partly in response to adverse findings associated with nonoxynol-9, which was linked to increased HIV transmission due to mucosal damage facilitating viral entry.

In contrast, ACIDFORM and Phexxi have demonstrated indirect microbicidal properties in vitro and in animal models by maintaining an acidic environment hostile to pathogens such as *Chlamydia trachomatis*, *Neisseria gonorrhoeae*, *Herpes simplex virus*, and HIV. In a murine model, ACIDFORM significantly reduced chlamydia and herpes infection rates compared with placebo gels or nonoxynol-based products.

In a recent clinical trial, Phexxi use was associated with a 50% reduction in chlamydia infections and a 78% reduction in gonorrhoea, suggesting additional protective potential that could be leveraged in public health strategies focused on dual protection. (Su & Vincent, 2022).

Other Emerging Agents in Development

In response to the growing demand for non-hormonal contraceptive methods that offer safety, efficacy, and user autonomy, new compounds and formulations with spermicidal function are currently in development:

Ovaprene ®

Ovaprene® is a non-hormonal intravaginal ring that combines a physical polymer barrier with the local release of ascorbic acid and ferrous gluconate. This dual system prevents sperm penetration and reduces their motility. It has successfully completed Phase II studies through postcoital testing and is expected to proceed to Phase III trials shortly (Mauck et al., 2024).

ZB-06 and MB66 (ZabBio)

ZB-06 is a vaginal film that delivers human antisperm antibodies, promoting sperm agglutination within cervical mucus. MB66, in contrast, contains monoclonal antibodies against HIV and HSV. Both are undergoing Phase I clinical trials, and their combined use aims to offer contraceptive protection alongside defence against sexually transmitted infections (Thurman et al., 2023).

Mandelic Acid

Mandelic acid and its polymeric derivative SAMMA act by reducing sperm motility through mitochondrial dysfunction. Mandelic acid induces minimal structural alteration in sperm and causes little vaginal irritation in animal models, while also demonstrating potential microbicidal activity against HIV. Its mechanism suggests a safer profile compared to traditional surfactants such as nonoxynol-9 (Xia et al., 2020).

Spermicides and Their Combination with Other Contraceptive Methods (Male and Female Condoms, Diaphragms, and Cervical Caps)

The diaphragm used in conjunction with a spermicide has demonstrated reasonable contraceptive efficacy. According to available data, its annual failure rate with perfect use is approximately 6%, while with typical use this figure rises to around 12%.

These estimates are largely based on studies in which the spermicidal agent used was nonoxynol-9, which is now discontinued in some countries. In comparative trials evaluating single-use diaphragms with N-9 versus cellulose-based placebo gels, no statistically significant differences in pregnancy rates were found (approximately 10.4%). Most participants achieved correct placement after a single session of medical counselling, and a high percentage expressed satisfaction with the method (Hassoun, 2018).

Cervical caps used with spermicides show variable pregnancy rates depending on the user's obstetric history. In nulliparous women, the pregnancy rate with perfect use reaches 26%, whereas in multiparous women it falls to 9%. These figures increase significantly with typical use, rising to 32% and 16% respectively (Hassoun, 2018; Trussell et al., 1994).

In direct comparative studies between caps and diaphragms, the cap has demonstrated higher pregnancy rates (13.5% versus 7.9%). Nonetheless, it has been associated with a lower incidence of urinary tract infections compared to the diaphragm. However, its use poses greater technical challenges, particularly regarding insertion and removal. Cytological evaluations after three months of use showed no significant differences in cervico-vaginal smears between the two methods (Trussell et al., 1994).

Conclusion

- *Spermicides* are local, non-hormonal contraceptive methods that act primarily by immobilising and destroying sperm through surfactant or acidifying agents.
- Nonoxynol-9 (N-9), although historically widely used, has been phased out in several countries due to its cytotoxic potential—particularly with frequent use—and its association with an increased risk of sexually transmitted infections (STIs), including HIV.
- *Benzalkonium chloride (BZK)* represents a safer alternative to N-9. Its spermicidal mechanisms include enzymatic inhibition, disruption of the sperm membrane, and alteration of cervical mucus. It is available in multiple pharmaceutical forms, generally well tolerated, with mild and transient adverse effects.
- *Vaginal pH-regulating gels* (ACIDFORM, Amphora, Phexxi) have introduced a significant innovation by maintaining an acidic vaginal pH after ejaculation, thereby impairing sperm motility without causing significant epithelial damage or disrupting the vaginal microbiota.
- *Spermicides* are more effective when used in combination with barrier methods, such as condoms, diaphragms, or cervical caps, substantially increasing contraceptive efficacy compared to their use alone.
- Research in the field of spermicides is progressing towards multipurpose formulations that not only prevent unintended pregnancies but also reduce the incidence of STIs, through non-hormonal, self-administered products with high bioadhesive properties and sustained vaginal retention.

References

Amaral, Eliana, Antero Perdigâo, Maria Helena Souza, Christine Mauck, Donald Waller, Lourens Zaneveld, y Anibal Faundes. 2004. "Postcoital Testing after the Use of a Bio-Adhesive Acid Buffering Gel (ACIDFORM) and a 2% Nonoxynol-9 Product." *Contraception* 70 (6): 492-97. https://doi.org/10.1016/j.contraception.2004.06.007.

American College of Obstetricians and Gynecologists. n.d. *Barrier Methods of Birth Control: Spermicide, Condom, Sponge, Diaphragm, and Cervical Cap.* Accessed May 21, 2025. https://www.acog.org/womens-health/faqs/barrier-methods-of-birth-control-spermicide-condom-sponge-diaphragm-and-cervical-cap.

Batár, István. 2010. "State-of-the-Art of Non-Hormonal Methods of Contraception: II. Chemical Barrier Contraceptives." *The European Journal of Contraception & Reproductive Health Care* 15, no. 2: 89–95. https://doi.org/10.3109/13625180903462326.

Bayer, Lisa L., y Jeffrey T. Jensen. 2014. "ACIDFORM: A Review of the Evidence." Contraception 90 (1): 11-18. https://doi.org/10.1016/j.contraception.2014.01.015.

Clarke, Gary N., Scott G. McCoombe, and Roger V. Short. 2006. "Sperm Immobilizing Properties of Lemon Juice." *Fertility and Sterility* 85, no. 5: 1529–30. https://doi.org/10.1016/j.fertnstert.2005.10.040.

Ferguson, Lisa L. "Contraception and Abortion." In Maternity and Women's Health Care, 8th ed., 143–64. Elsevier, n.d. Accessed May 21, 2025. https://www-clinicalkey-es.sescam.a17.csinet.es/#!/content/book/3-s2.0-B9780323810180000085?scrollTo=%23hl0000795.

Trussell, James. 2014. "Contraceptive Efficacy." *Global Library of Women's Medicine* (ISSN 1756-2228). Last updated February 2014. DOI: 10.3843/GLOWM.10375. Accessed May 21, 2025. http://www.glowm.com/section-view/heading/Contraceptive%20Efficacy/item/374.

Einarson, T. R., G. Koren, D. Mattice, and O. Schechter-Tsafriri. 1990. "Maternal Spermicide Use and Adverse Reproductive Outcome: A Meta-Analysis." *American Journal of Obstetrics and Gynecology* 162, no. 3: 655–60. https://doi.org/10.1016/0002-9378(90)90976-e.

Encyclopedia of Reproduction. 2018. Academic Press.

Gallaway, M. Shayne, D. Kim Waller, Mark A. Canfield, Angela Scheuerle, and National Birth Defects Prevention Study. 2009. "The Association between Use of Spermicides or Male Condoms and Major Structural Birth Defects." *Contraception* 80, no. 5: 422–29. https://doi.org/10.1016/j.contraception.2009.03.007.

Garg, S., R. A. Anderson, C. J. Chany, D. P. Waller, X. H. Diao, K. Vermani, and L. J. Zaneveld. 2001. "Properties of a New Acid-Buffering Bioadhesive Vaginal Formulation (ACIDFORM)." *Contraception* 64, no. 1: 67–75. https://doi.org/10.1016/s0010-7824(01)00217-7.

Grimes, David A., Laureen M. Lopez, Elizabeth G. Raymond, Vera Halpern, Kavita Nanda, and Kenneth F. Schulz. 2013. "Spermicide Used Alone for Contraception." *The Cochrane Database of Systematic Reviews* 2013, no. 12: CD005218. https://doi.org/10.1002/14651858.CD005218.pub4.

Hassoun, D. 2018. "Méthodes de contraception naturelle et méthodes barrières. RPC contraception CNGOF." *Gynécologie Obstétrique Fertilité & Sénologie*, Recommandations pour la pratique clinique élaborées par le CNGOF 46, no. 12: 873–82. https://doi.org/10.1016/j.gofs.2018.10.002.

"Historia evolutiva de la anticoncepción." 2018. *Anales de la Real Academia Nacional de Medicina de España* (blog). August 16, 2018. https://analesranm.es/revista/2018/135_01/rev09.

Ingram, Matthew J., Edel Zeller, Gary P. Moss, and Charlotte E. Hall. 2006. "A Potential Anti-Implantation and Spermicidal Strategy: Putative Derivatives of Nonoxynol-9 and Anti-Inflammatory Agents and Their Spermicidal Activity." *The European Journal of Contraception & Reproductive Health Care* 11, no. 4: 258–61. https://doi.org/10.1080/13625180600907487.

Iyer, Vidya, and S. S. Poddar. 2008a. "Update on Nonoxynol-9 as Vaginal Spermicide." *The European Journal of Contraception & Reproductive Health Care: The Official Journal of the European Society of Contraception* 13, no. 4: 339–50. https://doi.org/10.1080/13625180802263515.

Kuyoh, M. A., C. Toroitich-Ruto, D. A. Grimes, K. F. Schulz, and M. G. Gallo. 2002. "Sponge versus Diaphragm for Contraception." *The Cochrane Database of Systematic Reviews* 2002, no. 3: CD003172. https://doi.org/10.1002/14651858.CD003172.

Marinaro, Jessica A., and Marc Goldstein. 2025. "Non-Hormonal Contraception: Current and Emerging Targets." *Advances in Experimental Medicine and Biology* 1469: 245–72. https://doi.org/10.1007/978-3-031-82990-1_11.

Mauck, Christine, Andrea Thurman, Jeffrey T. Jensen, Courtney A. Schreiber, Jeff Baker, Melody Y. Hou, Steven Chavoustie, et al. 2024. "Safety Testing of Ovaprene: An Investigational Nonhormonal Monthly Vaginal Contraceptive." *Contraception* 135 (July): 110440. https://doi.org/10.1016/j.contraception.2024.110440.

Nelson, Anita L. 2018. "An Overview of Properties of Amphora (Acidform) Contraceptive Vaginal Gel." *Expert Opinion on Drug Safety* 17, no. 9: 935–43. https://doi.org/10.1080/14740338.2018.1515197.

Pendharkar, Sonal, Axel Skafte-Holm, Gizem Simsek, and Thor Haahr. 2023. "Lactobacilli and Their Probiotic Effects in the Vagina of Reproductive Age Women." *Microorganisms* 11, no. 3: 636. https://doi.org/10.3390/microorganisms11030636.

Riddle, John M. 1997. *Eve's Herbs: A History of Contraception and Abortion in the West*. Harvard University Press.

Roddy, Ronald E., Léopold Zekeng, Kelley A. Ryan, Ubald Tamoufé, and Kathryn G. Tweedy. 2002. "Effect of Nonoxynol-9 Gel on Urogenital Gonorrhea and Chlamydial Infection: A Randomized Controlled Trial." *JAMA* 287, no. 9: 1117–22. https://doi.org/10.1001/jama.287.9.1117.

Serfaty, D. 2017. "[Contraception during Perimenopause: The Spermicides Option]." *Journal of Gynecology Obstetrics and Human Reproduction* 46, no. 3: 211–18. https://doi.org/10.1016/j.jogoh.2016.10.007.

Su, Shanna, and Kathleen L. Vincent. 2022. "Lactic Acid, Citric Acid, and Potassium Bitartrate Non-Hormonal Prescription Vaginal pH Modulator (VPM) Gel for the Prevention of Pregnancy." *Expert Review of Clinical Pharmacology* 15, no. 6: 659–70. https://doi.org/10.1080/17512433.2022.2100347.

Suthutvoravut, Somsak, and Ourawan Kamyarat. 2016. "Spermicidal Effects of Lemon Juice and Juices from Other Natural Products." *Agriculture and Natural Resources* 50, no. 2: 133–38. https://doi.org/10.1016/j.anres.2015.09.004.

Thurman, Andrea R., Thomas R. Moench, Marshall Hoke, Joseph A. Politch, Howard Cabral, Emilie Mausser, Ellena Nador, et al. 2023. "ZB-06, a Vaginal Film Containing an Engineered Human Contraceptive Antibody (HC4-N), Demonstrates Safety and Efficacy in a Phase 1 Postcoital Test and Safety Study." *American Journal of Obstetrics and Gynecology* 228, no. 6: 716.e1–716.e12. https://doi.org/10.1016/j.ajog.2023.02.024.

Chapter 7

Combined Hormonal Contraceptives

A. Santos Fernández[1,*], MD
A. García Buendía[1], MD
C. García Fernández[1], MD
M. Juan Rodrigo1, MD
and C. Aparicio Martínez[2], MD

[1]Obstetrics and Gynecology Department, University and Hospital of Albacete, Albacete, Spain
[2]Obstetrics and Gynecology Department, Hospital of Tomelloso, Tomelloso, Spain

Abstract

Combined hormonal contraceptives (CHCs) are among the most widely used reversible contraceptive methods. They contain a synthetic estrogen and progestogen that work primarily by inhibiting ovulation and inducing endometrial and cervical changes that prevent implantation.

CHCs are available in various routes of administration—oral, transdermal, vaginal, and intramuscular—all of which exhibit similar pharmacokinetic profiles. Consequently, they share comparable metabolic effects, side effects, indications and contraindications, as well as safety and efficacy profiles. The choice of method should be tailored to the user's preferences.

In recent years, several clinical guidelines have been developed to improve adherence by adapting to individuals' daily routines and lifestyles. These efforts aim to reduce the gap between theoretical efficacy (>99%) and real-world effectiveness, which is estimated to result in approximately 8 unintended pregnancies per 1,000 women per year (Trussell 2011).

Keywords: combined hormonal contraceptives, vaginal ring, transdermal patch

---

* Corresponding Author's Email: aliciasantos7@gmail.com

In: Advances in Reproductive Health
Editors: Llanos Belmonte Andujar and Ana Fuentes Rozalen
ISBN: 979-8-90134-038-7

Introduction

Combined hormonal contraceptives, composed of a synthetic estrogen and progestogen, are a widely used contraceptive option worldwide. Their primary mechanism of action is the inhibition of ovulation, which confers high contraceptive efficacy and reversibility upon discontinuation. Over the years, formulations and dosages have evolved with the goal of improving adherence and narrowing the gap between theoretical efficacy (>99%) and real-world effectiveness, which is considerably lower (Trussell 2011).

Among their advantages are non-contraceptive benefits, such as regulation of the menstrual cycle and relief of various gynecological symptoms, including dysmenorrhea, mastalgia, and heavy menstrual bleeding. These contraceptives are available in several forms—pills, patches, and vaginal rings—with similar indications, allowing for adaptation to individual preferences and needs, thus promoting a more personalized and satisfactory use (FSRH 2019). It is essential that users receive clear, evidence-based information about the efficacy, safety, and potential risks of these methods, enabling them to make informed decisions in line with their personal needs and lifestyle.

Characteristics of the Method

Mechanism of Action of CHCs

CHC is based on the simultaneous administration of an oestrogen and a progestogen with the primary aim of inhibiting ovulation and, secondarily, inducing a series of changes in the endometrium and cervical mucus that hinder fertilisation and implantation.

Ovulation Inhibition

The main mechanism of CHCs is the suppression of gonadotropin release (LH and FSH) by the pituitary gland through negative feedback on the hypothalamic-pituitary axis. The progestogenic component is primarily responsible for inhibiting ovulation by suppressing the pulsatile secretion of gonadotropin-releasing hormone (GnRH) from the hypothalamus, leading to reduced luteinizing hormone (LH) secretion and thus preventing ovulation. It also modulates the effects of estrogen on the endometrium and hepatic metabolism. The estrogen component enhances contraceptive efficacy by further suppressing GnRH and follicle-stimulating hormone (FSH), preventing the selection of a dominant follicle (FSRH 2023; (Teal y Edelman 2021).

Effects on the Endometrium and Cervical Mucus

Progestogens induce a non-receptive secretory transformation of the endometrium, which impairs implantation. They also increase cervical mucus viscosity, creating a barrier to sperm penetration (Guillebaud 2017).

Estrogens Used in CHCs

Traditionally, the most commonly used estrogen in CHCs has been ethinylestradiol (EE), a high-potency synthetic estrogen typically used in doses of 15–35 μg in current formulations. Higher doses, such as the 50 μg formulations used in earlier decades, have been withdrawn due to their association with increased thromboembolic risk and other adverse effects (FSRH 2023; Guillebaud 2012).

More recently, formulations containing “natural” estrogens have been developed that lack the ethinyl group in their molecular structure. These include estradiol valerate, 17β-estradiol (identical to endogenous estrogen), and estetrol (E4), an estrogen naturally produced by the fetal liver. These compounds undergo less hepatic metabolism than EE and are associated with a lower impact on hepatic protein synthesis, including clotting factors, which may translate into a more favorable thromboembolic risk profile (Tulchinsky, Hobel, Yeh y Marshall 1975; Coelingh Bennink, Verhoeven y Zimmerman 2008; Duijkers, I. J., A. Verhoeven, H. J. Coelingh Bennink, y J. D. Zimmerman. 2015; FSRH 2023; IARC 2007).

Estetrol, in particular, is notable for its selective action on estrogen receptors—classified as a Native Estrogen with Selective action in Tissues (NEST). It activates estrogen receptors in the uterus, bone, and vagina, while inhibiting activity in the breast, liver, and vascular system, potentially resulting in an improved benefit-risk profile (Gemzell-Danielsson et al. 2022).

Progestogens Used in CHCs

Progestogens are potent antigonadotropins, providing high contraceptive efficacy through their progestogenic and antiestrogenic actions. Their pharmacological profiles vary depending on their affinity for different hormone receptors, which may result in androgenic, anti-androgenic, glucocorticoid, or antimineralocorticoid effects (Calaf 2005; Taylor, Pal, and Seli 2019) (see Table 1).

Progestogens can be classified according to the generation to which they belong (Calaf 2005) (FSRH 2023) (IARC 2007).

Table 1. Hormonal activity of the main progestogens used in combined hormonal contraceptives. Their relative efficacy as anti-estrogenic, oestrogenic, androgenic, anti-androgenic and glucocorticoid is indicated. (+) effective, (+/-) not very effective, (-) not effective (Calaf 2005) (Taylor, Pal and Seli 2019).

PROGESTAGEN	Anti-estrogenic	Estrogenic	Androgenic	Anti - Androgenic	Glucocorticoid
Chlormadinone	+	-	-	+	+
Cyproterone	+	-	-	++	+
Dienogest	+/-	+/-	-	+	-
Drosperinone	+	-	-	+	-
Etonorgestrel	+	-	+	-	-
Gestodene	+	-	+	-	+
Levonorgestrel	+	-	+	-	-
Medroxyprogesterone Ac.	+	-	+/-	-	+
Nomegestrol Ac.	+	-	-	+/-	-
Norestisterone	+	+	+	-	-
Norgestimate	+	-	+	-	-
Progesterone	+	-	-	+/-	+

The first progestogens were compounds derived from testosterone, so their androgenic activity is prominent. Within these compounds, they are classified into 3 generations (Reust et al. 2012):

- *First generation*: norethisterone and ethinodiol.
- *Second generation*: levonorgestrel and norgestrel.
- *Third generation:* gestodene, desogestrel, etonogestrel (active metabolite of desogestrel), norgestimate and its active metabolite, norelgestromin.

Subsequently, new compounds were developed with the aim of correcting the androgenicity of the previous compounds, classified as fourth generation.

- *Fourth generation and new gestagens*: these stand out as anti-androgenic, such as drospirenone (derived from spironolactone), cyproterone acetate, nomegestrol acetate (derived from progesterone) or dienogest (derived from testosterone) (van Vliet et al. 2005).

Interaction Between Oestrogen and Progestogen

It is important to note that the androgenic activity of certain progestogens not only contributes to dermatological side effects such as acne and hirsutism, but also modulates various systemic effects. Androgenic activity can influence fluid retention, potentially leading to weight gain or oedema, particularly in susceptible women. Moreover, it affects lipid and glucose metabolism. Progestogens with higher androgenic activity—such as norethindrone and levonorgestrel—may increase LDL cholesterol and reduce HDL cholesterol levels, potentially raising cardiovascular risk (Beck 1977). Effects on glucose metabolism have also been observed to be more pronounced in women with a history of diabetes or insulin resistance (Jick SS 2004).

When combined with estrogens, it is worth highlighting that androgenic progestogens may partially counteract the estrogen-induced procoagulant effect. In contrast, anti-androgenic progestogens do not, which could explain the higher thrombotic risk associated with certain newer-generation formulations (Van Vliet et al. 2005).

Available Formulations

Routes of Administration of Combined Hormonal Contraceptives

CHCs can currently be administered by four main routes: oral, transdermal, vaginal and intramuscular. All share a common mechanism of action based on suppression of the hypothalamic-pituitary-ovarian axis. The choice of one route or another depends on the user's preferences, clinical characteristics and adherence to treatment.

Oral Route

This is the most common route of administration. Preparations can be classified according to several criteria:

- *Type of hormonal regimen:* Most pills are monophasic, meaning they contain the same dose of estrogen and progestogen in all active tablets. Multiphasic (bi- or triphasic) preparations aim to mimic the natural hormonal fluctuations of the menstrual cycle but have declined in use due to their complexity in case of missed pills and a lack of clear benefits over monophasic regimens.
- *Type of estrogen:* Most commonly used pills contain ethinylestradiol (EE) in doses ranging from 15 to 40 µg, although formulations with natural estrogens—such as estradiol valerate, 17β-estradiol, or estetrol—are also available.
- *Cycle length*: the classical 21/7 regimen (21 days of active pills followed by a 7-day hormone-free interval, HFI) is still widely used. However, newer regimens include 24 or 26 active pills with shorter HFIs to improve symptoms related to hormone withdrawal (e.g. headache, mastalgia, dysmenorrhea) and maintain more consistent ovarian suppression. Some 28-day formulations include placebo pills to facilitate adherence by preserving a daily routine (FSRH 2019).
- *Extended or continuous regimens*: These regimens reduce or eliminate HFIs and consequently the frequency of withdrawal bleeds. They may follow fixed schedules (e.g. 84/7), flexible schedules (HFI only in case of persistent bleeding), or continuous schedules (365 days without interruption). These regimens show similar safety and efficacy to traditional regimens and may enhance adherence (Sánchez-Borrego 2010; FSRH 2019; Edelman et al. 2014).

Vaginal Route

Consists of monthly insertion of a flexible vaginal ring that releases 15 mcg EE and 120 mcg etonogestrel or 150 mcg segesterone acetate and 13 mcg EE daily for three weeks, followed by one week without a ring to allow withdrawal bleeding. It shares the efficacy and safety profile with the oral route (Barriga et al. 2020) (Herndon and Zieman 2004) Systemic absorption is higher than for the oral route, due to rapid and efficient absorption through the vaginal mucosa. Bioavailability for etonogestrel is about 100% (superior to the oral route), while for EE it is about 56% (similar to the oral route).

The ring has some advantages (Dieben, Roumen and Apter 2002) (Mulders and Dieben 2001) (Lopez et al. 2013):

- Avoidance of the first hepatic pass, which decreases the synthesis of procoagulant hepatic factors.
- Lower dose needed and more stable hormone levels due to the high absorption capacity of the vaginal mucosa, maintaining constant serum levels.
- Not affected by vomiting or diarrhoea. Nor is its effectiveness compromised by the use of spermicides or antifungals.
- Improves adherence by requiring only one monthly action.

In addition, insertion and removal are simple, and it does not interfere with sexual activity or other daily activities (Quílez Conde 2024) (FSRH 2023).

Transdermal Route

This consists of the use of weekly patches that release 150 mcg of norelgestromin and 20 mcg of ethinylestradiol per day. Three consecutive patches are applied with a week off, replicating the 21/7 schedule (Herndon and Zieman 2004). Its pharmacokinetics are similar to the oral route, although with somewhat higher systemic hormone exposure than the ring and oral route, with no evidence of relevant clinical repercussions (Zieman et al. 2022) (FSRH 2023) (Lopez et al. 2013).

Its main advantages are:

- It avoids first-pass hepatic metabolism.
- It is not affected by gastrointestinal disturbances.
- It improves compliance by requiring only one weekly action.
- It is well tolerated, although mild skin reactions may occur.

Parenteral Route

Less commonly used, there is a monthly intramuscular injectable preparation that combines 10 mg of estradiol enanthate and 150 mg of dihydroxyprogesterone (Herndon and Zieman 2004). It is applied between the 7th-8th day of each cycle (Quílez Conde 2024). Its use is restricted to specific situations where other routes are not feasible. It is not currently marketed in all countries, where it must be requested as a foreign medicine (FSRH 2023).

Contraceptive Efficacy

The Pearl index, which measures the number of pregnancies per 100 woman-years of use, varies according to the route of administration and, above all, the type of use:

- *Perfect use* (strict adherence to guidelines): efficacy close to 99-99.7%.
- *Typical use* (conditioned by forgetfulness, errors or misuse): slightly lower efficacy, but still high (Trussell, 2011).
  - Combined pill: 0.3% (perfect) / ~7% (typical)
  - Vaginal ring: 0.3% / ~7%.
  - Transdermal patch: 0.3% / ~7%.

Non-Contraceptive Indications and Benefits

In addition to their use as a method of contraception, CHCs have multiple therapeutic benefits. Common indications include the management of menstrual disorders, dermatological conditions, symptoms related to premenstrual syndrome and gynaecological diseases such as endometriosis or polycystic ovarian syndrome (PCOS), as well as the reduction of the risk of certain types of cancer.

Menstrual Cycle Disorders

CHCs have been shown to be effective in reducing heavy menstrual bleeding (HMB), improving both the volume and regularity of bleeding. They can also alleviate primary dysmenorrhoea, especially when given in an extended or continuous schedule (FSRH 2023) (Dragoman 2014).

Premenstrual Syndrome and Premenstrual Symptoms

The use of CHCs, particularly those with drospirenone, can alleviate symptoms of premenstrual syndrome and premenstrual dysphoric disorder. Continuous regimens appear to offer greater symptomatic improvement than cyclic regimens (Ma and Song 2023).

Acne and Hirsutism

Progestogen anti-androgen preparations block ovarian and adrenal secretion of sex hormones with a consequent decrease in testosterone.

A Cochrane review showed that CHCs significantly reduce the number and severity of acne lesions compared to placebo (Ma and Song 2023).

Polycystic Ovary Syndrome (PCOS)

CHCs are considered first-line treatment for the management of menstrual irregularity, acne and hirsutism in women with PCOS, including in adolescents. Although the optimal duration of treatment has not been defined, it has been observed that drospirenone preparations may be particularly beneficial because of their anti-androgenic effect (Legro et al. 2013).

Endometriosis

After conservative surgery, the use of CHCs, especially in continuous regimens, can significantly reduce the associated pain and decrease the risk of recurrence of endometriosis. An improvement in quality of life and sexual function has also been observed in these patients (Becker et al. 2022).

Vasomotor Symptoms in Perimenopause

Although hormone replacement therapy (HRT) is the standard approach, low-dose CHCs may be a useful alternative in perimenopausal women who also need contraception. However, the evidence is limited (FSRH 2023).

Bone Health

In perimenopausal women, the use of CHCs may contribute to preserving bone mineral density (BMD), although the available data are inconclusive regarding their impact on reducing fracture risk. In adolescents, some studies suggest that CHCs may decrease the expected BMD gain, particularly with 21/7 regimens (Scholes et al. 2016).

Cancer Risk Reduction

This topic is discussed in detail in its corresponding chapter.

How to Start Taking CHC

The method is usually started on the first day of the next menstrual period. However, it can also be started at any time during the cycle ("quick start") provided that pregnancy has been ruled out previously, with a negative pregnancy test or if there are no signs or symptoms of pregnancy and at least one of the following criteria is met:

- No sexual intercourse has occurred since the last normal period.
- A reliable contraceptive method has been used correctly.
- The initiation occurs within the first 7 days of a normal menstrual period.
- Initiation takes place within the first 4 weeds postpartum in non-breastfeeding women, or within the first 6 months postpartum in breastfeeding women with amenorrhea.
- It is found in the first 7 days after an abortion.

How to Change Methods

Table 2. Switching from method to ACH (Quilez Conde 2024) (FSRH 2023)

Previous method	When to start	
Other CHC	Day after last active pill, patch or ring	No
LNG IUD	Can start immediately if the previous method was used correctly and consistently	Yes (7 to 9 days if starting a method with natural oestrogen)
Progestogen-only (GS) method (implant, progestogen-only pill or)	Start at any time, if initiation is within the active period within the active period of the previous method. Also, after an active OS pill	No
Copper IUD	Up to the 5th day of the menstrual cycle. On the 1st day of the cycle if the preparation contains a natural oestrogen. The IUD can be removed at any time. At any other time during the cycle or if the client is amenorrhoeic.	No Yes (unless the IUD is kept in place for the first 7 or 9 days if a method with natural oestrogen is started).

In this case, if the method is started beyond the first 5 days of the cycle, another method of contraception should be used for the next 7 or 9 days, depending on the preparation.

Adverse Effects

Minor Adverse Effects

Many adverse effects do not pose a medical risk, but their importance lies in the lack of adherence to treatment and they are often the main reason for discontinuation of the method. Most of these effects decrease with continued use, and their occurrence is common during the hormone-free interval, so the use of continuous or extended regimens may improve tolerance (Ma and Song 2023) (Mendoza et al. 2014).

Nausea and Vomiting

This is mainly related to the oestrogen component and tends to disappear after the first few cycles. In oral administration, it should be noted that vomiting in the first two hours after intake may compromise efficacy, unlike other routes (Consensus Conference 2000) (Sánchez Borrego and Martínez 2003).

A recent study by Khalil et al. (2025) examined the relationship between the use of combined oral contraceptives and the risk of developing gastroparesis in premenopausal women. They found that the use of this method in premenopausal women was associated with a significantly increased risk of gastroparesis (OR 1.29, $p < 0.0001$), and this relationship was maintained up to five years of follow-up. In addition, AHC users had more gastrointestinal symptoms, increased use of prokinetics and more diagnostic tests such as endoscopy and gastric emptying studies. These results suggest that CHCs may affect gastric motility and contribute to digestive discomfort (Khalil et al. 2025).

Headache

It is one of the most commonly cited symptoms and may worsen during ILH. Although no clear association with the type of CHC or route of administration has been demonstrated, its initial presence tends to decrease over time (Loder, Buse, and Golub 2005) (MacGregor 2013). Catamenial migraine may improve with continued regimens, but migraine with aura remains an absolute contraindication because of the increased risk of ischaemic stroke. (Ma and Song 2023).

Intermenstrual Bleeding

Breakthrough bleeding is a relatively common side effect in CHC users with an incidence ranging from 10-18% per cycle, regardless of the route of administration (Merz et al., 2015; Endrikat et al., 2001). Vaginal rings appear to have a lower incidence of unscheduled bleeding, possibly because they maintain more stable serum oestrogen levels. Since stability in hormone exposure is associated with a reduction in bleeding frequency, continuous or extended patterns may contribute to a lower incidence of breakthrough bleeding, thus providing better tolerance to the method (Lopez et al., 2016; Dieben, Roumen, & Apter, 2002).

A 2013 Cochrane review, which analysed 22 randomised clinical trials (RCTs), found that combined oral contraceptive formulations containing 20 μg ethinylestradiol are associated with a higher incidence of unscheduled bleeding compared to those containing higher doses of oestrogen (Gallo et al., 2013). Regarding the type of oestrogen, studies comparing natural oestrogen preparations versus those containing ethinylestradiol show no clear differences in the incidence of breakthrough bleeding, although one study reported fewer days of bleeding in oestradiol preparations (Ahrendt et al., 2009).

Regarding the type of progestogens, a 2004 systematic review including 22 studies reported that two RCTs found a lower frequency of breakthrough bleeding with third generation progestogens compared to second generation progestogens (RR 0.71, 95% CI 0.55-0.91). However, these results are limited by the short duration of the studies. On the other hand, six RCTs showed that combined contraceptives with second generation progestogens offered better cycle control compared to those with first generation progestogens, both in monophasic (RR 0.69, 95% CI 0.52-0.91) and triphasic (RR 0.61, 95% CI 0.43-0.85) formulations.

Mood Changes

Although many women do not have clinically significant changes, some may notice changes, especially if they have a history of dysthymia. Evidence on the causal relationship with depression is limited. Drospirenone may have a more favourable profile (Skovlund et al. 2016).

Libido

This is a controversial issue as libido is influenced by multiple social and psychological factors. Current evidence is limited, mainly due to the heterogeneity of the preparations studied, the different assessment tools used and the absence of placebo groups or non-hormonal comparators in the studies. Overall, no clear association has been found between the use of CHCs containing ≥20 μg ethinylestradiol and changes in libido (Padragomanstor, Holla, and Chmel 2013).

Weight Gain

There is no strong evidence linking CHC use with significant weight gain in either adolescent or adult women. In the few cases where it does occur, it is usually related to fluid retention. Progestogens with antimineralocorticoid activity, such as drospirenone, may minimize this effect (Gallo et al. 2014).

Major Adverse Effects

Venous Thromboembolism

The incidence of venous thromboembolism (VTE), defined as the occurrence of deep vein thrombosis or pulmonary thromboembolism, during CHC use is estimated to be between 5 and 10 cases per 10,000 women/year (Heinemann and Dinger 2006). Approximately 1% of these events are fatal (European Medicines Agency 2013).

This risk is considerably lower than that observed during pregnancy and the puerperium, where the estimated annual incidence of VTE is 29 and between 300-400 cases per 10,000 women, respectively. The thrombotic risk is highest in the first few months after starting CHC or when resuming it after a suspension of at least one month. It tends to decrease during the first year of use and remains stable thereafter (European Medicines Agency 2013).

CHCs increase the risk of VTE by inducing a state of acquired hypercoagulability. The main agent responsible for this effect is oestrogen, although the type of progestogen present in the formulation also has a significant influence. Oestrogen increases levels of procoagulant factors such as factors VII, VIII and X, fibrinogen and prothrombin; reduces natural anticoagulants such as protein S; induces protein C resistance; and decreases antithrombin III activity and fibrinolysis (Tchaikovski and Eichinger 2021).

The type of progestogen modulates the magnitude of these procoagulant effects. CHCs containing levonorgestrel or norethisterone have been shown to produce less acquired resistance to activated protein C than those containing gestodene, desogestrel or norgestimate, as well as more discrete alterations in protein S and tissue factor pathway inhibitor levels. These differences could be attributed to their more androgenic profile (Martinez et al. 2012).

In a meta-analysis published by Dragoman et al. (2018), the risk of VTE associated with the use of combined oral contraceptives with oestrogen at doses <50 mcg of EE with cyproterone acetate, desogestrel, dienogest, drospirenone or gestodene was assessed. These preparations were associated with an increased risk of VTE (with a relative risk range between 1.5 and 2.0) compared to those containing levonorgestrel. This difference did not reach statistical significance for dienogest. (Dragoman et al. 2018).

In addition, the action of the progestogen may be enhanced by the oestrogen dose of the preparation. Therefore, low-dose ethinylestradiol formulations (<35 mcg) are recommended, as they are associated with a lower relative risk of venous thromboembolism (Consensus Conference 2000; FSRH 2023).

Route of administration alone does not significantly modify VTE risk when comparing oral vs. transdermal vs. vaginal (Martinez et al. 2012).

Arterial Thromboembolic Disease

The risk of arterial thromboembolic disease, such as acute myocardial infarction or stroke, is extremely low and would be related to high doses of oestrogen. However, because of the morbidity and mortality consequences of these events, any increased risk is important (FSRH 2023).

This risk is significantly increased in women with other associated risk factors for arterial disease and should not be prescribed in women with hypertension, aged over 35, smokers, high BMI, dyslipidaemia and diabetes, and in women with migraine with or without aura appearing after the introduction of CHCs.

In contrast, women who are neither smokers nor have other associated cardiovascular risk factors do not have an increased risk of AMI (Lidegaard et al. 2012).

A Cochrane review concluded that the risk of arterial thromboembolism is increased with increasing doses of oestrogen in preparations. No difference was seen in the type of progesterone used (Roach et al. 2015).

Contraindications: Eligibility Criteria

The World Health Organization (WHO) classifies different methods according to the restrictions these preparations have in the presence of certain conditions based on available evidence (last updated 2015, 5th edition, current).

Table 3. CHC eligibility criteria (based on WHO and CDC recommendations

CATEGORY 4 (contraindicative)	CATEGORY 3
Breastfeeding in the first 6 weeks postpartum*.	Breastfeeding between 6 weeks postpartum and 6 months.
Non-breastfeeding women in the first 3 weeks postpartum, if there are other risk factors for venous thromboembolism (immobility, transfusion, BMI > 30, caesarean delivery...).	Immediate postpartum without breastfeeding (first 3 weeks) or other risk factors. Between 21 and 42 days postpartum, if there are other risk factors for DVT.
Smoking more than 15 cigarettes/day in those over 35 years of age.	Smoking less than 15 cigarettes/day in those over 35 years of age.
Multiple cardiovascular risk factors (age, smoking, diabetes, hypertension, waist circumference >88 cm).	Diabetes Mellitus of more than 20 years of evolution or associated with vasculopathy, neuropathy or nephropathy.
Personal history of deep vein thrombosis (VTE) or pulmonary embolism (PE).	Controlled arterial hypertension or uncontrolled systolic hypertension of 140-159 mm Hg or diastolic hypertension of 90-99 mm Hg.
History of stroke.	Current active gallbladder disease and/or under medical treatment.
SLE with anti-P (+) or unknown anti-P (+) antibodies.	History of cholestasis associated with previous hormonal contraceptive use.
Valvulopathy complicated by pulmonary hypertension, atrial fibrillation, history of endocarditis or metallic prostheses**.	Taking drugs such as rifampicin-rifabutin and/or anticonvulsants. ****
Migraine headaches with aura.	Migraine without aura in initiating migraine sufferers over 35 years of age. Migraine without aura in patients under 35 years of age.
Current history of breast cancer (last 5 years).	Previous history of breast cancer (within the last 5 years).
Acute or exacerbated viral hepatitis.	The CDC also considers category 3: Superficial venous thrombosis (current or previous). Peripartum cardiomyopathy more than 6 months ago. Multiple sclerosis with prolonged immobilisation. Current or medically treated cholecystitis.
Decompensated cirrhosis.	
Current VTE/PE.	
Major surgery with prolonged immobility.	
Diagnosed familial thrombophilia: situations in which there are gene mutations with thrombogenic character. thrombogenic character.	
Current or past ischaemic heart disease.	

*CDC considers contraindication during lactation for the first 21 days if there are no other thromboembolic risk factors. If there are associated thromboembolic risk factors, it is considered category 3-4.

**According to the CDC, it is considered category 4 if you have had peripartum heart disease less than 6 months ago or with moderate or severe impairment of cardiac function (NYHASFC III or IV).

***According to the CDC, the following medical conditions are considered category 4: renal disease: current nephrotic syndrome, haemodialysis or peritoneal dialysis. diabetes with nephropathy, retinopathy or neuropathy, other vascular disease or >20 years of evolution (category 3 or 4). Sickle cell anaemia. Graft rejection.

The US Centers for Disease Control and Prevention MMWR has also published a risk/benefit stratification based on 4 categories (equivalent to those of the WHO) (WHO 2015) (Table 3) (Nguyen et al. 2024).

- Category 1: no restrictions
- Category 2: benefits outweigh risks

- Category 3: risks generally outweigh the benefits
- Category 4: use of OCPs is contraindicated.

Special Populations

High BMI

The safety and effectiveness of AHCs in women with BMI 35 kg/m2 has been controversial. Obesity doubles the risk of VTE; however, the absolute risk remains very low. Therefore, the WHO and CDC in the latest updates of the eligibility criteria consider obesity as category 2, indicating that it should be considered as a cardiovascular risk factor. But they warn that in the presence of additional thrombosis risk factors (such as smoking, dyslipidaemia, diabetes...), it could pose an unacceptable risk of thrombosis, which would force us to re-evaluate the indication. (WHO 2015) (FSRH 2023).

Regarding the effectiveness of these preparations, the evidence is limited and contradictory. It does not seem to be reduced, except for the patch in users with BMI>30 or >90 kg (Rocha et al. 2017) (López et al. 2016).

Inflammatory Bowel Disease

In women with inflammatory bowel disease (IBD), it is essential to consider both general risk factors and the particularities of this condition. Although IBD itself does not appear to increase the risk of VTE alone, during periods of moderate to severe activity or in the presence of other added factors, such as immobilisation, surgery, smoking, obesity, or a family history of VTE, the risk may be significantly increased (Nguyen et al. 2024).

According to the CDC, in women with IBD without other risk factors for VTE, the use of combined hormonal contraceptives (CHCs) is generally safe (category 2), with the benefits considered to outweigh the risks. However, in the presence of additional thrombotic risk factors, CHCs are classified as category 3, and their use should be carefully evaluated (Nguyen et al. 2024).

The Faculty of Sexual and Reproductive Healthcare (FSRH) guidelines agree that, although the overall risk is low in patients with stable, uncomplicated IBD, in those with active flares, severe disease, hospitalisation or a stoma, the use of combined contraceptives should be avoided because of the added risk of VTE and thrombotic complications. (FSRH 2023).

On the other hand, absorption of oral contraceptives may be compromised in patients with Crohn's disease who have undergone extensive bowel resections, especially of the ileum, as well as during episodes of severe diarrhoea or persistent vomiting, compromising the efficacy of the method. In these situations, alternative routes such as the transdermal patch or vaginal ring, whose absorption is not affected by gastrointestinal transit, are recommended (FSRH 2023).

In addition, current evidence has not shown that the use of combined hormonal contraceptives has a significant impact on IBD activity or the rate of exacerbations, so they can be used safely in women with well-controlled disease (FSRH 2023) (American Gastroenterological Association IBD Parenthood Project Working Group 2019).

Clinical Considerations

CHC is a widely used method that requires a targeted history taking to ensure safety and efficacy. Initial assessment should focus on personal and family history, with special emphasis on cardiovascular risk factors (smoking, obesity, hypertension, thrombophilias, previous episodes of deep vein thrombosis), history of migraine with aura, breast cancer or genetic predisposition, hepatobiliary disease, and obstetric-gynecological history, including previous contraceptive use.

Blood pressure measurement is essential at the first visit, as significant hypertension contraindicates the use of CHC. Elevated blood pressure (SBP ≥160/100 mmHg or SBP 140-159/90-99 mmHg with category 3) prompts the choice of alternative contraceptive methods and referral for monitoring. Although CHCs may raise blood pressure by 3-5 mmHg, this elevation is generally not clinically relevant.

Calculation of body mass index (BMI) is recommended to identify possible associated risks, although obesity alone does not contraindicate the use of CHCs.

Before starting the method, routine analyses are not required except in cases with a family history of thrombosis at a young age or in atypical locations, where a thrombophilia study will be indicated. Basic gynaecological examination, cervical screening, breast examination and screening for sexually transmitted infections are also not essential requirements.

Clear and personalised information about the method is key to improving adherence and continuity. Contraceptive counselling should include efficacy, risks and benefits, types of preparations and routes of administration, guidelines for use, follow-up, and addressing misconceptions. Non-contraceptive benefits and how to manage side effects should be highlighted, and dual protection to avoid sexually transmitted infections should be recommended.

Follow-up ideally takes place 3-6 months after initial prescription, assessing tolerance and risk factors, with annual check-ups recommended to monitor blood pressure and weight.

This comprehensive approach ensures a safe, effective prescription that is tailored to the individual characteristics of each user.

Drug Interactions

This topic is covered in its corresponding chapter.

How to Deal with Forgetfulness

The management of errors and oversights described in this chapter follows the recommendations set out by the FSRH (FSRH 2020).

Oral Route

In case of a missed pill in a monophasic regimen, it is recommended to take it immediately and continue with the regimen as usual, without the use of an additional method.

If two or more tablets are missed, it is recommended to take the last pill immediately and continue with the usual regimen. It is recommended to use an additional barrier method for 7 days.

- If the missed pill is between the 1st-7th day, emergency contraception should be considered.
- If it is between 8th-14th day, emergency contraception is not recommended.
- If between 15-21 days, it is recommended to skip the hormone-free period and continue with a new pack.

If the regimen is multiphasic, follow each manufacturer's instructions.

If vomiting or diarrhoea occurs within 2-4 hours of taking the pill, a new tablet can be taken. If it persists, it is advisable to use a barrier method for up to 7 days afterwards.

After discontinuation of CHC treatment, many women regain normal menstrual cycles within 30 days, and fertility within 90 days (Allen 2024).

Transdermal Route

The main advantage of the transdermal contraceptive patch is that it can improve adherence to treatment compared to the oral route by avoiding the need for daily administration. The usual schedule consists of a weekly patch application for three consecutive weeks, followed by a one-week break during which hormonally deprived bleeding occurs.

To minimise the risk of skin irritation or sensitisation to the adhesive, it is recommended to alternate application sites, always avoiding areas with previously applied creams, oils or lotions, as these may interfere with proper adhesion. Once the patch is in place, cosmetics can be used on the area without compromising its efficacy.

Management of forgetfulness and slippage:

- Delaying patch placement after the hormone-free interval (>7 days):
  - Apply a new patch after ruling out pregnancy and use a barrier method for the next 7 days.
- Forgetting at the start of a new cycle:
  - Apply the patch as soon as possible, considering it as the first day of the cycle.
- Delay in changing the second or third patch (>7 days since the last change):
  - If the delay is less than 48 hours, apply a new patch without further action, maintaining the usual weekly change day.
  - If the delay is more than 48 hours, apply a new patch, use a barrier method for 7 days and consider that day as the new start of the cycle.
- Patch detachment:

- If less than 24 hours have passed, replace the same patch or a new one, considering it as a new change day, without compromising contraceptive efficacy.
- If more than 24 hours have passed or there is any doubt about the time of detachment, apply a new patch and add a barrier method for the next 7 days.

It should be noted that as a transdermal route, the efficacy of the patch is not affected by vomiting or diarrhoea.

Transvaginal Route

It is essential to inform users that the vaginal ring does not act as a barrier method, so its correct insertion is inside the vagina, without the need to reach a specific position, as its effectiveness depends on the continuous release of hormones and not on its precise location.

The regimen of use consists of keeping the ring in place for three consecutive weeks, after which it is removed and a one-week rest is taken, a period in which hormonal withdrawal bleeding usually occurs.

The method remains effective even if removal of the ring is delayed for up to seven days, without requiring the additional use of a barrier method.

If the ring is dislodged or accidentally removed, it can be washed with lukewarm water (avoiding hot water, which may disrupt hormone release) and reinserted into the vagina. Removal for less than three hours does not affect contraceptive efficacy. If the ring remains outside the vagina for more than three hours, it is recommended to reinsert it as soon as possible and use an additional method of contraception, such as a condom, for the next seven days.

As it is a local route of administration, contraceptive efficacy is not affected by episodes of vomiting or diarrhoea.

Conclusion

Combined hormonal contraceptives represent a fundamental tool in reproductive health, not only because of their high contraceptive efficacy, but also because of their multiple additional benefits in the management of various gynaecological conditions. Their versatility in routes of administration and formulations allows for individualisation of treatment that favors adherence and user satisfaction.

Over the years, advances in the types of oestrogens and progestogens, as well as the development of more flexible patterns of use, have improved both the safety profile and tolerability. Despite the associated risks, such as venous or arterial thromboembolism, the benefit-risk balance is favourable in most healthy women, provided that an adequate clinical assessment is made beforehand.

The choice of the ideal preparation should be based on the clinical characteristics, preferences and lifestyle of each woman, ensuring clear, evidence-based information. Medical care should include proper indication, regular follow-up and management of adverse effects or special situations, such as use in women with obesity or inflammatory bowel disease.

In short, CHCs remain a safe and effective option when used in an appropriate and personalised way, and their prescription should be integrated into a client-centred sexual and reproductive health strategy.

References

Allen, Rebecca H. 2024. "Anticonceptivos orales combinados de estrógeno y progestina: selección de pacientes, asesoramiento y uso." *UpToDate*. Actualizado por Mary M. Gallenberg. Consultado en abril de 2025. https://www.uptodate.com.

Ahrendt, H.-J., D. Makalová, S. Parke, et al. 2009. "Bleeding Pattern and Cycle Control with an Estradiol-Based Oral Contraceptive: A Seven-Cycle, Randomized Comparative Trial of Estradiol Valerate/Dienogest and Ethinyl Estradiol/Levonorgestrel." *Contraception 80: 436–444.* https://doi.org/10.1016/j.contraception.2009.04.004.

American Gastroenterological Association IBD Parenthood Project Working Group. 2019. "Inflammatory Bowel Disease in Pregnancy Clinical Care Pathway: A Report From the American Gastroenterological Association IBD Parenthood Project Working Group." *PubMed.* Consultado en mayo de 2025.

Barriga Pooley, Patricio, Andrea Von Hoveling, Guillermo Galán, y Jorge López Berroa. 2020. "Analysis and New Contraception Frontiers with Combined Vaginal Rings." *Gynecological Endocrinology.* https://doi.org/10.1080/09513590.2020.1729730.

Becker, Christian M., Attila Bokor, Oskari Heikinheimo et al. 2022. "ESHRE Guideline: Endometriosis." *Human Reproduction Open (2): hoac009.* https://doi.org/10.1093/hropen/hoac009.

Beck, Paul. 1977. "Effect of Progestins on Glucose and Lipid Metabolism." *Annals of the New York Academy of Sciences* 286: 434–45. https://doi.org/10.1111/j.1749-6632.1977.tb29435.x.

Calaf J. 2005. *Manual básico de Anticoncepción. 3ª ed. Masson: 91-107.*

Coelingh Bennink, H. J., A. Verhoeven, y J. D. Zimmerman. 2008. "Pharmacology and Clinical Profile of Estetrol, a New Natural Estrogen for Oral Use." *Climacteric 11 (suppl 1): 47–58.*

Dieben, Thom O. M., Frans J. M. E. Roumen, y Dan Apter. 2002. "Efficacy, Cycle Control, and User Acceptability of a Novel Combined Contraceptive Vaginal Ring." *Obstetrics & Gynecology 100 (3): 585–93.* https://doi.org/10.1016/S0029-7844(02)02124-5.

Dragoman, Monica V. 2014. "The Combined Oral Contraceptive Pill: Recent Developments, Risks and Benefits." *Best Practice & Research: Clinical Obstetrics & Gynaecology 28 (6): 825–834.* https://doi.org/10.1016/j.bpobgyn.2014.06.003.

Dragoman, M. V., Tepper, N. K., Fu, R., Curtis, K. M., Chou, R., y Gaffield, M. E. 2018. A systematic review and meta-analysis of venous thrombosis risk among users of combined oral contraception. *International Journal of Gynaecology and Obstetrics 141 (3): 287–294.* https://doi.org/10.1002/ijgo.12455.

Duijkers, I. J., A. Verhoeven, H. J. Coelingh Bennink, y J. D. Zimmerman. 2015. "A Pharmacodynamic Study on Estetrol, a Natural Estrogen, in Combined Oral Contraceptives." *European Journal of Contraception and Reproductive Health Care 20 (6): 476–89.*

Edelman, Alison, Elizabeth Micks, Makalapua L. Motu'apuaka, Lyndsey S. Benson, y Fiona Stewart. 2014. "Continuous or Extended Cycle vs. Cyclic Use of Combined Hormonal Contraceptives for Contraception." *Cochrane Database of Systematic Reviews, no. 7: CD004695.* https://doi.org/10.1002/14651858.CD004695.pub3.

Endrikat, J., R. Hite, R. Bannemerschult, C. Gerlinger, y W. Schmidt. 2001. "Multicenter, Comparative Study of Cycle Control, Efficacy and Tolerability of Two Low-Dose Oral Contraceptives Containing 20 Microg Ethinylestradiol/100 Microg Levonorgestrel and 20 Microg Ethinylestradiol/500 Microg Norethisterone." *Contraception 64 (1): 3–10.* https://doi.org/10.1016/s0010-7824(01)00221-9.

Faculty of Sexual & Reproductive Healthcare (FSRH). 2020. Recommended Actions after Incorrect Use of Combined Hormonal Contraception. *Revisión 2021. London: FSRH Clinical Effectiveness Unit.* https://www.fsrh.org/…incorrect-use…

Faculty of Sexual & Reproductive Healthcare. January 2019. Combined Hormonal Contraception. *Amended October 2023. London: Faculty of Sexual & Reproductive Healthcare.* https://www.fsrh.org/…combined-hormonal-contraception/

Frank Gallo, Maria F., Laureen M. Lopez, David A. Grimes, Florence Carayon, Kenneth F. Schulz, y Frans M. Helmerhorst. 2014. "Anticonceptivos Combinados: Efectos sobre el Peso." *Cochrane Database of Systematic Reviews, 29 de enero*. https://doi.org/10.1002/14651858.CD003987.pub5.

Gallo, M. F., K. Nanda, D. A. Grimes, et al. 2013. 20 μg versus >20 μg estrogen combined oral contraceptives for contraception. *Cochrane Database of Systematic Reviews, no. CD003989.* https://doi.org/10.1002/14651858.CD003989.pub3.

Grandi, Giovanni, Fabio Facchinetti, y Johannes Bitzer. 2022. "Confirmation of the Safety of Combined Oral Contraceptives Containing Oestradiol on the Risk of Venous Thromboembolism." *European Journal of Contraception & Reproductive Health Care 27 (2): 83–84.* https://doi.org/10.1080/13625187.2022.2029397.

Gemzell-Danielsson, Kristina, Nathalie Massai, Jean-Luc Donnez, Santiago Palacios, Johannes Bitzer, y Pedro-Antonio Regidor. 2022. "A Novel Estetrol-Containing Combined Oral Contraceptive: European Expert Panel Review." *European Journal of Contraception & Reproductive Health Care 27 (3): 215–22. https://doi.org/10.1080/13625187.2022.2089830.*

Guillebaud, John. 2012. Contraception: Your Questions Answered. 6ª ed. London: *Elsevier.* https://shop.elsevier.com/books/…/978-0-7020-4619-3.

Heinemann, Lothar A. J., y Jürgen C. Dinger. 2006. "Range of Published Estimates of Venous Thromboembolism Incidence in Young Women." *Contraception 75 (4): 328–36.* https://doi.org/10.1016/j.contraception.2006.12.019.

Herndon, Emily J., y Miriam Zieman. 2004. "New Contraceptive Options." *American Family Physician 69 (4): 853–60.*

IARC (International Agency for Research on Cancer). 2007. Combined Estrogen-Progestogen Contraceptives and Combined Estrogen-Progestogen Menopausal Therapy. *IARC Monographs on the Identification of Carcinogenic Hazards to Humans. Accessed May 12, 2025.* https://publications.iarc.fr/…/Combined-Estrogen-Progestogen…

Kulier, R., F. M. Helmerhorst, N. Maitra, et al. 2004. "Effectiveness and Acceptability of Progestogens in Combined Oral Contraceptives: A Systematic Review." *Reproductive Health 1 (1): 1.* https://doi.org/10.1186/1742-4755-1-1.

Legro, Richard S., Seema A. Arslanian, David A. Ehrmann, Kathleen M. Hoeger, Mohamad H. Murad, Roberto Pasquali, Christos K. Welt, y Endocrine Society. 2013. "Diagnosis and Treatment of Polycystic Ovary Syndrome: An Endocrine Society Clinical Practice Guideline." *Journal of Clinical Endocrinology and Metabolism 98 (12): 4565–92.* https://doi.org/10.1210/jc.2013-2350.

Lidegaard, Øjvind, Lotte H. Nielsen, Charlotte W. Skovlund, Finn Egil Skjeldestad, y Ellen Løkkegaard. 2011. "Risk of Venous Thromboembolism from Use of Oral Contraceptives Containing Different Progestogens and Oestrogen Doses: Danish Cohort Study, 2001–9." *BMJ 343 (julio): d6423.* https://doi.org/10.1136/bmj.d6423.

Lidegaard, Øjvind, Ellen Løkkegaard, Anna Jensen, Charlotte Wessel Skovlund, y Niels Keiding. 2012. "Thrombotic Stroke and Myocardial Infarction with Hormonal Contraception." *New England Journal of Medicine 366 (24): 2257–66.* https://doi.org/10.1056/NEJMoa1111840.

Loder, Elizabeth W., Dawn C. Buse, y Jill R. Golub. 2005. "Headache as a Side Effect of Combination Estrogen-Progestin Oral Contraceptives: A Systematic Review." *American Journal of Obstetrics and Gynecology 193 (3 Pt 1): 636–649.* https://doi.org/10.1016/j.ajog.2004.12.089.

Lopez, Laureen M., David A. Grimes, Maria F. Gallo, Laura L. Stockton, y Kenneth F. Schulz. 2013. "Skin Patch and Vaginal Ring versus Combined Oral Contraceptives for Contraception." *Cochrane Database of Systematic Reviews 4: CD003552.* https://doi.org/10.1002/14651858.CD003552.pub4.

Lopez, L. M., A. Bernholc, M. Chen, T. W. Grey, C. Otterness, C. Westhoff, A. Edelman, y F. M. Helmerhorst. 2016. "Hormonal Contraceptives for Contraception in Overweight or Obese Women." *Cochrane Database of Systematic Reviews 2016 (8): CD008452.* https://doi.org/10.1002/14651858.CD008452.pub4.

Khalil, J., Hill, H., Einstadter, D., & Fass, R. (2025). Combined oral contraceptives are associated with increased risk of developing gastroparesis in pre-menopausal women. *Digestive and Liver Disease, 57(5), 604–610.* https://doi.org/10.1016/j.dld.2025.01.190

Ma, Siyan, y Sae Jin Song. 2023. Oral contraceptives in the central nervous system: Basic pharmacology, methodological considerations, and current state of the field. *Frontiers in Neuroendocrinology, 68, 101040.* https://doi.org/10.1016/j.yfrne.2022.101040

Ma, Siyan, y Sae Jin Song. 2023. "Oral Contraceptives Containing Drospirenone for Premenstrual Syndrome." *Cochrane Database of Systematic Reviews, no. 6: CD006586.* https://doi.org/10.1002/14651858.CD006586.pub5.

MacGregor, E. A. 2013. "Contraception and Headache." *Headache 53, no. 2: 247–76.* https://doi.org/10.1111/head.12035.

Mendoza, N., P. Lobo, R. Lertxundi, M. Correa, E. Gonzalez, A. Salamanca, y R. Sánchez-Borrego. 2014. "Extended Regimens of Combined Hormonal Contraception to Reduce Symptoms Related to Withdrawal Bleeding and the Hormone-Free Interval: A Systematic Review of Randomised and Observational Studies." *The European Journal of Contraception & Reproductive Health Care 19, n.° 5: 321–39.* https://doi.org/10.3109/13625187.2014.927423.

Martínez, Francisca, Isabel Ramírez, Ezequiel Pérez-Campos, Kepa Latorre, e Iñaki Lete. "Venous and Pulmonary Thromboembolism and Combined Hormonal Contraceptives. Systematic Review and Meta-Analysis." *The European Journal of Contraception & Reproductive Health Care 17, no. 1 (2012): 7–29.* https://doi.org/10.3109/13625187.2011.643836.

Merz, M., R. Kroll, R. Lynen, y K. Bangerter. 2015. "Bleeding Pattern and Cycle Control of a Low-Dose Transdermal Contraceptive Patch Compared with a Combined Oral Contraceptive: A Randomized Study." *Contraception 91 (2): 113–120.* https://doi.org/10.1016/j.contraception.2014.10.004.

Mulders, T. M., y T. O. Dieben. 2001. "Use of the Novel Combined Contraceptive Vaginal Ring NuvaRing for Ovulation Inhibition." *Fertility and Sterility 75 (5): 865–70.* https://doi.org/10.1016/S0015-0282(01)01689-2.

Nguyen, Antoinette T., Kathryn M. Curtis, Naomi K. Tepper, Katherine Kortsmit, Anna W. Brittain, Emily M. Snyder, Megan A. Cohen, Lauren B. Zapata, y Maura K. Whiteman. 2024. U.S. Medical Eligibility Criteria for Contraceptive Use, 2024. R*ecommendations and Reports 73 (4): 1–126 (8 de agosto de 2024).*

Pastor, Zdenek, Katerina Holla, y Roman Chmel. 2013. "The Influence of Combined Oral Contraceptives on Female Sexual Desire: A Systematic Review." *The European Journal of Contraception & Reproductive Health Care 18, no. 1: 27–43.* https://doi.org/10.3109/13625187.2012.728643.

Reust, Charles E., Sandra A. Espinoza, Julie Ruplinger, y Scott Swofford. 2012. "What Is the Approach to Intermenstrual Bleeding in a Woman Taking a Combined Oral Contraceptive?" *Evidence-Based Practice 15: 29.*

Roach, Rachel E. J., Frans M. Helmerhorst, Willem M. Lijfering, Theo Stijnen, Ale Algra, y Olaf M. Dekkers. 2015. "Combined Oral Contraceptives: The Risk of Myocardial Infarction and Ischemic Stroke." *Cochrane Database of Systematic Reviews 27 de agosto.* https://doi.org/10.1002/14651858.CD011054.pub2.

Rocha, A. L. L., R. R. Campos, M. M. S. Miranda, L. B. P. Raspante, M. M. Carneiro, C. S. Vieira, y F. M. Reis. 2017. "Safety of Hormonal Contraception for Obese Women." *Expert Opinion on Drug Safety 16 (12): 1387–93.* https://doi.org/10.1080/14740338.2018.1389893.

Sánchez Borrego, R. 2010. "Prog Obstet Ginecol." *Prog Obstet Ginecol 53 (5): 189–93.*

Sánchez Borrego, R., y O. Martínez, eds. 2003. Guía práctica de anticoncepción oral basada en la evidencia. *Madrid: Emisa.*

Scholes, Deborah, Andrea Z. LaCroix, Rebecca A. Hubbard, Laura E. Ichikawa, Lori Spangler, Brian H. Operskalski, Nancy Gell, y Susan M. Ott. 2016. "Oral Contraceptive Use and Fracture Risk around the Menopausal Transition." *Menopause 23 (2): 166–74.* https://doi.org/10.1097/GME.0000000000000595.

Skovlund, Catherine W., Lina S. Mørch, Lars V. Kessing, y Øjvind Lidegaard. 2016. "Association of Hormonal Contraception With Depression." *JAMA Psychiatry 73 (11): 1154–62.* https://doi.org/10.1001/jamapsychiatry.2016.2387.

Taylor, Hugh S., Lubna Pal, y Emre Seli. 2019. Clinical Gynecologic Endocrinology and Infertility. *9.ª ed. Philadelphia: Lippincott Williams & Wilkins.*

Tchaikovski, Sergei, y Sabine Eichinger. 2021. "Combined Oral Contraceptives and Venous Thromboembolism: Review and Perspective to Mitigate the Risk." *Frontiers in Endocrinology 12: 769187*. https://doi.org/10.3389/fendo.2021.769187

Teal, Sarah, y Alison Edelman. 2021. "Contraception Selection, Effectiveness, and Adverse Effects: A Review." *JAMA 326 (24): 2507–18.* https://doi.org/10.1001/jama.2021.21392.

Trussell, James. 2011. "Contraceptive Failure in the United States." Contraception 83 (5): 397–404.

Tulchinsky, D., D. K. Hobel, T. Yeh, y S. M. Marshall. 1975. "Plasma Estrone, Estradiol, Estriol, Progesterone and 17-Hydroxyprogesterone in Human Pregnancy." *Journal of Clinical Endocrinology and Metabolism 40 (3): 560–67.*

van Vliet, H. A. A. M., M. Frolich, M. Christella, L. G. D. Thomassen, C. J. M. Doggen, F. R. Rosendaal, J. Rosing, y F. M. Helmerhorst. 2005. "Association between Sex Hormone-Binding Globulin Levels and Activated Protein C Resistance in Explaining the Risk of Thrombosis in Users of Oral Contraceptives Containing Different Progestogens." *Human Reproduction 20 (2): 563–68.* .https://doi.org/10.1093/humrep/deh612.

World Health Organization. 2015. Medical Eligibility Criteria for Contraceptive Use. WHO/RHR/15.07. Accedido en mayo de 2025. https://iris.who.int/…/WHO_RHR_15.07_eng.pdf.

Zieman, M., M. Guillebaud, E. Weisberg, et al. 2002. "Contraceptive Efficacy and Cycle Control with Evra Transdermal System: The Analysis of Pooled Data." *Fertility and Sterility 77 (suppl 2): 13–18.*

Chapter 8

Progestin-Only Hormonal Contraception

A. García Buendía[1,*], MD
C. García Fernández[1], MD
A. Santos Fernández[1], MD
A. Tello Delsors[2], MD
and L. Gómez Muñoz[3], MD

[1]Obstetrics and Gynaecology Department, University and Hospital Complex of Albacete, Spain
[2]Obstetrics and Gynecology Department, University and Hospital of Santa Lucía, Cartagena, Murcia, Spain
[3]Obstetrics and Gynaecology Department, Hospital of Tomelloso, Tomelloso, Ciudad Real, Spain

Abstract

Progestogen-only contraception is nowadays an effective and safe option with a wide range of tools available. In this chapter we will provide a comprehensive review of the different methods of progestogen-only contraception, including the oral pill, the levonorgestrel-releasing IUD, the etonogestrel implant, the injectable medroxyprogesterone acetate depot, and other methods that are less widely used. We will discuss their mechanism of action, effectiveness, indications and contraindications, their non-contraceptive benefits, side effects, and some clinical considerations to take into account, among other relevant aspects.

Keywords: progestin-only pill, levonorgestrel intrauterine device, etonogestrel implant, medroxyprogesterone acetate injectable, effectiveness, side effects

Introduction

Progestogen-only contraception represents a key option in the broad spectrum of contraceptive methods available today. Its importance lies in its safety profile, versatility and adaptability to different women's needs and health conditions. These methods, which include pills, implants, injections and intrauterine devices, offer an effective alternative for those who cannot use oestrogen-containing methods. In addition, their use can contribute to improving the quality of

* Corresponding Author's Email: anagarciauendia23@gmail.com

In: Advances in Reproductive Health
Editors: Llanos Belmonte Andujar and Ana Fuentes Rozalen
ISBN: 979-8-90134-038-7

life for many women by providing effective control over their fertility with few side effects, as well as many other beneficial effects, such as reduced menstrual bleeding or dysmenorrhoea. In this chapter, we will discuss the characteristics, advantages and disadvantages, and clinical considerations of progestogen-only contraceptives.

The contraceptive efficacy of hormonal methods depends primarily on the progestogenic component through different mechanisms of action. At the central level, progestogen inhibits follicle maturation and ovulation in the ovary through homogeneous and sustained negative feedback of gonadotropin secretion. In the endometrium, progestogen prevents endometrial proliferation and induces early secretory transformation. In the fallopian tubes, progestogen alters the motility and secretion of the tubal epithelium, which hinders sperm transport. Finally, at the level of the cervical mucus, it increases its volume and viscosity, preventing sperm penetration into the upper reproductive tract (Bastianelli et al., 2018).

When estrogen is combined with a progestogen, as in the case of combined hormonal contraceptives (discussed in Chapter 7), its action is enhanced by stimulating the synthesis of progesterone receptors in the cell in all its target tissues (Valdés-Bango, Castelo-Branco, 2020).

Over time, generations of synthetic progestogens have emerged, with the aim of reducing side effects and achieving other beneficial actions.

Classification of Synthetic Progestogens

- *First generation:* rarely used today because of side effects. Norethindrone acetate, ethinodiol diacetate, linestrenol, norethinodrel.
- *Second generation*: They have androgenic activity. They increase LDL (low-density lipoprotein) and triglycerides, and decrease HDL (high-density lipoprotein). They are associated with a low thromboembolic risk, and due to their androgenic action, have a reduced impact on libido. Levonorgestrel, norgestrel.
- *Third generation:* they appear later, to mitigate androgenic effects and effects on the lipid profile. Gestodene and its active metabolite, etonogestrel: less androgenic activity and less impact on the lipid profile, but a higher thromboembolism risk compared to levonorgestrel. Norgestimate and norelgestromin: behave like gestodene in terms of lipid profile, but similar thromboembolic risk to levonorgestrel.
- *Fourth generation:* most are progesterone derivatives, and their main characteristic is their anti-androgenic action.
  - Progesterone derivatives:
    - Cyproterone acetate: a progestogen with the strongest anti-androgenic effect, with great efficacy in the treatment of acne, hirsutism and hypertrichosis. Little used due to risk of thromboembolism.
    - Chlormadinone acetate: 2nd progestogen with the greatest anti-androgenic effect. Useful as a contraceptive in situations of hyperandrogenism.
    - Nomegestrol acetate: actions similar to progesterone.
    - Spironolactone derivatives: drospirenone. Marked anti-androgenic action, less potent than cyproterone acetate. It has an antimineralocorticoid action, which helps reduce of fluid retention.

- Testosterone derivatives: dienogest. Medium-high anti-androgenic effect (Wiegratz, Kuhl, 2006).

Table 1. Comparison of gestagens according to their different actions

Progestagen	Anti-estrogen	Estrogenic	Androgenic	Anti-androgenic	Glucocorticoid	Anti-mineralcorticoid
Progesterone	+	-	-	+/-	+	+
Levonorgestrel	+	-	+	-	-	-
Norgestimate	+	-	+	-	-	?
Etonorgestrel	+	-	+	-	-	?
Gestodene	+	-	+	-	+	+
Chlormadinone	+	-	-	+	+	-
Cyproterone	+	-	-	++	+	-
Dienogest	+/-	+/-	-	+	-	-
Drospirenone	+	-	-	+	-	+
Nomegestrol ac.	+	-	-	+/-	-	-
Norethisterone	+	+	+	-	-	?
Desogestrel	+	-	+	-	+	-

(-) no action; (+/-) little or no action; (+) no action; (++) strong action]. Table adapted from 'Metabolic and clinical effects of progestogens. (Wiegratz, Kuhl, 2006).

Progestogen-Only Pill

Progestogen-only pills are a highly effective method of contraception. They have fewer adverse effects than combined contraceptives, without significantly affecting coagulation parameters and treatment tolerance. Several preparations are currently available, the most common being:

- *Drospirenone.* It is available as 24 pills of 4 mg + 4 placebo pills. Its main contraceptive mechanism of action is the inhibition of ovulation in up to 97% of cycles. Drospirenone has antimineralocorticoid activity comparable to 25 mg of spironolactone, so patients with hyperkalaemia should use it with caution. The Pearl index of drospirenone is 0.7, which makes it similar to combined hormonal contraceptives. However, more studies are needed, as it is a relatively new formulation on the market (Archer, David, Ahrendt, Drouin, 2015).
- *Desogestrel,* in presentation of 28 active 75 µg pills. It has been on the market for years and has extensive clinical use, although it provides less cycle control compared to drospirenone. Suppresses ovulation in over 90% of cycles (Korver et. al, 2005).
- Other progestogen-only pill formulations include *norethindrone* (35 µg), in 28 active tablet form, taken without a break. Norethindrone users ovulate in 30-40% of cycles ('Norethindrone' 2006). The *norgestrel* pill comes in 28 tablets of 75 µg norgestrel (Glasier et al., 2022).

The main mechanism of action of these two contraceptive pills, except norethindrone, is the inhibition of ovulation, which occurs in about 90-97% of cycles (Bastianelli et al., 2020). Like all progestogen-only contraceptives, other important mechanisms of action are the increase in volume and viscosity of cervical mucus, which occurs shortly after starting to take it and is considered complete protection in this respect two days after starting to take it, although the effect is short-lived and disappears after 24 hours; decreased endometrial thickness and conversion to secretory endometrium, which makes it unsuitable for blastocyst implantation and explains the low volume of bleeding in users of progestogen-only contraceptives; and decreased fallopian tube motility.

Norethindrone, on the other hand, acts by increasing the viscosity of cervical mucus and thinning the endometrium, as well as inhibiting sperm migration, decreasing the mid-cycle peak of FSH and LH, and slowing fallopian tube motility. In this case, ovulation occurs irregularly, occurring in about half of the cycles (National Institute of Child Health and Human Development, 2006).

Indications and Contraindications

Most patients of any age can use the progestogen-only pill. In fact, most clinical contraceptive guidelines recommend its use in patients with comorbidities, especially those who are contraindicated for taking oestrogen-containing contraceptives, or who prefer to avoid their use (Curtis et al., 2024). It is especially indicated in patients who must avoid oestrogen, either temporarily as during lactation, or permanently, such as smokers over 35 years of age or women with other risk factors for thromboembolic disease. In the case of migraine patients, both with and without aura, there is no contraindication for the progestogen-only pill, unlike the combined pill.

The progestogen-only pill is also indicated for women who have had an abortion, whether spontaneous or voluntary, in the postpartum period, and during breastfeeding.

In general, the main contraindications for taking the progestogen-only pill are: suspected pregnancy, current breast cancer, and liver disease, either benign or malignant tumours, severe decompensated cirrhosis, or acute liver failure (Curtis et al., 2024).

Effectiveness

The effectiveness of the progestogen-only pill varies according to the sources consulted, and according to the compound used. In general, it is considered to be 95-99.5% effective, with a Pearl Index of 0.5-5 gestations per year of use, the average being 2. (Glasier, 2022) (Archer, David, Ahrendt, Drouin, 2015) (Zuniga, 2023).

Specifically, desogestrel and drospirenone have the highest effectiveness rates within this group, since if used correctly (every day at the same time) they reach an effectiveness of 99%, close to that of combined oral contraceptives (Zuniga, 2023). The comparison with the effectiveness of combined oral contraceptives is complex, as it must be taken into account that the progestogen-only pill is generally chosen by populations with characteristics associated with lower fertility, such as breastfeeding, older age, or comorbidities, which may result in lower method failure rates.

Factors That Can Alter Effectiveness

Drug Interactions

Taking certain medications can reduce the effectiveness of the progestogen-only pill. This is especially true for drugs that induce CYP liver enzymes, which are responsible for the metabolism of many drugs with a first- pass metabolism through the liver, as well as hormonal contraceptives (Schoretsanitis, 2022). Patients being treated with some antiepileptic drugs such as phenytoin, carbamazepine, topiramate and barbiturates, or antibiotics such as rifampicin and rifabutin should consider using another method of contraception that is not affected by the induction of liver metabolism caused by these drugs, such as injectables or levonorgestrel intrauterine device (Edelman, 2014). Patients who are to receive short-term treatment (less than 2 months) with these enzyme-inducing drugs while using gestagen-only pills may continue with this method if they use additional precautions during treatment and for up to 28 days after the last enzyme-inducing drug administration (Edelman, 2014). This will be discussed in more detail in a separate chapter of this book.

Obesity

Obesity may decrease the effectiveness of the progestogen-only pill, although data are limited. Adjustment strategies, such as increasing hormone dose, are available, but more studies in severely obese women are needed to establish definitive recommendations (Harris, 2019). On the other hand, women who have undergone bariatric surgery with procedures that decrease absorption, such as Roux-en-Y gastric bypass or biliopancreatic diversion, it is thought that the absorption of the drug may also be decreased, reducing its efficacy and making the progestogen-only pill not recommended in these cases (Curtis, 2016).

Intestinal Transit Disorders

Due to decreased absorption of the pill in cases of vomiting or severe diarrhoea within 3-4 hours of taking the tablet, a new tablet should be taken as if it were a missed pill, and following the recommendations for missed pills (explained below). If the vomiting or diarrhoea is due to a chronic condition, another method of contraception that does not require intestinal absorption should be recommended.

Non-Contraceptive Benefits

The use of progestogen-only contraceptives may help in the management of abnormal uterine bleeding, dysmenorrhoea, and mid-cycle ovulatory pain by suppressing ovulation. Their use in the management of pelvic pain secondary to endometriosis has classically had more limited evidence (Weiderpass, 1999). However, more recent reviews comparing the efficacy of progestogens versus placebo conclude that progestogens significantly reduce pain. Specifically, Dienogest, a fourth-generation progestogen, has been the most studied because it has been shown to reduce the intensity of chronic pelvic pain also in cases of deep endometriosis. However, it is not accepted as a contraceptive pill, and its main disadvantage is poor cycle control, which is the main cause of treatment abandonment (Brown, Kives, Akhtar, 2012) (Strowitzki, Faustmann, Gerlinger, Seitz, 2012).

The use of progestogens also plays a rolc in reducing the risk of endometrial cancer (see Chapter Cancer and contraception).

In no case should the use of progestogen-only hormonal contraceptives be considered a replacement for barrier methods in the prevention of sexually transmitted diseases. However, the increased volume and thickening of cervical mucus appear to hinder the ascent of bacteria into the upper genital tract, reducing the risk of developing pelvic inflammatory disease. (Workowski et al., 2021).

Side Effects

Bleeding Pattern Alterations

The main adverse effect of the use of progestogen-only contraceptives, in general, is the change in bleeding pattern, which is the main cause of method discontinuation (Palacios, Colli, Regidor, 2020). Before starting any of the progestogen-only contraceptive methods, the bleeding pattern of individual users is unknown, but it appears that behaviour during the first 3 months is predictive of future bleeding trends. Users should be informed of possible changes in bleeding pattern, with irregular bleeding and spotting being the two most common patterns with gestagen-only pill use, and prolonged bleeding and amenorrhoea the least likely (Worly, Brett, Gur, Schaffir, 2018). Informing women can help reduce discontinuation rates. The drospirenone pill, meanwhile, causes fewer bleeding episodes compared to the desogestrel pill, with up to 70% of users experiencing breakthrough bleeding, prolonged bleeding, or spotting in one or more cycles (Palacios, Colli, Regidor, 2020) (Zigler, Rachel, McNicholas, 2017). Other causes of bleeding should be considered, especially when there is a sudden change in the patient's usual bleeding pattern.

Follicular Cysts

During continued use of progestogen-only contraceptives there may be an increased occurrence of follicular cysts or persistent follicles, probably due to the increased suppression of LH over FSH. In the vast majority of cases, these cysts are asymptomatic and resolve spontaneously. However, on some occasions they may persist and worry patients or be painful. In these cases, women should be advised to use other contraceptive methods, or in those who do not wish to change methods, a dose increase may be prescribed, although there is a lack of data to support this management (Beerthuizen et al., 2000).

Weight Gain

Here too, the scientific evidence is limited. Recent evidence suggests that the use of progestogen-only contraceptives may be associated with a slight weight gain, less than 2 kg during the first year of use, and with no differences between comparison groups using other contraceptive methods. The progestogen-only pill does not appear to be associated with significant weight gain (Beksinska et al., 2021). In addition, oral contraceptives containing drospirenone have a more favourable effect weight maintenance or reduction, attributed to their antimineral-corticoid activity (Zigler, Rachel, McNicholas, 2017).

Increased Thromboembolic Risk

There is not a significantly increased risk of venous thromboembolism associated with the use of progestogen-only contraceptives compared to non-users of hormonal contraceptives (Bergendal et al., 2014) (Furlong, Lesley, 2002) (Furlong, Lesley, 2002). However, medroxyprogesterone acetate depot, as discussed below, is considered to increase thromboembolic risk, particularly in women with additional risk factors, although the association is not as robust as with combined contraceptive methods, contributing half the risk of the latter.

Ectopic Gestation
The progestogen-only pill decreases the overall risk of ectopic pregnancy by preventing conception. The use of this contraceptive method does not increase the overall risk of ectopic pregnancy (Am, Kaunitz, 1997). However, if the method fails, the likelihood of ectopic gestation is higher than in women who do not use contraception (5 vs. 2%) (Vercellini et al., 2016).

Controversial Side Effects

Libido
Current evidence is limited on the effects of progestogen-only contraceptives on libido. This possible adverse effect cannot be excluded, although no significant association has been demonstrated.

Depression and Mood Swings
Available evidence suggests that, in some women, progestogen-only contraceptives may be associated with depressive changes and symptoms, although most studies do not find a significant association (Lopez et al., 2016).

Breast Cancer
The relationship of hormonal contraceptives to increased cancer risk is a topic that will be addressed in another chapter of this book. In general, the evidence does not support an association between breast cancer and use of progestogen-only hormonal contraception, and any increase in risk would be small and likely to decrease over time after discontinuation of the method (Girum, Tadele, Wasie, 2018).

Headaches
The relationship of progestogen-only contraceptives with migraine is a widely studied topic due to the drawback of increased thromboembolic risk of oestrogen contraceptives, as migraine, especially with aura, is associated with increased risk of ischaemic stroke (Warhust et al., 2018). Progestogen-only contraceptives are considered a safe and effective method for these patients, as they generally do not increase thromboembolic risk, and also provide benefits in reducing migraine frequency and intensity, especially those that inhibit ovulation (Samson et al., 2016).

Return of Fertility
In terms of fertility return, the available evidence is unanimous that any temporary method of contraception and its duration does not have a negative effect on fertility (Tepper et al., 2016).

Bone Mineral Density
Evidence is also limited in this regard, but suggests that the use of the progestogen-only pill does not affect bone mineral density in young women, unlike medroxyprogesterone acetate depot. For adult women, some studies have observed a decrease in bone density with prolonged use, although there is no evidence of an increased risk of fractures (Machado et al., 2010).

Breastfeeding

Available evidence shows that progestogen-only contraceptives do not appear to affect a woman's ability to breastfeed her child, or the growth and development of her child (Bouquier et al., 2012).

Clinical Considerations

Stating Contraception and Pre-Testing

No medical examination is recommended prior to taking the progestogen-only contraceptive pill, other than a detailed medical history. In addition, we should inform the patient about the method chosen, and about possible changes in the bleeding pattern, which will increase adherence to the method.

The pill should be taken at the same time every day, whether or not there is vaginal bleeding. This not only ensures maximum effectiveness of the method, but also increases adherence to treatment.

There are several options for starting the progestogen-only pill. If the user starts taking the pill between day 1 and 5 of the menstrual cycle (first-day start), no additional protection is necessary. Alternatively, she can start any day of the cycle (any-day-start), as long as she is certain that she is not pregnant. In this case, additional contraceptive protection should be used for the first 48 hours. If the user is amenorrhoeic and is certain that she is not pregnant, the pill can be started on any day, and in this case additional protection is also recommended for the first 48 hours ("Norethindrone, 2006). If started immediately after childbirth or post-abortion, additional protection is not required until 21 days postpartum or post-abortion (Curtis et al., 2016).

Action to Be Taken in the Event of Forgetfulness

In general, the recommendation in case of a missed dose with any of the progestogen-only pills is to take it as soon as possible, even if this means taking two pills on the same day. The difference is the missed interval at which an additional method is needed, which is different for each formulation.

- In the case of norethindrone, if intake is delayed by 3 hours or longer, additional barrier protection will be necessary for 2 days, as it decreases its action on cervical mucus (Korver et al., 2005).
- In the case of desogestrel, additional precautions are necessary if the missed dose lasts 12 hours or longer, and are recommended for 7 days. If the missed pill is less than 12 hours, the patient will take the pill as soon as she remembers it, and no additional protection is needed. This is because the suppression of ovulation is maintained until 12 hours later, as well as the thickening of cervical mucus (Duijkers et al., 2016).
- Drospirenone, on the other hand, defers the need for additional methods to 24 hours of forgetting. If this happens, an additional method must be used for 7 days. In the case of both desogestrel and drospirenone, if the missed pills are missed more than 12 hours or 24 hours, respectively, during the first week, the patient should consider taking emergency contraception (Duijkers, 2016). If the forgetting occurs in the third week of taking drospirenone tablets, the risk of contraceptive failure is very high, as it is

very close to 4 days of taking inactive tablets. In this case, the user can prevent this risk by avoiding the inactive tablets and continuing with the next blister pack of hormone-containing tablets (Batur, Pelin, Kransdorf, Casey, 2016).

Indications for Emergency Contraception During Gestagen-Only Pill Use

Emergency contraception should be recommended in cases where sexual intercourse has occurred during the time when additional protection is recommended, if the initiation protocol was not followed or if the user is taking medications that interact with the pill. If the unsafe intercourse occurred 3-5 days ago, Ulipristal Acetate 30 mg may be administered, or an IUD may be inserted. If the woman chooses to take Ulipristal Acetate, additional precautions should be recommended for 14 days, as it is a selective progesterone receptor modulator and may decrease the efficacy of the progestogen-only pill. If intercourse occurred less than 3 days ago, levonorgestrel can be taken, which will require additional protection for the following two days (Mansour et al., 2008).

Management of Bleeding Disorders

Bleeding disturbance is the main cause of method discontinuation for progestogen-only contraceptives.

If the user has amenorrhoea, she should be reassured and informed that it is not harmful to her health. However, if tolerance is poor, another method of contraception should be recommended. On the other hand, in the case of irregular bleeding, spotting or prolonged bleeding, it should be reported that they generally improve with time of use, but if they persist, possible gynaecological causes should be ruled out, as well as ensuring the correct use of the method in the case of the pill.

There are a number of treatments that can be used in conjunction with progestogens to reduce bleeding, although their effect is usually limited to the duration of the treatment.

On the one hand, the combination of any progestogen-only method with oestrogens, either by combined pill or conjugated oestrogen, can reduce bleeding by stabilising the endometrium. It can be used cyclically or continuously for at least 3 months, with the regimen being individualised according to response (Apter et al., 2014).

Nonsteroidal anti-inflammatory drugs have shown some efficacy in reducing bleeding. The most studied are ibuprofen and mefenamic acid, 2 or 3 times a day for 5 days.

Doxycycline may also be useful, due to its anti-inflammatory action and inhibition of matrix metalloproteinases. However, there are no recommendations as to the optimal regimen (Apter et al., 2014).

Switching to a progestogen-only pill formulation has not been shown to help with improvement in the bleeding pattern, although it may help some women. The drospirenone pill appears to improve the bleeding pattern over the desogestrel pill (Apter et al., 2014).

Follow-Up

A follow-up visit 3-6 months after starting the progestogen-only pill is recommended to assess adherence to the method and resolve questions about bleeding patterns.

Levonorgestrel-Releasing IUDs

The levonorgestrel-releasing intrauterine device (IUD) performs its contraceptive action in two ways. On the one hand, the device acts, like the copper IUD, as a foreign body in the uterus, triggering an inflammatory reaction that reduces sperm motility. On the other hand, the constant release of small amounts of levonorgestrel directly into the target organ causes several local effects: thickening of cervical mucus, intense endometrial antiproliferative effect due to insensitivity to circulating oestradiol, decidualisation of the endometrium, and a decrease of endometrial receptors (Apter et al., 2014). In addition, it has anti-estrogenic activity, and can produce negative feedback on LH and inhibit ovulation, although this does not appear to be the primary contraceptive mechanism of this method. Ovulation rates are higher the lower the LNG load (Faculty of Sexual & Reproductive Healthcare, 2023).

Indications and Contraindications

The use of the LNG IUD is indicated for all women who want a long-lasting and highly effective method of contraception. This method has few contraindications, which are similar to those previously described in the section on the progestogen-only pill, to which are added those inherent to the use of an intrauterine device, which are as follows: (Curtis et al., 2024).

- Uterine abnormalities with gross distortion of the cavity.
- Current or recurrent pelvic inflammatory disease (at least 3 months must pass).
- Gestational trophoblastic disease: increased risk of uterine perforation and tumour dissemination.
- Pelvic tuberculosis.
- Uterine infection after childbirth or septic abortion within the last 3 months.
- Cancer of the cervix or uterus.
- Systemic lupus erythematosus with positive antiphospholipid antibodies: contraindicated or careful evaluation due to risk of infections.

In addition to its primary use as a contraceptive, the LNG IUD is indicated for the treatment of heavy menstrual bleeding, whether or not secondary to fibroids. In the case of patients with uterine fibroids, cases should be selected where there is no distortion of the endometrial cavity due to the myoma in order to recommend safe use (Francis, Jenny, Gold, 2017), (Mittermeier, Theresa, Farrant, Wise, 2020). On the other hand, the LNG IUD is also useful in the treatment of primary dysmenorrhoea, or that associated with adenomyosis or endometriosis (Wattanayingcharoenchai et al., 2021) (Alcalde et al., 2021) ('National Guideline Alliance', 2018). The non-contraceptive benefits of contraceptives are addressed in a specific chapter of this book.

Effectivenes

Effectiveness depends on the amount of LNG in the different presentations (Figure 1).
In the case of the LNG 52 mg IUD (MIRENA, LEVOSERT - not approved in the United States), with a release of 20 μg/day, its contraceptive efficacy is maintained for 8 years, although in the case of insertion in women over 45 years of age, its use could be extended until menopause or up to 55 years of age. Its Pearl rate is 0.21% in the first year and 0% after 8 years,

taking into account pregnancies due to undetected expulsions and perforations (Rattray et al., 2015) (Creinin, Mitchell, 2014).

The 19.5 mg LNG IUD (KYLEENA), which releases 12 µg/day, maintains contraceptive efficacy for up to 5 years. The Pearl rate is 0.16% in the first year and 0.29% at 5 years (Creinin, Mitchell, 2014).

The LNG 13.5 mg IUD (JAYDESS -trade name in Spain-, SKYLA -trade name in the USA), releases 8 µg/day, with contraceptive effect for up to 3 years. It has a Pearl index during the first year of 0.41%, and after 3 years of 0.33% (Creinin, Mitchell, 2014).

Side Effects

Although the LNG IUD is generally a well-tolerated method and only a small amount of progestogen is released, some hormone-related side effects, such as acne, headache, breast tension and mood swings, have been described, although the available evidence is limited.

Changes in Bleeding Pattern

Changes in the menstrual pattern are the most frequent side effect, as with other progestogen-only contraceptive methods, which should be explained to patients prior to IUD insertion, which will improve tolerance to the IUD. During the first three months of use, spotting is common, which usually improves over time. There is no consensus on the pharmacological management of unsatisfactory bleeding patterns in LNG IUD users (Gemzell et al., 2017).

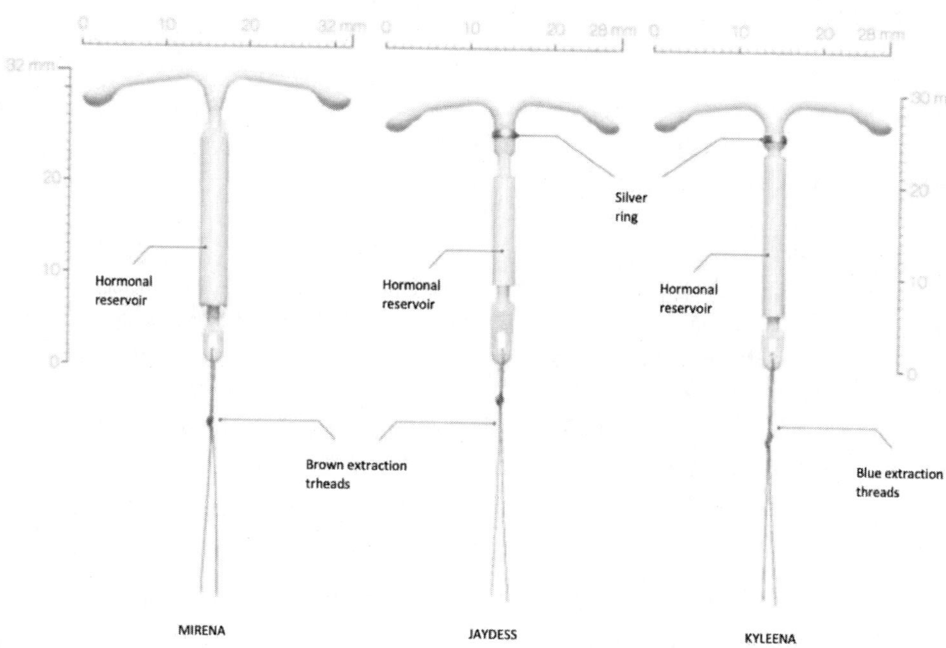

Figure 1. Comparison of the different LNG-IUDs available, according to some characteristics (Perelló, Guillén, 2024).

Occurrence of Ovarian Cysts

The frequency of occurrence of benign functional ovarian cysts is dose-dependent, being higher with increasing LNG dose, up to 22% with LNG 52 mg IUD. Most are asymptomatic and resolve spontaneously (Mol et al., 2005).

Ectopic Pregnancy

The absolute risk is decreased compared to women not using contraception (0.3% per year vs. 1.5% per year). Moreover, the risk decreases with higher LNG dose (Brown et al., 2024).

Expulsion

The incidence of expulsion is considered low, between 3-6%. The risk of expulsion is higher in women with dysmenorrhoea, heavy menstrual bleeding, adolescents, postpartum insertion, or recent second trimester abortion, fibroids, and in menstrual cup users (Brown et al., 2024).

Uterine Perforation and Malposition of the Device

Uterine perforation occurs in 1-2/1000 IUD insertions, depending on the series. It occurs more frequently in women with any of the following risk factors: distorted uterine cavity, immobile uterus, stenotic cervix, or insertion postpartum, after second-trimester abortion, or during breastfeeding. In case of suspected perforation during insertion, the procedure should be stopped, broad-spectrum antibiotherapy should be considered, and at least 6 weeks should be allowed for insertion of a new device (Pakarinen et al., 1997).

Device malposition is a less severe complication than uterine perforation, but may be associated with decreased effectiveness as it may result in less uniform endometrial suppression. However, the evidence is very limited. If a woman has symptoms, such as prolonged spotting, and wants to remove the device, she should wait at least 7 days after the last unprotected intercourse, and if she wants to replace it with another one, pregnancy should be ruled out before doing so (Tepper et al., 2013).

Pelvic Inflammatory Disease

The risk of developing PID is similar in women who use LNG IUDs as in women who do not use them, and they also have a protective effect against PID due to the thickening of cervical mucus, which makes it more difficult for microorganisms to enter the cervix (Workowski, Bachmann, 2021).

However, the risk of developing PID is highest during the first 21 days after insertion, probably due to cervical-uterine manipulation, and is directly related to the likelihood of having a pre-existing sexually transmitted disease. Therefore, although STI testing is not recommended for all women, it is important to assess for signs of infection prior to insertion, to assess sexual history, and screening is indicated in the presence of risk factors. In the case of management of PID in an IUD user, the evidence supports that antibiotic treatment is equally effective if the IUD is retained, and removal is recommended only if there is no clinical improvement 48-72 hours after initiation of treatment (Workowski, Bachmann, 2021).

Meningiomas

All progestogens could influence the growth of meningiomas, due to the presence of progesterone receptors (Bergin et al., 2012).

Clinical Considerations

Start of the Method and Pre-Testing

No health screening is required prior to IUD insertion, except for STI testing for women with risk factors ('Long-Acting Reversible Contraceptive Expert Work Group', 2016).

IUD insertion can be done at any time during the menstrual cycle, having ruled out pregnancy. This is important to know, as approximately half of women who schedule an appointment for IUD insertion do not attend the appointment, same-day insertion is recommended to increase the rate of use and decrease the rate of unplanned pregnancies (Ampatzis, Zervoudis, Iatrakis, Mastorakos, 2022).

Additional method use should be recommended for the first 7 days after IUD insertion unless it is inserted immediately after a curettage abortion, in the first 21 days postpartum, in transition from another contraceptive method or during the first 7 days of the menstrual cycle (Curtis, et al., 2024).

Post-Abortion Insertion

IUD insertion immediately after abortion is safe and effective, and guidelines (Perelló, Guillén, 2024) recommend its routine use for first-trimester abortions, both induced and spontaneous, either by medical treatment or curettage. It is considered a category 1 in the medical eligibility criteria after a first trimester abortion, and a category 2 in second trimester abortions, due to an increased risk of expulsion. The only contraindication to immediate insertion after abortion is the presence of signs of infection (Perelló, Guillén, 2024).

Postpartum Insertion

Immediate postpartum insertion of a LARC method is recognised as good practice due to the prevention of unintended pregnancy (Sothornwit et al., 2022). The timing of postpartum IUD insertion has been extensively studied, and immediate postpartum insertion has been found to be safer in terms of uterine perforation risk than late insertion during the 4-6 weeks postpartum period (Phillips et al., 2016). In contrast, early insertion has a higher risk of expulsion (Ogburn et al., 2005). The use of progestogen-only contraceptive methods has little or no negative effect on breastfeeding (Sothornwit et al., 2022) (Phillips et al., 2016).

Follow-Up

This contraceptive method does not require specific follow-up, except for a check-up after 6 weeks to detect possible alarm symptoms, according to the WHO.

LNG IUDs and Emergency Contraception

After the use of emergency contraception, the use of LNG IUDs can be initiated, but it should be noted that after the use of ulipristal acetate 30 mg, IUD insertion should be deferred for 5 days to avoid reducing the effectiveness of the emergency contraceptive, unlike the use of oral levonorgestrel 1.5 mg, which can be inserted immediately.

The Cu IUD is the only intrauterine device approved for emergency contraception, while the use of the LNG 52 mg IUD is under investigation, and studies support its use. This topic will be addressed in another chapter of this book.

Special Populations

- Adolescents: Adolescent girls with no medical contraindications can safely use IUDs, and in fact they are recommended by several societies (McNicholas et al., 2012).
- Nulliparous: Nulliparous women have high rates of acceptability and continuation of IUDs, and there is no contraindication to their use. They are well tolerated, although more pain at insertion has been reported compared to multiparous women (Imai, Matsunami, Takagi, Ichigo, 2014).

Etonogestrel Implant

The contraceptive implant is a long-acting contraceptive method consisting of a rod placed subdermally in the upper arm. It contains 68 mg of etonogestrel, with a release rate of 60-70 μg/day in the first weeks, and 25-30 μg/day in the last year, and lasts for 3 years (Figure 2).

The mode of action of the implant is mainly due to two effects: on the one hand, like all progestogens, the change in cervical mucus and the decrease in tubal motility, which hinders sperm migration and thus prevents fertilisation. On the other hand, high-dose progestins inhibit gonadotropin secretion, thereby inhibiting follicular maturation and ovulation (serum etonogestrel levels of more than 90 pg/ml inhibit ovulation in 97% of cases). This dual effect allows contraceptive efficacy to be maintained when norgestrel release is lower during the third year, and ovulation inhibition is inconsistent (Funk et al., 2005).

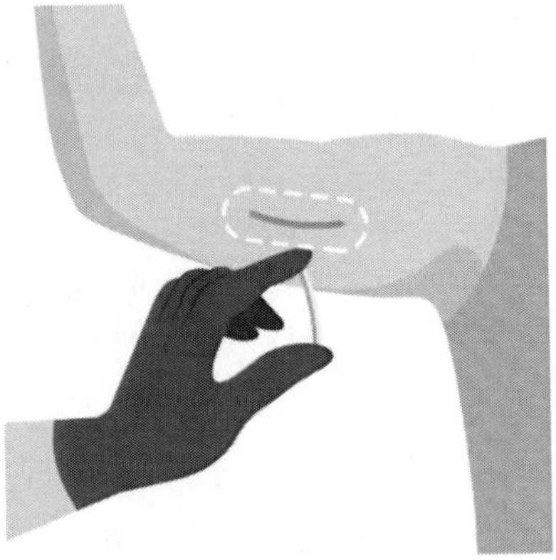

Figure 2. Location etonogestrel implant.

Indications and Contraindications

Most women are candidates for the use of the subdermal implant, as there are few medical contraindications to its use.

It is especially indicated for use in women at high risk of unintended pregnancy, including adolescents, patients undergoing induced abortions, or socially excluded patients, as these women are at higher risk of discontinuing other methods (Floyd et al., 2020).

Contraindications for use include hypersensitivity to the active substance or excipients, active venous thromboembolism, sex hormone-sensitive neoplasms, diagnosis or history of liver tumours, severe liver disorders until the values have normalised, or undiagnosed vaginal bleeding. Continuation of the method in case of ischaemic heart disease and migraine with or without aura is also considered that the risks outweigh the benefits. Past venous thromboembolic disease is not a contraindication for use (Apatzis, Zervoudis, Iatrakis, Mastorajos, 2022).

Use During Breastfeeding and Postpartum

The etonogestrel implant can be used during lactation and the postpartum period. There is no need to delay its use. The risk of thromboembolic disease does not appear to be high (Carmo et al., 2017), and small amounts of etonogestrel are excreted in breast milk (approximately 0.2% of the maternal daily dose), and no differences in growth and development have been detected.

Effectiveness

The etonorgestrel implant is over 99% effective, with a Pearl index of 0.38. It is one of the most effective contraceptives available, with lower failure rates than definitive sterilisation surgery and without the risks of invasive surgery.

Factors That May Decrease Effectiveness

The contraceptive effect is related to plasma concentrations of etonogestrel, which are inversely proportional to body weight and decrease with time. Thus, the effectiveness in the third year in overweight women is unknown, it cannot be ruled out that the contraceptive effect is lower than in women of normal weight, and therefore early implant replacement should be considered (Abraham, Margaret, Zhao, Peipert, 2015). Interactions with microsomal enzyme inducing drugs, in particular cytochrome P450, which increases renal clearance of sex hormones, may also occur with the use of the implant.

Side Effects

Alterations in Bleeding Pattern

78% of users report irregular bleeding. Amenorrhoea is not usually achieved with the implant. Those who achieve a favourable pattern during the first 3 months seem to continue with the method, while those who have an unfavourable pattern during the first 3 months have a 50% chance of improvement. Between 6 and 23% of users abandon the method because of bleeding problems (Aleem et al., 2013). Acceptance of these changes can be improved by pre-insertion information, and by making a bleeding schedule (Halpern et al., 2014).

All other side effects are similar to other gestagen-only contraceptive methods

Clinical Considerations

Start of the Method

In order to start this contraceptive method safely, pregnancy must be ruled out by means of anamnesis. If the woman has not used any contraceptive method during the previous month and has had unprotected intercourse, pregnancy must be ruled out with certainty. Otherwise, insertion can be performed between days 1 and 5 of the cycle without the need for an additional method, or on any day of the cycle, using a barrier method for the following seven days.

In women with previous use of another contraceptive method, in the case of pills, the implant should be inserted the day after the last tablet taken (maximum 24 hours after the last pill was taken). When switching from other methods (LNG IUD, injectable, vaginal ring, transdermal patch), the implant should be inserted on the day of withdrawal of these methods (Funk et al., 2005).

Post-Abortion or Post-Partum Use of the Method
The implant can be inserted immediately after a planned or spontaneous abortion. In first-trimester abortions, if inserted within the first 5 days, no complementary method is necessary; in cases of second-trimester abortions, the window is extended to 21 days, as in postpartum insertion (Carmo et al., 2017).

Follow up
Routine follow-up of women using an etonogestrel implant is not necessary, although they should be consulted if the implant is no longer palpable, if they notice changes in the insertion site, if they have any medical problems or start treatment with any medication that interacts with the method, or if they become pregnant (Perelló, Guillén, 2024).

Pregnancy
Actual method failure is rare; possible causes are insertion failure, drug interactions, or failure to use additional precautions. Unless the woman decides to terminate her pregnancy, it is recommended that, if it occurs, the implant should be removed (Perelló, Guillén, 2024).

Medroxyprogesterone Acetate Injectable

Effectiveness
Depot medroxyprogesterone acetate (DMPA) is a progesterone-only injectable method of contraception with a duration of 3 months, which confers high effectiveness and, as an added advantage, provides privacy to the user. The unintended pregnancy rate is 6% in the first year of use with typical use. In studies of women with ideal use, the failure rate is 0.7%, comparable to the failure rate of intrauterine devices (Winner et al., 2012).

DMPA is available in two formulations, which are administered every 3 months. First, the 150 mg/1 ml intramuscular injection, which reaches peak blood concentration (7 ng/ml) within a few days of administration and lasts for about 3 weeks, after which levels decrease to undetectable levels 120-200 days after administration. Ovulation is inhibited at DMPA levels below 0.1 ng/ml. On the other hand, the formulation for subcutaneous administration contains 104 mg/0.65 ml, a lower dose than the formulation for intramuscular administration, as subcutaneous administration provides slower and more sustained absorption than intramuscular injection (Mishell et al., 1996). However, it has more local side effects, such as lipoatrophy, although another advantage is that women can self-administer it, which may favour its continuity over time, according to the WHO.

Serum oestradiol levels decrease after several months of DMPA (depot medroxyprogesterone acetate) use, but although this leads to endometrial atrophy, vasomotor symptoms are infrequent, and the vaginal epithelium does not appear to be altered (Winner et al., 2016).

DMPA's primary method of contraceptive action is the inhibition of gonadotropin secretion, thereby inhibiting follicular maturation and ovulation. In addition, like other gestagen-only contraceptives, it produces changes in cervical mucus and tubal motility.

By providing high doses of progestogen, the efficacy of the method is not reduced in women with higher body weight, nor with concurrent use of other drugs (Winner et al., 2016).

Indications and Contraindications

The indications for this gestagen-only contraceptive method are basically the same as for the rest of the options in this class, with the particularity that they are especially indicated in cases where the woman has a physical or intellectual disability that makes the use of other methods difficult, or where social circumstances require a discreet method of contraception.

Contraindications are also generally the same as for the other gestagen-only methods, but the risk is considered to outweigh the benefits in women with venous thromboembolic disease at high risk of recurrence, with or without anticoagulant therapy. On the other hand, diabetes mellitus is not a contraindication per se for the use of these methods, but in the case of DMPA the risks are considered to outweigh the benefits if there is vascular disease or if the woman has had diabetes mellitus for more than 20 years, unlike the other gestagen-only contraceptive methods (Ampatzis, Zervoudis, Iatrakis, Mastorakos, 2022). On the other hand, its use is also contraindicated in women with a personal history of or risk factors for pathological bone fractures, as will be discussed below.

Side Effects

It is important to inform users of possible side effects, especially changes in bleeding patterns, as this has been shown to encourage continued use.

Local Reactions

2-20% of patients using subcutaneous injection experience local reactions such as granuloma or skin atrophy, or other minor reactions such as pruritus or erythema. Intramuscular injection, on the other hand, produces no local reactions (Hubacher et al., 2009).

Menstrual Changes

All women using this contraceptive method will have menstrual disturbances, which are the main reason for discontinuation of the method, and approximately 8% of users will not take a second injection (Hubacher et al., 2009). The most common pattern with continued use is amenorrhoea, which together with spotting occurs in 50 and 80%, respectively, of users with 1-5 years of use. The frequency and duration of irregular bleeding decreases with time of use. After the first few months of use, if irregular bleeding continues, potentially responsible causes, such as cervical or endometrial pathology, should be ruled out. Once ruled out, no further testing is necessary unless new symptoms appear, such as pelvic pain or foul-smelling discharge. If the client is still dissatisfied with the method, another method of contraception should be recommended.

Amenorrhoea becomes more prevalent as the duration of DMPA use increases. According to the series consulted, approximately 50% of users will achieve amenorrhoea after one year of use, and 70% with a longer duration of use (Arias et al., 2006).

Return of Fertility
Although there is no permanent impact on endocrine function, recovery of fertility may be delayed because anovulation is maintained. However, around 50% of women seeking pregnancy after the last injection become pregnant within 10 months of administration ("Winner et al., 2016).

Weight Changes
As with all other hormonal contraceptive methods, weight gain is a highly debated adverse effect. It appears that the contraceptive method most associated with weight gain is injectable medroxyprogesterone acetate depot, which has been shown to increase fat mass to the detriment of lean mass, compared to the other contraceptive methods. However, weight gain has not been shown to be directly attributed to the use of these methods (Martin, Vincent, Behbehani, 2006).

Headaches
Among the side effects of DMPA, it has been reported that it may help trigger headaches in susceptible women. However, it is not contraindicated in women with migraine both with and without aura (Curtis et al., 2024).

Metabolic Effects

Reduced Bone Mineral Density
The advantages of DMPA use outweigh the risks in terms of decreased bone mineral density, according to the different societies consulted (ACOG, CDC, WHO). This should not be a reason to restrict the initiation or continuation of DMPA use in adolescents, women aged 18-45 years, or older women. Current evidence does not justify limiting the use of DMPA, it can be continued for decades (Ampatzis, Zervoudis, Iatrakis, Mastorakos, 2022).

As discussed in this chapter, the method of action of this contraceptive is the suppression of gonadotropin secretion, which results in the inhibition of ovarian oestradiol production (Cockrum et al., 2022). In states of hypoestrogenism, bone resorption exceeds bone formation, leading to a decrease in bone mineral density, which is not linear, but is greatest during the first one to two years of use (0.5-3.5% and 5.7-7.5% decrease, respectively). Subsequently, the loss becomes similar to the rest of the population, and, moreover, with the abandonment of the method, the loss is recovered (Curtis et al., 2024). Nevertheless, a risk-benefit balance should be taken into account, and its use should be avoided in women with risk factors for osteoporosis, such as prolonged treatment with corticosteroids, or with a personal history of pathological fractures.

Cardiovascular Risk
DMPA should be avoided in women with additional cardiovascular risks (hypertension, diabetes mellitus with vascular involvement), and also in women at increased risk of venous thromboembolic disease, as this method has been shown to provide twice the risk of thrombosis

in users compared to non-users, unlike other progestogen-only hormonal contraceptive methods, which provide lower doses (Curtis et al., 2024).

Changes in Insulin Resistance

DMPA use has been associated with an increased risk of diabetes in women at increased baseline risk (Berenson et al., 2011). In addition, also in low-risk women, its use has been associated with increased insulin resistance, although this is probably not clinically significant (Sönmezer et al., 2005). This does not contraindicate its use in diabetic women, but they should closely monitor their blood glucose levels.

Clinical Considerations

Start of the Method

According to clinical guidelines, routine medical testing is not necessary prior to starting this method of contraception (Raymond et al., 2016).

The first injection of DMPA can be given at any time during the cycle as long as pregnancy has been reasonably ruled out, although there is no evidence that this drug increases the risk of congenital anomalies. In menstruating women, the ideal option is to start between day 1-7 of the cycle, as it avoids the need for a barrier back-up method. If administered after the 71st day of the cycle, a barrier method should be used for an additional 7 days.

For switching from a short-acting hormonal method (pill, patch, ring), it is recommended to continue with this method for an additional 7 days from the first injection.

In the case of abortion or postpartum, it may be administered immediately afterwards.

For changeover from an intrauterine device, DMPA administration should be performed 7 days prior to IUD removal (Raymond et al., 2016).

Continuation of the Method

DMPA should be administered every 3 months (maximum 13 weeks).

If the woman comes late for the injectable administration, if less than 14 weeks have passed, the next injection will be administered, since, with a dose of 150 mg, ovulation does not recover until at least 14 weeks have passed. In women who come after more than 15 weeks, pregnancy must be ruled out again in order to administer the method again.

Follow Up

No specific monitoring of the method is necessary, although as with other contraceptive methods, it is important that the woman has access to a health professional to clarify possible questions during use.

Use in Special Populations

Anticoagulated patients:

In addition to decreasing the volume of bleeding, DMPA, by inhibiting ovulation, may prevent the development of haemorrhagic cysts.

Adolescence and Perimenopause:
As previously discussed, decreased bone mineral density is not a reason to contraindicate the use of DMPA in adolescent women or in the perimenopause. There is no age limit for the use of DMPA.

Post-Abortion
This method is acceptable in patients who have just had an abortion, regardless of the method of treatment. It should be noted that, if medical treatment is performed, DMPA administration may affect the efficacy of mifepristone, so delayed administration should be chosen (Nguyen et al., 2024).

Postpartum
This contraceptive method is compatible with breastfeeding. Depending on the guidelines consulted, it is indicated that it can be used at any time postpartum, and is compatible with breastfeeding (Ampatzis, Zervoudis, Iatrakis, Mastorakos, 2022), or after 6 weeks postpartum (Draper et al., 2006).

Other Gestagen-Only Methods

Levonorgestrel Implant
The levonorgestrel implant was the first effective system approved for reversible contraception. Specifically, the first levonorgestrel (LNG) implant on the market was a six-rod device with 36 mg of levonorgestrel each, releasing 50-80 µg of LNG per day, transitioning to 30-35 µg until the 5th year, when it should be withdrawn or changed. However, after the 5th year, about 70% of the drug remains in the rods, ensuring contraceptive security in women who delay refill. Its main mechanism, as with the etonogestrel implant, is suppression of ovulation, and it also reduces tubal motility, endometrial changes and changes in cervical mucus. Contraindications for the use of this device are the same as for the etonogestrel implant. The gestation rate in one year is 0.6/100, and 1-3.9/100 in 5 years, slightly higher than the etonogestrel implant (Sivin, 2003).

Norethisterone Oenanthate (NET-EN) Injectable
This injectable provides contraception for two months, effectively. Like the other available injectable, DMPA (discussed above), its main action is to suppress ovulation, and it also produces the cervical mucus and endometrial changes that aid contraception. NET-EN injectable is much less widely used than DMPA, and therefore fewer studies are available. However, according to a 2012 Cochrane review comparing the two methods, there is no difference in rates of accidental pregnancy, metabolic disturbances or weight change. However, a higher rate of amenorrhoea has been seen with DMPA than with NET-EN injectable (Draper et al., 2006).

Progesterone Releasing Vaginal Ring
Lactational amenorrhoea is a contraceptive method available to women who choose to breastfeed, which is 98% effective, as long as women meet the following criteria: menstruation

has not returned, exclusive or near-exclusive breastfeeding is chosen, or less than 6 months postpartum. However, an additional method should be offered as most women do not meet these criteria.

The progesterone vaginal ring is a contraceptive method specifically designed for use during lactation to continue lactational amenorrhoea, without affecting the duration of lactation or the infant's weight gain. This ring contains micronised progesterone, which is released at a rate of approximately 10 mg per day for 90 days, after which it should be replaced. It is indicated for continuous use for 6 months in women who breastfeed at least 4 times a day (Carr et al., 2016).

Conclusion

- Progestogen-only contraception is an effective and safe option for women who cannot or do not wish to use estrogen, as it reduces the risk of certain side effects associated with estrogen.
- These methods work primarily by thickening the cervical mucus, which makes it more difficult for sperm to enter the uterus, and in some cases, they also inhibit ovulation.
- The effectiveness of progestogen-only contraception is high when used correctly, with the etonogestrel implant being the most effective, followed by the 52 mg levonorgestrel IUD and the injectable medroxyprogesterone depot.
- One of the benefits of this method is that it can be used by most women, even if they have some medical conditions, such as hypertension, smoking or increased risk of thrombosis, as well as in postpartum or immediate postabortion, where estrogens are not recommended.
- Their use may cause some side effects, the most frequent being altered bleeding patterns, which are a problem for some users.
- Their availability in the form of LARCs (subdermal implants and IUDs) and the absence of age-related restrictions on their use means that they are increasingly chosen by users due to their many advantages.

References

Abdel-Aleem, Hany, Catherine d'Arcangues, Kirsten M. Vogelsong, Mary Lyn Gaffield, and A. Metin Gülmezoglu. 2013. "Treatment of Vaginal Bleeding Irregularities Induced by Progestin Only Contraceptives." *Cochrane Database of Systematic Reviews*, no. 10: CD003449. https://doi.org/10.1002/14651858.CD003449.pub5.

Abraham, Margaret, Qiuhong Zhao, and Jeffrey F. Peipert. 2015. "Young Age, Nulliparity, and Continuation of Long-Acting Reversible Contraceptive Methods." *Obstetrics and Gynecology* 126 (4): 823–29. https://doi.org/10.1097/AOG.0000000000001036.

Alcalde, A. M., M. A. Martínez-Zamora, and F. Carmona. 2021. "Adenomiosis. Una gran desconocida: ¿Qué debemos saber?" *Clinica e investigacion en ginecologia y obstetricia* 48 (2): 184–89. https://doi.org/10.1016/j.gine.2020.08.007.

Am, Kaunitz. 1997. "Revisiting Progestin-Only OCs." *Contemporary Ob Gyn* 42. https://www.semanticscholar.org/paper/d201767855d0218e43743802d933524b76cb46d2.

American College of Obstetricians and Gynecologists' Committee on Gynecologic Practice, and Long-Acting Reversible Contraceptive Expert Work Group. 2016. "Committee Opinion No 672: Clinical Challenges of Long-Acting Reversible Contraceptive Methods." *Obstetrics and Gynecology* 128 (3): e69-77. https://doi.org/10.1097/AOG.0000000000001644.

Ampatzis, C., S. Zervoudis, G. Iatrakis, and G. Mastorakos. 2022. "Effect of Oral Contraceptives on Bone Mineral Density." *Acta Endocrinologica (Bucharest)* 18 (3): 355–60. https://doi.org/10.4183/aeb.2022.355.

Apter, Dan, Kristina Gemzell-Danielsson, Brian Hauck, Kimberly Rosen, and Christian Zurth. 2014. "Pharmacokinetics of Two Low-Dose Levonorgestrel-Releasing Intrauterine Systems and Effects on Ovulation Rate and Cervical Function: Pooled Analyses of Phase II and III Studies." *Fertility and Sterility* 101 (6): 1656-62.e1-4. https://doi.org/10.1016/j.fertnstert.2014.03.004.

Archer, David F., Hans-Joachim Ahrendt, and Dominique Drouin. 2015. "Drospirenone-Only Oral Contraceptive: Results from a Multicenter Noncomparative Trial of Efficacy, Safety and Tolerability." *Contraception* 92 (5): 439–44. https://doi.org/10.1016/j.contraception.2015.07.014.

Arias, Raquel D., John K. Jain, Cosima Brucker, Doug Ross, and Amrit Ray. 2006. "Changes in Bleeding Patterns with Depot Medroxyprogesterone Acetate Subcutaneous Injection 104 Mg." *Contraception* 74 (3): 234–38. https://doi.org/10.1016/j.contraception.2006.03.008.

Bastianelli, Carlo, Manuela Farris, Vincenzina Bruni, Elena Rosato, Ivo Brosens, and Giuseppe Benagiano. 2020. "Effects of Progestin-Only Contraceptives on the Endometrium." *Expert Review of Clinical Pharmacology* 13 (10): 1103–23. https://doi.org/10.1080/17512433.2020.1821649.

Bastianelli, Carlo, Manuela Farris, Elena Rosato, Ivo Brosens, and Giuseppe Benagiano. 2018. "Pharmacodynamics of Combined Estrogen-Progestin Oral Contraceptives 3. Inhibition of Ovulation." *Expert Review of Clinical Pharmacology* 11 (11): 1085–98. https://doi.org/10.1080/17512433.2018.1536544.

Batur, Pelin, Lisa N. Kransdorf, and Petra M. Casey. 2016. "Emergency Contraception." *Mayo Clinic Proceedings. Mayo Clinic* 91 (6): 802–7. https://doi.org/10.1016/j.mayocp.2016.02.018.

Beerthuizen, R., A. van Beek, R. Massai, L. Mäkäräinen, J. Hout, and H. C. Bennink. 2000. "Bone Mineral Density during Long-Term Use of the Progestagen Contraceptive Implant Implanon Compared to a Non-Hormonal Method of Contraception." *Human Reproduction (Oxford, England)* 15 (1): 118–22. https://doi.org/10.1093/humrep/15.1.118.

Beksinska, Mags, Rodal Issema, Ivana Beesham, Tharnija Lalbahadur, Katherine Thomas, Charles Morrison, G. Justus Hofmeyr, et al. 2021. "Weight Change among Women Using Intramuscular Depot Medroxyprogesterone Acetate, a Copper Intrauterine Device, or a Levonorgestrel Implant for Contraception: Findings from a Randomised, Multicentre, Open-Label Trial." *EClinicalMedicine* 34 (100800): 100800. https://doi.org/10.1016/j.eclinm.2021.100800.

Berenson, Abbey B., Patricia van den Berg, Karen J. Williams, and Mahbubur Rahman. 2011. "Effect of Injectable and Oral Contraceptives on Glucose and Insulin Levels." *Obstetrics and Gynecology* 117 (1): 41–47. https://doi.org/10.1097/AOG.0b013e318202ac23.

Bergendal, Annica, Ingemar Persson, Jacob Odeberg, Anders Sundström, Margareta Holmström, Sam Schulman, Ola Björgell, and Helle Kieler. 2014. "Association of Venous Thromboembolism with Hormonal Contraception and Thrombophilic Genotypes." *Obstetrics and Gynecology* 124 (3): 600–609. https://doi.org/10.1097/AOG.0000000000000411.

Bergin, Ashlee, Sigrid Tristan, Mishka Terplan, Melissa L. Gilliam, and Amy K. Whitaker. 2012. "A Missed Opportunity for Care: Two-Visit IUD Insertion Protocols Inhibit Placement." *Contraception* 86 (6): 694–97. https://doi.org/10.1016/j.contraception.2012.05.011.

Bouquier, Julie, Virginie Fulda, Anne-Sophie Bats, Fabrice Lécuru, and Cyrille Huchon. 2012. "A Life-Threatening Ectopic Pregnancy with Etonogestrel Implant." *Contraception* 85 (2): 215–17. https://doi.org/10.1016/j.contraception.2011.07.008.

Brown, Jill E., Mitchell D. Creinin, Hongsheng Wu, David Hubacher, Courtney A. Schreiber, Bliss Kaneshiro, Kavita Nanda, and Diana L. Blithe. 2024. "Menstrual Cup Use and Intrauterine Device Expulsion in a Copper Intrauterine Device Randomized Trial." *Contraception* 134 (110415): 110415. https://doi.org/10.1016/j.contraception.2024.110415.

Brown J., Kives S., Akhtar M. 2012. "Progestagens and anti-progestagens for pain associated with endometriosis." Cochrane Database Syst Rev. 2012;(3):CD002122. DOI: 10.1002/14651858.CD002122.pub2

Carmo, Lilian Sheila de Melo Pereira, Giordana Campos Braga, Rui Alberto Ferriani, Silvana Maria Quintana, and Carolina Sales Vieira. 2017. "Timing of Etonogestrel-Releasing Implants and Growth of Breastfed Infants: A Randomized Controlled Trial." *Obstetrics and Gynecology* 130 (1): 100–107. https://doi.org/10.1097/AOG.0000000000002092.

Carr, Shannon L., Mary E. Gaffield, Monica V. Dragoman, and Sharon Phillips. 2016. "Safety of the Progesterone-Releasing Vaginal Ring (PVR) among Lactating Women: A Systematic Review." *Contraception* 94 (3): 253–61. https://doi.org/10.1016/j.contraception.2015.04.001.

Cicali, Brian, Lais Da Silva, Amir Sarayani, Karthik Lingineni, Michelle Pressly, Soyoung Kim, Thomas Wendl, et al. 2022. "Development of a Translational Exposure-Bracketing Approach to Streamline the Development of Hormonal Contraceptive Drug Products." *Clinical Pharmacology and Therapeutics* 112 (4): 909–16. https://doi.org/10.1002/cpt.2690.

Cockrum, Richard H., Jackie Soo, Sandra A. Ham, Kenneth S. Cohen, and Shari G. Snow. 2022. "Association of Progestogens and Venous Thromboembolism among Women of Reproductive Age." *Obstetrics and Gynecology* 140 (3): 477–87. https://doi.org/10.1097/AOG.0000000000004896.

Committee on Gynecologic Practice Long-Acting Reversible Contraception Working Group. 2015. "Committee Opinion No. 642: Increasing Access to Contraceptive Implants and Intrauterine Devices to Reduce Unintended Pregnancy." *Obstetrics and Gynecology* 126 (4): e44–48. https://doi.org/10.1097/AOG.0000000000001106.

Creinin, Mitchell D. 2014a. "Effects of Age, Parity, and Device Type on Complications and Discontinuation of Intrauterine Devices." *Obstetrics and Gynecology* 123 (6): 1356. https://doi.org/10.1097/AOG.0000000000000313.

"Extended Use of the Intrauterine Device: A Literature Review and Recommendations for Clinical Practice." *Contraception* 90 (1): 104. https://doi.org/10.1016/j.contraception.2014.04.002.

Curtis, Kathryn M., Antoinette T. Nguyen, Naomi K. Tepper, Lauren B. Zapata, Emily M. Snyder, Kendra Hatfield-Timajchy, Katherine Kortsmit, Megan A. Cohen, Maura K. Whiteman, and Contributors. 2024. "U.S. Selected Practice Recommendations for Contraceptive Use, 2024." *Recommendations and Reports: Morbidity and Mortality Weekly Report* 73 (3): 1–77. https://doi.org/10.15585/mmwr.rr7303a1.

"DailyMed." n.d. Nih.gov. Accessed May 24, 2025. https://www.dailymed.nlm.nih.gov/dailymed/index.cfm.

Draper, B. H., C. Morroni, M. Hoffman, J. Smit, M. Beksinska, J. Hapgood, and L. Van der Merwe. 2006. "Depot Medroxyprogesterone versus Norethisterone Oenanthate for Long-Acting Progestogenic Contraception." *Cochrane Database of Systematic Reviews* 2012 (3): CD005214. https://doi.org/10.1002/14651858.CD005214.pub2.

Duijkers, Ingrid J. M., Doris Heger-Mahn, Dominique Drouin, Enrico Colli, and Sven Skouby. 2016. "Maintenance of Ovulation Inhibition with a New Progestogen-Only Pill Containing Drospirenone after Scheduled 24-h Delays in Pill Intake." *Contraception* 93 (4): 303–9. https://doi.org/10.1016/j.contraception.2015.12.007.

Edelman, Alison B., Ganesh Cherala, Myrna Y. Munar, Martha McInnis, Frank Z. Stanczyk, and Jeffrey T. Jensen. 2014. "Correcting Oral Contraceptive Pharmacokinetic Alterations Due to Obesity: A Randomized Controlled Trial." *Contraception* 90 (5): 550–56. https://doi.org/10.1016/j.contraception.2014.06.033.

Faculty of Sexual & Reproductive Healthcare. 2023. Intrauterine Contraception March 2023 (Amended Jan 2025). BMJ Sexual & Reproductive Health 2023; 49: Suppl 1. doi: 10.1136/bmjsrh-2023-IUC.

Floyd, Jessica L., Anitra D. Beasley, Laurie S. Swaim, Mark A. Turrentine, and J. Biba Nijjar. 2020. "Association of Immediate Postpartum Etonogestrel Implant Insertion and Venous Thromboembolism." *Obstetrics and Gynecology* 135 (6): 1275–80. https://doi.org/10.1097/AOG.0000000000003760.

Fox, Michelle C., Julia Oat-Judge, Kathryn Severson, Roxanne M. Jamshidi, Rameet H. Singh, Raegan McDonald-Mosley, and Anne E. Burke. 2011. "Immediate Placement of Intrauterine Devices after First and Second Trimester Pregnancy Termination." *Contraception* 83 (1): 34–40. https://doi.org/10.1016/j.contraception.2010.06.018.

Francis, Jenny K. R., and Melanie A. Gold. 2017. "Long-Acting Reversible Contraception for Adolescents: A Review: A Review." *JAMA Pediatrics* 171 (7): 694–701. https://doi.org/10.1001/jamapediatrics.2017.0598.

Funk, Sidney, Michael M. Miller, Daniel R. Mishell Jr, David F. Archer, Alfred Poindexter, Juergen Schmidt, Edio Zampaglione, and Implanon US Study Group. 2005. "Safety and Efficacy of Implanon, a Single-Rod Implantable Contraceptive Containing Etonogestrel." *Contraception* 71 (5): 319–26. https://doi.org/10.1016/j.contraception.2004.11.007.

Furlong, Lesley-Anne. 2002. "Ectopic Pregnancy Risk When Contraception Fails. A Review." *The Journal of Reproductive Medicine* 47 (11): 881–85.

Gemzell-Danielsson, Kristina, Dan Apter, Sylvia Dermout, Thomas Faustmann, Kimberly Rosen, Thomas Schmelter, Martin Merz, and Anita Nelson. 2017. "Evaluation of a New, Low-Dose Levonorgestrel Intrauterine Contraceptive System over 5 Years of Use." *European Journal of Obstetrics, Gynecology, and Reproductive Biology* 210: 22–28. https://doi.org/10.1016/j.ejogrb.2016.11.022.

Girum, Tadele, and Abebaw Wasie. 2018. "Return of Fertility after Discontinuation of Contraception: A Systematic Review and Meta-Analysis." *Contraception and Reproductive Medicine* 3: 9. https://doi.org/10.1186/s40834-018-0064-y.

Glasier, Anna, Stephanie Sober, Robin Gasloli, Anupam Goyal, and Irene Laurora. 2022. "A Review of the Effectiveness of a Progestogen-Only Pill Containing Norgestrel 75 Mg/Day." *Contraception* 105: 1–6. https://doi.org/10.1016/j.contraception.2021.08.016.

Hage, Mirella, Oana Plesa, Isabelle Lemaire, and Marie Laure Raffin Sanson. 2022. "Estrogen and Progesterone Therapy and Meningiomas." *Endocrinology* 163 (2). https://doi.org/10.1210/endocr/bqab259.

Halpern, Vera, Stephanie L. Combes, Laneta J. Dorflinger, Debra H. Weiner, and David F. Archer. 2014. "Pharmacokinetics of Subcutaneous Depot Medroxyprogesterone Acetate Injected in the Upper Arm." *Contraception* 89 (1): 31–35. https://doi.org/10.1016/j.contraception.2013.07.002.

Hubacher, David, Laureen Lopez, Markus J. Steiner, and Laneta Dorflinger. 2009. "Menstrual Pattern Changes from Levonorgestrel Subdermal Implants and DMPA: Systematic Review and Evidence-Based Comparisons." *Contraception* 80 (2): 113–18. https://doi.org/10.1016/j.contraception.2009.02.008.

Imai, A., K. Matsunami, H. Takagi, and S. Ichigo. 2014. "Levonorgestrel-Releasing Intrauterine Device Used for Dysmenorrhea: Five-Year Literature Review." *Clinical and Experimental Obstetrics & Gynecology* 41 (5): 495–98. https://doi.org/10.12891/ceog17042014.

Jackson, Emily, and Anna Glasier. 2011. "Return of Ovulation and Menses in Postpartum Nonlactating Women: A Systematic Review: A Systematic Review." *Obstetrics and Gynecology* 117 (3): 657–62. https://doi.org/10.1097/AOG.0b013e31820ce18c.

Kaunitz, Andrew M., Paul D. Miller, Valerie Montgomery Rice, Doug Ross, and Michael R. McClung. 2006. "Bone Mineral Density in Women Aged 25-35 Years Receiving Depot Medroxyprogesterone Acetate: Recovery Following Discontinuation." *Contraception* 74 (2): 90–99. https://doi.org/10.1016/j.contraception.2006.03.010.

Korver, Tjeerd, Christine Klipping, Doris Heger-Mahn, Ingrid Duijkers, Gonnie van Osta, and Thom Dieben. 2005. "Maintenance of Ovulation Inhibition with the 75-Microg Desogestrel-Only Contraceptive Pill (Cerazette) after Scheduled 12-h Delays in Tablet Intake." *Contraception* 71 (1): 8–13. https://doi.org/10.1016/j.contraception.2004.07.016.

Lopez, Laureen M., Shanthi Ramesh, Mario Chen, Alison Edelman, Conrad Otterness, James Trussell, and Frans M. Helmerhorst. 2016. "Progestin-Only Contraceptives: Effects on Weight." *Cochrane Database of Systematic Reviews* 2016 (8): CD008815. https://doi.org/10.1002/14651858.CD008815.pub4.

Machado, Rogério Bonassi, Alice Pinheiro Pereira, Geórgia Perez Coelho, Larissa Neri, Larissa Martins, and Daniele Luminoso. 2010. "Epidemiological and Clinical Aspects of Migraine in Users of Combined Oral Contraceptives." *Contraception* 81 (3): 202–8. https://doi.org/10.1016/j.contraception.2009.09.006.

Mansour, Diana, Tjeerd Korver, Maya Marintcheva-Petrova, and Ian S. Fraser. 2008. "The Effects of Implanon on Menstrual Bleeding Patterns." *The European Journal of Contraception & Reproductive Health Care: The Official Journal of the European Society of Contraception* 13 Suppl 1 (supl): 13–28. https://doi.org/10.1080/13625180801959931.

Martin, Vincent T., and Michael Behbehani. 2006. “Ovarian Hormones and Migraine Headache: Understanding Mechanisms and Pathogenesis--Part I.” *Headache* 46 (1): 3–23. https://doi.org/10.1111/j.1526-4610.2006.00309.x.

McNicholas, Colleen P., Tessa Madden, Qiuhong Zhao, Gina Secura, Jenifer E. Allsworth, and Jeffrey F. Peipert. 2012. “Cervical Lidocaine for IUD Insertional Pain: A Randomized Controlled Trial.” *American Journal of Obstetrics and Gynecology* 207 (5): 384.e1-6. https://doi.org/10.1016/j.ajog.2012.09.018.

Medicamentos y Productos Sanitarios, Agencia Española de. n.d.”.:: CIMA ::. FICHA TECNICA JAYDESS 13,5 MG SISTEMA DE LIBERACION INTRAUTERINO.” Aemps.es. Accessed May 24, 2025a. https://cima.aemps.es/cima/dochtml/ft/77169/FichaTecnica_77169.html.

Miles, R. A., R. J. Paulson, R. A. Lobo, M. F. Press, L. Dahmoush, and M. V. Sauer. 1994. “Pharmacokinetics and Endometrial Tissue Levels of Progesterone after Administration by Intramuscular and Vaginal Routes: A Comparative Study.” *Fertility and Sterility* 62 (3): 485–90. https://doi.org/10.1016/s0015-0282(16)56935-0.

Mittermeier, Theresa, Charlotte Farrant, and Michelle R. Wise. 2020. “Levonorgestrel-Releasing Intrauterine System for Endometrial Hyperplasia.” *Cochrane Database of Systematic Reviews* 9 (9): CD012658. https://doi.org/10.1002/14651858.CD012658.pub2.

Mol, B. W., W. M. Ankum, P. M. Bossuyt, and F. Van der Veen. 1995. “Contraception and the Risk of Ectopic Pregnancy: A Meta-Analysis.” *Contraception* 52 (6): 337–41. https://doi.org/10.1016/0010-7824(95)00221-9.

Moray, Kusum V., Himanshu Chaurasia, Oshima Sachin, and Beena Joshi. 2021. “A Systematic Review on Clinical Effectiveness, Side-Effect Profile and Meta-Analysis on Continuation Rate of Etonogestrel Contraceptive Implant.” *Reproductive Health* 18 (1): 4. https://doi.org/10.1186/s12978-020-01054-y.

National Guideline Alliance (Great Britain). 2018. *Heavy Menstrual Bleeding: Assessment and Management.* National Institute for Health and Care Excellence.

Nguyen, Antoinette T., Kathryn M. Curtis, Naomi K. Tepper, Katherine Kortsmit, Anna W. Brittain, Emily M. Snyder, Megan A. Cohen, Lauren B. Zapata, Maura K. Whiteman, and Contributors. 2024. “U.S. Medical Eligibility Criteria for Contraceptive Use, 2024.” *Recommendations and Reports: Morbidity and Mortality Weekly Report* 73 (4): 1–126. https://doi.org/10.15585/mmwr.rr7304a1.

“Norethindrone.” 2006. In *Drugs and Lactation Database (LactMed®)*. Bethesda (MD): National Institute of Child Health and Human Development.

Ogburn, Joseph A. Tony, Eve Espey, and Jody Stonehocker. 2005. “Barriers to Intrauterine Device Insertion in Postpartum Women.” *Contraception* 72 (6): 426–29. https://doi.org/10.1016/j.contraception.2005.05.016.

Pakarinen, P. I., J. Suvisaari, T. Luukkainen, and P. Lähteenmäki. 1997. “Intracervical and Fundal Administration of Levonorgestrel for Contraception: Endometrial Thickness, Patterns of Bleeding, and Persisting Ovarian Follicles.” *Fertility and Sterility* 68 (1): 59–64. https://doi.org/10.1016/s0015-0282(97)81476-8.

Palacios, S., E. Colli, and P. A. Regidor. 2020. “Bleeding Profile of Women Using a Drospirenone-Only Pill 4 Mg over Nine Cycles in Comparison with Desogestrel 0.075 Mg.” *PloS One* 15 (6): e0231856. https://doi.org/10.1371/journal.pone.0231856.

Phillips, Sharon J., Naomi K. Tepper, Nathalie Kapp, Kavita Nanda, Marleen Temmerman, and Kathryn M. Curtis. 2016. “Progestogen-Only Contraceptive Use among Breastfeeding Women: A Systematic Review.” *Contraception* 94 (3): 226–52. https://doi.org/10.1016/j.contraception.2015.09.010.

Perelló J., Guillén A. 2024. “Levonorgestrel-releasing intrauterine device.” Contraception Spanish Society.

Rattray, Carole, Jeffrey Wiener, Jennifer Legardy-Williams, Elizabeth Costenbader, Karen Pazol, Natalie Medley-Singh, Margaret C. Snead, et al. 2015. “Effects of Initiating a Contraceptive Implant on Subsequent Condom Use: A Randomized Controlled Trial.” *Contraception* 92 (6): 560–66. https://doi.org/10.1016/j.contraception.2015.06.009.

Raymond, Elizabeth G., Mark A. Weaver, Karmen S. Louie, Yi-Ling Tan, Manuel Bousiéguez, Ana Gabriela Aranguré-Peraza, Elba M. Lugo-Hernández, et al. 2016. “Effects of Depot Medroxyprogesterone Acetate Injection Timing on Medical Abortion Efficacy and Repeat Pregnancy: A Randomized Controlled Trial.” *Obstetrics and Gynecology* 128 (4): 739–45. https://doi.org/10.1097/AOG.0000000000001627.

Regidor, P-A, and E. Colli. 2022. "Drospirenone 4 Mg in a 24/4 Regimen Maintains Inhibition of Ovulation Even after a 24-h Delay Pill Intake - Pharmacological Aspects and Comparison to Other Progestin-Only Pills." *European Review for Medical and Pharmacological Sciences* 26 (6): 1994–99. https://doi.org/10.26355/eurrev_202203_28348.

Samson, Marsha, Nancy Porter, Olubunmi Orekoya, James R. Hebert, Swann Arp Adams, Charles L. Bennett, and Susan E. Steck. 2016. "Progestin and Breast Cancer Risk: A Systematic Review." *Breast Cancer Research and Treatment* 155 (1): 3–12. https://doi.org/10.1007/s10549-015-3663-1.

Schoretsanitis, Georgios, Kristina M. Deligiannidis, Michael Paulzen, Edoardo Spina, and Jose de Leon. 2022. "Drug-Drug Interactions between Psychotropic Medications and Oral Contraceptives." *Expert Opinion on Drug Metabolism & Toxicology* 18 (6): 395–411. https://doi.org/10.1080/17425255.2022.2106214.

Segall-Gutierrez, Penina, Deshawn Taylor, Xinwen Liu, Frank Stanzcyk, Stanley Azen, and Daniel R. Mishell Jr. 2010. "Follicular Development and Ovulation in Extremely Obese Women Receiving Depo-Medroxyprogesterone Acetate Subcutaneously." *Contraception* 81 (6): 487–95. https://doi.org/10.1016/j.contraception.2010.01.021.

Sivin. 2003. "Risks and benefits, advantages and disadvantages of levonorgestrel-releasing contraceptive implants." *Drug Safety. 26(5):303-35. doi: 10.2165/00002018-200326050-00002.*

Sönmezer, M., C. Atabekoğlu, B. Cengiz, F. Dökmeci, and S. D. Cengiz. 2005. "Depot-Medroxyprogesterone Acetate in Anticoagulated Patients with Previous Hemorrhagic Corpus Luteum." *The European Journal of Contraception & Reproductive Health Care: The Official Journal of the European Society of Contraception* 10 (1): 9–14. https://doi.org/10.1080/13625180400020952.

Sothornwit J., Kaewrudee S., Lumbiganon P., Pattanittum P., Averbach S. 2022. "Immediate versus delayed postpartum insertion of contraceptive implant and IUD for contraception." Cochrane Database Syst Rev. 10(10):CD011913. doi: 10.1002/14651858.CD011913.pub3.

Strowitzki T., Faustmann T., Gerlinger C., Seitz C. 2010. "Dienogest in the treatment of endometriosis-associated pelvic pain: a 12-week, randomized, double-blind, placebo-controlled study." *Eur J Obstet Gynecol Reprod Biol*. 2010;151(2):193-8. DOI: 10.1016/j.ejogrb.2010.04.002.

Tepper, Naomi K., Maria W. Steenland, Mary E. Gaffield, Polly A. Marchbanks, and Kathryn M. Curtis. 2013. "Retention of Intrauterine Devices in Women Who Acquire Pelvic Inflammatory Disease: A Systematic Review." *Contraception* 87 (5): 655–60. https://doi.org/10.1016/j.contraception.2012.08.011.

Tepper, Naomi K., Maura K. Whiteman, Polly A. Marchbanks, Andra H. James, and Kathryn M. Curtis. 2016. "Progestin-Only Contraception and Thromboembolism: A Systematic Review." *Contraception* 94 (6): 678–700. https://doi.org/10.1016/j.contraception.2016.04.014.

Tsevat, Danielle, Rebecca Mercier, Camryn Bernheimer, Stephanie Lin, and Beth Schwartz. 2024. "Amenorrhea in Adolescents Using the Etonogestrel Contraceptive Implant." *Contraception* 133 (110413): 110413. https://doi.org/10.1016/j.contraception.2024.110413.

Vercellini, Paolo, Benedetta Bracco, Paola Mosconi, Anna Roberto, Daniela Alberico, Dridi Dhouha, and Edgardo Somigliana. 2016. "Norethindrone Acetate or Dienogest for the Treatment of Symptomatic Endometriosis: A before and after Study." *Fertility and Sterility* 105 (3): 734-743.e3. https://doi.org/10.1016/j.fertnstert.2015.11.016.

Warhurst, Samantha, Christopher J. Rofe, Bruce J. Brew, Deborah Bateson, Kevin McGeechan, Gabriele S. Merki-Feld, Raymond Garrick, and Susan E. Tomlinson. 2018. "Effectiveness of the Progestin-Only Pill for Migraine Treatment in Women: A Systematic Review and Meta-Analysis." *Cephalalgia: An International Journal of Headache* 38 (4): 754–64. https://doi.org/10.1177/0333102417710636.

Wattanayingcharoenchai, R., S. Rattanasiri, C. Charakorn, J. Attia, and A. Thakkinstian. 2021. "Postoperative Hormonal Treatment for Prevention of Endometrioma Recurrence after Ovarian Cystectomy: A Systematic Review and Network Meta-Analysis." *BJOG: An International Journal of Obstetrics and Gynaecology* 128 (1): 25–35. https://doi.org/10.1111/1471-0528.16366.

Weiderpass, E., H. O. Adami, J. A. Baron, C. Magnusson, R. Bergström, A. Lindgren, N. Correia, and I. Persson. 1999. "Risk of Endometrial Cancer Following Estrogen Replacement with and without Progestins." *Journal of the National Cancer Institute* 91 (13): 1131–37. https://doi.org/10.1093/jnci/91.13.1131.

Wiegratz I., Kuhl H. 2006. "Metabolic and clinical effects of progestogens." The European Journal of Contraception and Reproductive Health Care. 11(3):153-161. Doi: 10.1080/13625180600772741

Winner B., Peipert. F, Zhao Q., Buckel C., Madden T., Allsworth J., Secura GM. 2012. "Effectiveness of long-acting reversible contraception." N Engl J Med. 2012;366(21):1998. DOI: 10.1056/NEJMoa1110855
Workowski K., Bachmann L., Chan P., Johnston C., Muzny C., Park I., Reno H., Zenilma J., n, Bolan G. 2021. "Sexually Transmitted Infections Treatment Guidelines." *MMWR Recomm Rep 2021;70.*
Worly, Brett L., Tamar L. Gur, and Jonathan Schaffir. 2018. "The Relationship between Progestin Hormonal Contraception and Depression: A Systematic Review." *Contraception* 97 (6): 478–89. https://doi.org/10.1016/j.contraception.2018.01.010.
Zigler, Rachel E., and Colleen McNicholas. 2017. "Unscheduled Vaginal Bleeding with Progestin-Only Contraceptive Use." *American Journal of Obstetrics and Gynecology* 216 (5): 443–50. https://doi.org/10.1016/j.ajog.2016.12.008.
Zuniga, Carmela, Kelly Blanchard, Cynthia C. Harper, Alexandra Wollum, Katherine Key, and Jillian T. Henderson. 2023. "Effectiveness and Efficacy Rates of Progestin-Only Pills: A Comprehensive Literature Review." *Contraception* 119 (109925): 109925. https://doi.org/10.1016/j.contraception.2022.109925.

Chapter 9

Copper Intrauterine Device

Ll. Belmonte Andújar[1,2,*], PhD
A. M. Fuentes Rozalén[3], MD
M. M. Pérez Haro[1,3], MD
I. Sánchez Nieto[4], MD
and M. T. Gómez García[1,2]
[1]Obstetrics and Gynaecology Department, University and Hospital of Albacete, Spain
[2]Medical Science Department, School of Medicine of Albacete, Universidad de Castilla-La Mancha, Spain
[3]Bernabeu Institute, Alicante, Spain
[4]Obstetrics and Gynaecology Department, Hospital Can Misses, Ibiza, Spain

Abstract

The copper intrauterine device is considered the third most effective reversible method currently available, and the most cost effective of them. Despite this, its use varies greatly in different regions of the world, and it has been a source of controversy at certain times in history since its emergence. Different factors influence IUD efficacy, such as user age and IUD type. It is important to know these factors in order to make a realistic and safe contraceptive advise.

In general, it is a method that is very well accepted by users, with high continuation rates, although it is not without side effects and complications. There are also contraindications for its use that are important to know for proper contraceptive advice and management.

This chapter provides an update on the scientific evidence surrounding the use of copper IUDs and certain aspects to consider prior to, during, and after insertion that may be key to adequate tolerance and acceptance by users and, especially, to avoiding associated complications that in some cases can be serious, with the aim of optimizing contraceptive care.

Keywords: copper IUD, intrauterine device, LARC, long-acting reversible contraceptive

---

* Corresponding Author's Email: belmonte.llanos@gmail.com

In: Advances in Reproductive Health
Editors: Llanos Belmonte Andujar and Ana Fuentes Rozalen
ISBN: 979-8-90134-038-7

Introduction

Long-acting reversible contraceptives (LARCs) are a category of contraceptive methods that are reversible, have a long-lasting contraceptive effect (at least more than two menstrual cycles), and do not require compliance on the part of the user, while also being highly cost-effective. LARCs have few contraindications and should be offered routinely as safe and effective contraceptive options for most women. These include contraceptive implants and intrauterine devices. The latter are divided into levonorgestrel-releasing devices and copper intrauterine devices (IUD-Cu). In this chapter, we will focus exclusively on Cu-IUDs. Another chapter of this book discusses in detail all progestin-only contraceptive methods, including the levonorgestrel-releasing intrauterine device.

The copper IUD is the most widely used reversible contraceptive method worldwide, although its use varies greatly between different countries and regions. It is estimated that there are 169 million Cu-IUD users worldwide (United Nations 2024). In addition, it is considered the third most effective reversible method currently available and the most cost-effective of all, with an average failure rate of 0.8 pregnancies per 100 users in one year of Cu-IUD use, compared to a failure rate of 0.5 per 100 women who undergo irreversible bilateral tubal ligation (Trussell et al. 2015).

Cu-IUDs are also highly effective emergency contraception (EC) that can be retained to provide ongoing contraception. (This aspect of the IUD will be discussed in detail in the chapter on emergency contraception).

Despite all the advantages of using this contraceptive method, its use is not uniform across different regions of the world. Depending on the country, the proportion of women using IUDs varies widely. On average, 15% of women of reproductive age in developing countries and 8% in developed countries use this contraceptive method (d'Arcangues 2007). In the United States and Canada, only 10.5% (2017) and 4.3% (2006) of contraceptive users use IUDs, respectively. However, in countries such as Uzbekistan, Turkmenistan, North Korea, China, Egypt, Sweden, France, Tunisia and Cuba, the percentages of married women using contraception who use the copper IUD reach 49.7% (2006), 65.4% (2019), 44.2% (2017), 34.1% (2017), 30.1% (2014), 27.5% (2017), 21.5% (2010), 21. 3% (2018) and 20.1% (2019) respectively (United Nations, 2022).

These differences in the use of the Cu-IUD may be influenced by personal, political, economic, and social factors, and above all by medical-legal issues, which are often based on myths regarding the use of this method.

In this chapter, we conduct an exhaustive review of the literature on the main aspects of this contraceptive method, such as its history, its mechanism of action, aspects to consider before starting to use it, contraindications that discourage its use, and other aspects of interest, in order to provide clinicians with the knowledge necessary for its optimal use based on current scientific evidence.

Definition and Structure of the IUD-Cu

The IUD is the most widely used reversible contraceptive method for women worldwide. It is a device that is temporarily inserted into the uterus to provide contraception for as long as it remains in place, depending on the duration specified in the technical data sheet for each model. Threads that pass through the uterine cervix connect the IUD to the vagina, facilitating its removal when required.

The main structure of the device is made of a polymer that must be biocompatible, non-absorbable and viscoelastic. It also includes a substance that makes it radiopaque so that it can be seen on X-rays. IUDs are inserted into the uterus as a contraceptive method and can remain in place for 5 to 10 years continuously, or even longer in certain situations.

There are different types of copper IUDs, classified according to various parameters:

- *According to its design*: The most common format is modified T-shaped or Y-shaped. Other commercially available formats are anchor-shaped and circular. The GyneFix® model has been gaining popularity in many countries. GyneFix is a frameless IUD that is commonly used in Europe and Asia but is not available in North America. It consists of six 5 mm long copper sleeves threaded onto a monofilament polypropylene thread. The proximal end of the thread contains a knot that is anchored into the myometrium of the uterine fundus using a special inserter, thereby securing the device in the uterine cavity (Cheung 2006). Because of its frameless design, flexibility, and reduced size, the GyneFix is well tolerated in most women, with low removal rates for abnormal menstrual bleeding and pain (Wildemeersch et al. 2003).
- *According to their dimensions*: IUDs come in different sizes, depending on the dimensions of the uterine cavity and the woman's parity. The most common dimensions of the standard T-shaped IUD, which is the most widely used today, are approximately 3 cm for the vertical arm and 3 cm for the horizontal arm.
- *According to their composition*: The devices have an active copper surface area ranging from 250 to 380 mm2, which is usually coiled along the body of the IUD.
- *According to the arrangement of the copper:* In the case of T-shaped IUDs, the copper may also be coiled around the transverse arms. There are IUDs that, in addition to copper content, have cores of other metals, such as silver or gold, which confer greater resistance to fragmentation of the copper wire (Margulies 1975).

History of Intrauterine Devices

Devices placed in the cervix or uterus to prevent pregnancy predate hormonal methods.

Throughout the history of contraception, there have been multiple models of IUDs in different forms. These range from biological IUDs made of silk thread, inert IUDs made solely of plastic, metal IUDs (silver, nickel, copper, zinc, etc.), to hormone-releasing IUDs, specifically levonorgestrel.

The documented history of the IUD begins in the early 20th century. Previously, Hippocrates (5th century BC) referred in his writings to reproductive control through cervical and uterine manipulation, inserting a lead tube through the cervix through which certain medications were instilled, which is possibly the first reference to the IUD (McKay, W. J. S, n.d.).

Subsequently, there are various legends dating back to the Middle Ages that could be the origin of the idea of inserting an object into the uterus as a method of contraception. According to these legends, Arab nomads used objects that they inserted into the uterus of female camels through a hollow tube to prevent them from becoming pregnant during long journeys through the desert (Wessel 2014). Other legends tell that, later on, women began to insert small objects, such as buttons, silver or horsehair, for contraceptive purposes.

However, it was not until 1909 that the first article on the first modern IUD, Richter's silk ring (Richter, R. 1909), was published. This device consisted of a flexible ring made from silkworm gut. This material, in the form of two strands of thread linked together to form a ring 27 mm in diameter, was inserted into the uterus using a probe, leaving one end protruding from the vagina through the external cervical os to facilitate its removal. Once inside the uterus, it functioned as an effective contraceptive method for months or years. Prior to this discovery, all known contraceptive methods were related to intercourse, sexually frustrating and relatively ineffective. Richard Richter made possible, for the first time in history, a contraceptive method that was completely reversible and independent of sexual intercourse.

Almost two decades later, Richter's ring was revived by Pust (1923) and Grafenberg (1928). The former added a glass button that remained in the vagina with the intention of blocking the ascent of sperm towards the uterus (Pust, K 1923). The latter added silver to its composition to make it visible on X-rays. These devices met with strong opposition from gynaecologists at the time, so it took decades for new advances in intrauterine contraception to be made. In 1958, Lazar Marguiles created a coil made of radiopaque material, and in 1962, Lippes' loop appeared, which added the novelty of a plastic thread at its distal end to facilitate removal of the device (Tietze 1966)

In 1968, the Food and Drug Administration (FDA) published a comprehensive report on the intrauterine device, stating that 'the committee found adequate scientific data to support the effectiveness and usefulness of uterine contraceptives,' which was a new milestone in the dissemination of this method as a fully accepted contraceptive (FDA 1968).

Subsequently, in 1969, Jaime Zipper added copper to its composition, finding that this significantly increased its effectiveness. From then on, different models of copper IUDs appeared with various shapes and copper arrangements, gaining popularity and credibility in scientific societies (Zipper, Medel, and Prager 1969) (Zipper 1969) (Zipper 1971).

The transition to medicated IUDs marked the beginning of a new era, and by the end of 1973, multiple copper IUDs of different types and shapes had been tested: the copper T, the copper 7, and the Lippes Loop with copper. The studies were consistent in their results, confirming the increased effectiveness of the devices after the integration of copper into their designs (Tatum 1972) (Tietze C; Lewit S 1972).

Hormones were also incorporated into intrauterine devices. In 1971, Scommegna and colleagues designed Progestasert, similar in shape to the copper T, but consisting of a permeable polymer membrane that released progesterone in a predictable and controlled dose of 65 μg per day (Scommegna et al. 1970). Its effectiveness was described as similar to that of the copper IUD, although decades later its development would be perfected and it would prove to be a contraceptive method with greater effectiveness than the Cu-IUD.

In that same year, 1971, the Dalkon shield was marketed in the United States, advertised as having excellent intrauterine retention and low expulsion and removal rates. Its popularity grew, but despite its low expulsion rates, the device began to be suspected of being associated with a high risk of fatal septic abortion compared to other IUD models (Huber, 1975).

A review by the FDA Advisory Committee suggested that the Dalkon Shield could cause an increase in septic abortion for various reasons, including the multifilament thread that connected the shield to the vagina for removal and location. Nevertheless, since then, public reaction and certain negative scientific reports led to the Dalkon device becoming a commercial disaster, and it was withdrawn from the market in the USA in 1974 (Lee et al. 1983).

The consequences of these events with the standard Dalkon shield spread to other IUDs, especially in the USA, where their distribution and placement fell by 50% from 1973 to 1974, and the marketing of different IUD models ceased between 1982 and 1985 (Jennings, 1974). Rising legal liability costs led researchers to abandon the promotion of other IUD models.

In the late 1970s and throughout the 1980s, various DIUs -Cu IUDs (T-Cu 220C, T-Cu 380A, Nova-T, etc.) were developed, mainly in Europe—a continent where the Dalkon shield disaster did not cause as much damage as it did in the United States—by adding a copper surface, which had been shown to increase their effectiveness and durability. One of the most popular devices, developed in 1977 by the Dutchman Van Os, which combined the advantages of the Dalkon shield and the copper T, was the Multiload-250 (van Os et al. 1977), which later had 375 mm2 of copper surface area and is still available on the market today.

On the other hand, among the possible drawbacks of intrauterine devices, the possibility of expulsion stood out, which occurred with variability depending on the shape and type of device. In order to reduce the expulsion rate, in 1984, Wildemeersch devised a linear device model with six 5 mm copper tubes, threaded onto a polyethylene monofilament, with a knot at its proximal end that anchored it to the endometrium during insertion, thus minimising the possibility of expulsion. This IUD, with a total copper exposure area of 390 mm2, was named Cu-Fix, and its first results were seen in a study published in 1988, which showed a considerable reduction in expulsion rates (Wildemeersch 1988).

In 1986, the WHO organised a panel of experts to review the various aspects of intrauterine contraception in detail, concluding that the IUD was a safe and highly effective method with high continuation rates and numerous advantages. Another important conclusion regarding its mechanism of action was the denial of its anti-implantation capacity, which helped to calm opponents who claimed that these devices had an abortive effect (WHO 1987).

Subsequently, in 1988, the T380A copper IUD was marketed in the United States, marking the return of the device to family planning in that country, and its use spread worldwide due to its low pregnancy rates and long durability. This device remains one of the most widely used intrauterine contraceptives today (Pitkin 1988).

Two years later, in 1990, the levonorgestrel-releasing IUD was marketed in Europe, specifically in Finland. Based on the Nova-T model, it released 20 μg of hormone daily into the uterus. Various studies showed results that exceeded the effectiveness of the copper IUD, with pregnancy rates of 0.1%, and even added non-contraceptive benefits such as reduced menstrual bleeding (Chi 1991). These devices revolutionised the field of contraception and gynaecology in general, as they added multiple non-contraceptive benefits and were considered a treatment for multiple gynaecological conditions as well as a contraceptive. Subsequently, IUDs with different levonorgestrel loads have been marketed and widely accepted by users.

More recently, in the 2010s, a novel Cu IUD design was marketed under the name IUBTM SCu 300 (IUB Ballerine). Available in three different sizes (12, 15 and 18 mm) and lasting up to five years, the device consisted of seventeen 2.1-millimetre copper beads in a special memory alloy that, once inserted into the uterine cavity, took on a spherical shape that adapted completely to it without sharp edges or angles. Its total copper surface area is 304 mm2. Due to its shape and size, it could be assumed that its insertion would be less uncomfortable and would have lower rates of expulsion, bleeding and abdominal pain compared to traditional

IUDs, but there are no comprehensive studies analysing its results in terms of efficacy and safety, and those that do exist, with small sample sizes, have yielded mixed results to date (Wiebe and Trussell 2016). This device is no longer on the market.

Currently, there is a phase III trial in the US with a new device with a unique structure called Veracept (hormone-free), composed of nitinol and 175 mm2 of copper exposure surface, and another phase II trial with a hormone-releasing device, LevoceptTM, with no results yet.

At the present time, the only copper IUD available in the United States is Paragard.

In short, since their inception, intrauterine devices have been highly effective contraceptive methods, with a brilliant evolution, to the point of becoming one of the cheapest, most effective and longest-lasting methods, peppered with controversy and sometimes mistreated by the more conservative sectors of the population, certain exaggerated scientific publications and, consequently, by public opinion.

Mechanism of Action

The specific mechanism of action of the IUD is not precisely known. Numerous studies have been published, conducted on different animal species, investigating this aspect; however, the different mechanisms of action of the IUD vary considerably among the different animal species analysed.

Traditionally, based on the results of studies conducted on different animal species, and even studies analysing the intracavitary fluid of human uteri from hysterectomy specimens, it was thought that the main mechanism of action of the IUD was to prevent the implantation of the fertilised egg (Parr and Shirley 1976) (Hilgers 1974).

Thus, this belief that embryos reaching the uterine cavity occupied by an IUD were destroyed before, during, or after implantation became very popular among healthcare professionals, the media, the church, and the general population.

Today, it is known that its main effect is actually to inhibit fertilisation, although it is known that the IUD exerts a contraceptive effect through multiple possible mechanisms of action (Ortiz, Croxatto, and Bardin 1996) (Ortiz and Croxatto 1987) (Sivin 1989) (Jonsson et al. 1991). These can be classified into two groups, depending on whether they occur before or after fertilisation:

The known pre-fertilisation effects are (Hagenfeldt 1972) (Stanford and Mikolajczyk 2002):

- inhibition of sperm migration and viability at the level of the cervix, endometrium and fallopian tubes,
- slowing or acceleration of egg transport through the fallopian tubes,
- damage or destruction of the egg prior to fertilisation, accelerating the process of egg apoptosis.

On the other hand, the possible post-fertilisation effects of the IUD are (Stanford and Mikolajczyk 2002):

- slowing or acceleration of embryo transport through the fallopian tubes,

- damage or destruction of the embryo prior to its arrival in the uterus and prevention of implantation (Hagenfeldt 1972).

Therefore, the contraceptive effect of the copper IUD does not respond exclusively to the supposed model of endometrial inflammatory response, with the addition of copper apparently being the main contraceptive agent. Thus, we could think of a cascade of effects occurring after inserting the IUD into the uterus, where once inside the cavity and in contact with bodily fluids, the copper undergoes a process of oxidation, releasing cupric ions, which alter the metabolism of endometrial cells, producing a release of prostaglandins, which modifies tubal motility, hindering the encounter between sperm and eggs. Likewise, the endometrial wall and uterine cervix would be impregnated with copper ions with spermicidal action and a thickening of the cervical mucus that would hinder the migration of sperm towards the uterine cavity (Ortiz, Croxatto, and Bardin 1996).

All of this, combined with the inflammatory reaction to foreign bodies caused by the presence of a foreign body in the endometrial cavity, whose inflammatory reaction appears to be exacerbated by the presence of copper, produces the final contraceptive effect (Cuadros and Hirsch 1972).

In short, the active substances released by Cu-IUDs, together with the products derived from the inflammatory reaction to foreign bodies present in the fluids of the female genital tract, are toxic to sperm and oocytes, preventing the encounter of healthy gametes and the consequent formation of viable embryos (Ortiz and Croxatto 2007).

Cost-Effectiveness of the Copper IUD

Studies conducted in different regions of the world show the high cost-effectiveness of the copper IUD. While it is true that cost-effectiveness depends on the healthcare model, most published studies confirm the high cost-effectiveness of the intrauterine device.

A study published in 2015 by Trusell et al, which aimed to estimate the annual cost of different reversible methods in the U.S. and quantify the minimum duration of use of long-acting methods to achieve cost-effective neutrality compared to short-acting methods, was conducted on a sample of 1,000 women aged 20 to 29 over a period of five years. Taking into account the costs associated with the purchase of the method, its administration and failure (considered as unwanted pregnancy), concluded that the most cost-effective method of all those analysed over a 5-year period of use was the DIU -Cu IUD ($304 per year), followed by the LNG IUD ($308 per year), compared to short-acting methods such as the vaginal ring ($730 per year) or the patch ($748 per year) (Trussell et al. 2015).

Another study published in 2008 by Mavranezouli, which aimed to establish the cost-effectiveness of long-acting contraceptive methods from the perspective of the British National Health Service (NHS), concluded that long-acting contraceptive methods were cost-effective for this health system, with the IUD -Cu being the cheapest contraceptive method, although its cost-effectiveness varied depending on the years of use, being surpassed by the subdermal implant after 15 years of use and by permanent tubal sterilisation after 6 years of use (Mavranezouli and LARC Guideline Development Group 2008).

Previously published studies agree with those described regarding the high cost-effectiveness of the Cu IUD, such as the one published by Chiou et al in 2003, which analysed the cost-effectiveness of nine contraceptive methods in the US over 5 years of use, including modern methods such as the -Cu IUD, the LNG IUD, the quarterly injectable, oral contraceptives, and others such as tubal ligation, the diaphragm, spermicides, the female condom, and the cervical cap. It concluded that the most cost-effective methods were the LNG IUD and the Cu IUD, with bilateral tubal ligation being slightly more effective but at a much higher cost than IUDs (Chiou et al. 2003). However, the Cu IUD as an emergency contraceptive method does not appear to be cost-effective initially, but it is if its use continues beyond emergency contraception (Trussell et al. 1997).

Effectiveness of the Cu IUD

The Cu IUD is considered the third most effective reversible method currently available, with an average failure rate of 0.8 pregnancies per 100 users in one year of Cu-IUD use (Illustration), compared to a failure rate of 0.5 per 100 women who undergo irreversible bilateral tubal ligation (Trussell et al. 2015).

In addition, the copper IUD is the most effective emergency contraception method currently available (Mierzejewska et al. 2024) and is not affected by enzyme-inducing drugs or weight/body mass index (BMI). However, higher BMI is associated with an increased risk of IUD expulsion (Anthony et al. 2022).

The effectiveness of the IUD, measured as the percentage of unwanted pregnancies among users of the device, varies in published studies depending on the IUD model, the size of the sample analysed, and the follow-up period. In general, and for high-dose Cu IUDs, these figures range from 0% to 2.9% (Thonneau et al. 2008). In other studies that analyse this percentage in a non-randomised manner, we find figures of up to 5% for unwanted pregnancies during use (Tugrul et al. 2005).

According to a review conducted by the Cochrane Database Systematic Reviews in 2007, which compared 10 different types of IUDs in approximately 48,000 women, the most effective Cu-IUDs were T-shaped with 380 mm2 of copper, with additional copper bands on the arms, mainly the TCu-380 A and S models. The cumulative pregnancy rates of the different IUDs analysed were 0.5% to 2.2% for those with a copper surface area of less than 300 mm2, and 0.1% to 1.0% for those with a copper surface area greater than or equal to 300 mm2 during the first year of use. After 12 years of use, the cumulative pregnancy rate was 5.8% for the TCu220 compared to 2.2% for the TCu380A. Of all the IUDs analysed, the TCU380 A and S had the lowest pregnancy rates and the greatest durability, minimising the need for replacement and therefore the problems associated with it (Kulier et al. 2006).

On the other hand, it appears that the Cu-IUD is as effective and safe in nulliparous women as in women who have given birth at least once (Dueñas et al. 1996). Furthermore, the safety and efficacy of the method has been demonstrated in women who have recently given birth or had an abortion (Sonalkar and Kapp 2015) and even in those who have had immediate insertion during a caesarean section (Al Safty et al. 2022).

Factors That Can Alter the Effectiveness of the IUD

There are several factors that can influence the contraceptive effectiveness of copper intrauterine devices. The main ones are:

- Surface area and distribution of copper in the device: the higher the copper content of the device, the greater its contraceptive effectiveness and the longer it lasts. Copper IUDs with a copper surface area equal to or greater than 380 mm2 are, after LNG IUDs, the most effective intrauterine devices. The distribution of copper on the surface of the device also seems to influence its effectiveness, with maximum effectiveness in T-shaped devices in which the copper is not only wound around the central stem but also around the vertical arms, reaching the edges of their distal ends (O'Brien et al. 2008).
- Age of the user. Generally, the spontaneous fertility rate decreases as a woman's age increases. Fertility declines mainly from the age of 32 and exponentially from the age of 37 (Johnson, Tough, and SOGC Genetics committee 2012), from which we can deduce that any method is more likely to fail at younger ages, and the IUD does not appear to be an exception. Therefore, from the age of 40 onwards, the effectiveness of the Cu IUD is considered to be at its maximum, and it is justified to keep a Cu IUD in place until the patient no longer requires contraception (extended use).
- On the other hand, there is limited evidence reporting an increased risk of Cu-IUD expulsion in young women and adolescents, regardless of parity, these being possible factors influencing the effectiveness of the device in these age groups (Madden et al. 2014).
- Parity: there is consistent scientific evidence to suggest that the effectiveness of Cu IUDs is similar in nulliparous or nulligravid women compared to those who have already had children, with no increased risk of pelvic inflammatory disease or expulsion, although there is a risk of pain and difficulty during insertion. Despite this, most insertions in this group are successful and well tolerated. Similarly, menstrual bleeding in nulliparous users of copper IUDs may be heavier, without increasing the risk of perforation during insertion (Madden et al. 2014).
- Training or experience of the healthcare personnel performing the insertion: the device should be inserted in the presence of a trained clinician who can supervise and monitor the woman's specific characteristics or conditions and who can assist her in the event of a complication during insertion (FSRH 2023).
- Expulsion rate. This rate may vary depending on the type or model of the Cu IUD. In the Cochrane review published in 2010, which analysed 35 studies comparing 10 IUD models in more than 48,000 users, the Tcu380A model had a higher expulsion rate than other models. However, this particular model proved to be the most effective of all those compared in the review (O'Brien et al. 2008). In a secondary analysis of the ongoing, prospective, non-interventional European Active Surveillance Study on LCS12 (EURAS-LCS12), it was concluded that the risk of expulsion after insertion of a copper IUD is related to the shape, with the Nova-T and Tatum models presenting the lowest risk (Boehnke et al. 2024).

Extended Use of Copper IUD

The Cu-IUDs currently available are licensed for either 5 or 10 years of use. Most scientific societies support extended use of the Cu-IUD when inserted at age 40 years or over and in some IUD models this age is set at 35 years old. A Cu-IUD containing ≥300 mm^2 copper inserted at or after age 40 years can be used for contraception until menopause. Menopause can be diagnosed 1 year after the final menstrual period if this occurs when the individual is age 50 years or older (NICE 2014) ('FSRH 2023) (Black et al. 2016).

This recommendation is based on observations made by different authors, who confirm the effectiveness of multiple models of copper IUDs beyond the manufacturer's recommendations. Thus, a published review of the extended or prolonged use of different existing IUD models concluded that there is evidence to recommend extended use in parous (or multiparous) women aged at least 25 years at the time of insertion of the TCu 380 A and TCu 220 models for at least 12 years, the Multiload Cu-375® for 10 years, and the GyneFix® for 9 years. On the other hand, women aged at least 35 years at the time of insertion of the TCu 380 A model could continue with the same device until menopause without needing to change to a new device (Wu and Pickle 2014).

This conservative approach to prolonged IUD use offers multiple advantages, such as user comfort, cost savings, and the extension of the non-contraceptive benefits of the devices, as well as those derived from avoiding the various possible risks associated with reinserting a new device, as described above.

Recommendations Prior to Insertion

Time of Insertion

The copper IUD can be inserted at any time during the menstrual cycle, provided that pregnancy can be reasonably ruled out, as pregnancy is an absolute contraindication for its insertion. In fact, a systematic review published in 2013 concluded that continuation rates, effectiveness, and safety were not better when a copper IUD was inserted during menstruation, and requiring a woman to be menstruating could represent a barrier to access (Whiteman et al. 2013).

The criteria for reasonably ruling out pregnancy, according to the British Faculty of Sexual and Reproductive Health ('FSRH Guideline (March 2023) Intrauterine Contraception' 2023a) and the US Selected Practice Recommendations for Contraceptive Use (Curtis et al. 2024), include one or more of the following criteria, provided there are no symptoms or signs of pregnancy:

- Has no sexual intercourse since the start of the last normal (natural) menstrual period, since childbirth, abortion, miscarriage, ectopic pregnancy or uterine evacuation for gestational trophoblastic disease.
- Is, correctly and consistently, using a reliable method of contraception. (Barrier methods of contraception can be considered reliable providing that they have been used consistently and correctly for every episode of intercourse.)
- Is ≤ 7 days of the onset of a normal (natural) menstrual period. They are less than 21 days postpartum (non-breastfeeding individuals*)*.
- Is fully breastfeeding or nearly fully breastfeeding (exclusively breastfeeding or the vast majority [≥85%] of feeds are breastfeeds), amenorrhoeic ***and*** less than 6 months' postpartum.
- Is ≤ 7 days after spontaneous or induced first or second trimester abortion, miscarriage, ectopic pregnancy or uterine evacuation for gestational trophoblastic disease.

- No sexual intercourse for >21 days ***and*** have a negative high-sensitivity urine pregnancy test (able to detect human chorionic gonadotrophin (hCG) levels around 20 mIU/ml).

Medical History, Examination and Information Prior to Insertion

Prior to IUD insertion, the user should be asked about her menstrual pattern (amount and duration of bleeding) and whether she suffers from dysmenorrhoea, including aspects of her sexuality and that of her current partner, in order to assess the risk of sexually transmitted infections (STIs). The user should also be examined to rule out genital malformations and signs of active genital infection that would contraindicate insertion. It is also important to measure the uterine cavity (either by ultrasound or hysterometry) to reduce the risk of perforation and low insertion of the device. In addition, she should be properly informed about:

- Characteristics of the method.
- Type of IUD: choose one that offers longer-lasting contraceptive efficacy, as this will reduce the risks associated with the reinsertion process (infection, perforation, and expulsion) (Lee et al. 1983).
- Insertion process and complications that may arise during it, follow-up, duration of its effect. All of this will be adequately specified in the informed consent form.
- Possible changes in menstrual patterns such as prolonged and heavy menstruation, irregular bleeding and cramps or pain during menstruation, which are usually temporary and usually disappear after 3-6 months of use (Tietze C; Lewit S 1972). Conveying this information to the user is essential to encourage adherence to the method.
- All users should be warned that the IUD does not protect against the transmission of sexually transmitted infections.

We must explain and complete the informed consent form correctly. The patient must read and sign it to legitimise the insertion. The implementation of the informed consent form in the clinical process of IUD insertion is essential to respect the patient's autonomy, minimise risks, address clinical consequences, and comply with legal responsibilities (Enjezab et al. 2023).

Potential users should be warned that, although most insertions are associated with mild to moderate pain or discomfort, pain can range from none to severe. Analgesia options should be discussed and offered to all patients, and an assistant should be present to help the person during the insertion procedure and monitor them for any signs of pain or distress. Although there is no optimal anaesthesia/analgesia option for IUD insertion, paracervical block, intracervical injection of local anaesthetic, 10% lidocaine spray, or a cream containing 2.5% lidocaine plus 2.5% prilocaine applied to the cervix appear to be beneficial in reducing pain related to insertion ('FSRH Guideline (March 2023) Intrauterine Contraception' 2023a).

Screening for Sexually Transmitted Infections

Screening for sexually transmitted infections (mainly Chlamydia trachomatis and Neisseria gonorrhoeae) in asymptomatic women is not routinely necessary prior to IUD insertion, except in users at high risk for STIs: women ≤ 25 years of age who have not been screened in the previous year or women 25 years of age or older who are at increased risk for chlamydial and gonococcal infections (if they have a new partner, more than one sex partner, a sex partner with concurrent partners, or a sex partner who has an STI; practice inconsistent condom use when not in a mutually monogamous relationship; have a previous or coexisting STI; have a history of exchanging sex for money or drugs; or have a history of incarceration) (US Preventive Services Task Force et al. 2021) (Workowski et al. 2021).

In cases where genital cultures are taken prior to insertion, it would not be justified to delay insertion while awaiting the results. If the results are positive for chlamydial infection or gonorrhoea, the infection should be treated without removing the IUD (Committee on Practice Bulletins-Gynecology, Long-Acting Reversible Contraception Work Group 2017) ('FSRH 2023).

The insertion of an intrauterine device is contraindicated in women with current purulent cervicitis or known infection with chlamydia or gonorrhoea (US MEC Category 4) (Nguyen et al. 2024) (Curtis et al. 2024). Although the optimal timing for IUD insertion among women treated for cervical infections is unclear, it is advisable to delay IUD insertion until treatment is complete, symptoms have resolved, cervical examination results appear normal, and bimanual examination reveals no masses or tenderness. Due to the high risk of reinfection, the CDC recommends repeat testing at 3 months for women who have been treated for gonorrhoea or chlamydia (Workowski et al. 2021).

Antibiotic prophylaxis prior to insertion is not necessary except in users with complicated valvular disease (pulmonary hypertension, risk of atrial fibrillation, or history of subacute bacterial endocarditis), in which case prophylactic antibiotic therapy is recommended (Grimes and Schulz 2001) (ACOG 2017).

Recommendations After Insertion

No additional contraceptive method is required after insertion of a copper IUD (Committee on Practice Bulletins-Gynecology, LARC Work Group 2017).

In general, routine checks are not necessary after insertion of a Cu-IUD. The WHO and other organisations recommend a single follow-up visit after the first menstruation or 3-12 weeks after insertion (FSRH March 2023). This follow-up visit allows for the exclusion of infection and expulsion, an assessment of bleeding patterns, an assessment of patient and partner satisfaction, a clinical examination and string check, and an opportunity to reinforce the issue of condom use for protection against STIs and HIV. After this visit, a woman using an IUC should continue well-woman care as for any sexually active woman. An exception would be cases of IUDs inserted within 48 hours of delivery, where a follow-up visit with a clinician is recommended 4-6 weeks after insertion, as insertion during this period is associated with a higher risk of expulsion and long or non-visible strings. This visit also serves to clarify doubts or discomforts related to the IUD. Vaginal examination is not necessary unless infection or IUD expulsion is suspected to verify it. Subsequently, no further routine visits are necessary, only those recommended by the current health programs.

However, it is desirable to be able to consult a doctor at any time if you notice a problem or have any questions about the use of the IUD. Women who use an intrauterine device should be advised to contact their healthcare provider if any of the following occurs: She cannot feel the IUD strings:

- She or her partner can feel the lower part of the IUD.
- She thinks she is pregnant. She uses a Cu-IUD and is amenorrheic.
- She experiences persistent abdominal pain, fever, or unusual vaginal discharge.
- She or her partner feel pain or discomfort during intercourse.
- She experiences a sudden change in her menstrual periods.
- She wishes to have the device removed or wishes to conceive.

If a woman using an IUC wishes to switch from an IUC to a hormonal method of contraception, she should start the hormonal contraceptive 1 week before removing the IUC. If a woman wishes to have a new IUC inserted, the new IUC can be inserted at the same time that the old IUC is being removed. Women using an IUC who request a tubal ligation should be advised to use condoms and/or abstain from vaginal intercourse for 7 days prior to the tubal ligation if the IUC is to be removed at the same time.

If the user experiences abdominal discomfort or pain in the days following insertion, this can be treated with standard painkillers (paracetamol, metamizole, ibuprofen or any commonly used non-steroidal anti-inflammatory drug).

Contraindications for IUD Use

Contraindications are defined as conditions in which the use of contraception may be more harmful than an unwanted pregnancy. The use of IUDs as a method of contraception has few contraindications (Nelson 2007).

The WHO and the CDC have developed guidelines that classify different medical conditions into four categories, based on the level of risk posed by the use of different contraceptive methods in each case (WHO 2015) (Nguyen et al. 2024) (Curtis et al. 2024).

Thus, according to the WHO classification, for the use of the Cu IUD, these would be:

Category 4, and therefore absolute contraindications for IUD use (in cases marked with an asterisk, if the woman already has a copper IUD when each specific situation arises, it is not necessary to remove the IUD immediately, but rather the device can continue to be used, even if it would be a contraindication for starting the method in these cases):

- Pregnancy.
- Pelvic inflammatory disease (chlamydia or gonorrhoea) or purulent cervicitis at present*.
- Puerperal sepsis.
- Immediately after a septic abortion.

- Anatomical abnormality or myomatosis distorting the uterine cavity*.
- Abnormal vaginal bleeding that has not been identified, when a serious condition is suspected*.
- Endometrial or cervical cancer awaiting treatment*.
- Malignant gestational trophoblastic disease or persistently elevated
- βhCG levels: until human chorionic gonadotropin (hCG) levels are normal because of a theoretical increased risk of uterine perforation and dissemination of the tumour by the insertion of the IUC
- Pelvic tuberculosis*.
- Wilson's disease or allergy to any of the components of the Cu IUD.

Category 3, and therefore situations in which the method is not recommended unless other more appropriate methods are not available or are not accepted:

- Solid organ transplant with complications.
- Gestational trophoblastic disease with decreasing or undetectable βhCG levels.
- Severe or advanced HIV disease*.
- Postpartum (after the first 48 hours up to 4 weeks). (If the woman already has a Cu IUD, it is not necessary to remove the IUD immediately, and she may continue to use it).

Risks, Complications, and Side Effects of the Copper IUD

The main drawbacks of using this contraceptive method are the possible side effects or complications that may arise during and after insertion.

Complications During Insertion of the Device

Vasovagal Reaction

Cervical stimulation during IUD insertion may cause a vasovagal response, presyncope, syncope, nausea, bradycardia, and hypotension. The frequency of occurrence of these phenomena is estimated to be around 1 in 100 insertions. In healthy women, most reactions are transient and resolve spontaneously. The Trendelenburg position, a cold compress or cloth on the head, neck or chest, and an alcohol pad under the nose to distract and treat nausea may be beneficial. In rare circumstances, the vasovagal reaction may be severe enough to require intravenous (IV) fluid support and/or atropine (0.4 to 0.6 mL IV) to improve symptoms and vital signs. In these circumstances, continuous individualised monitoring should be performed (Gillian Dean G, Goldberg AB., n.d.).

Uterine Perforation

Uterine perforation is a rare complication with a high potential for severity, occurring in 0.3 to 2.2 per 1,000 insertions according to published data. It can be partial (if it does not penetrate the uterine serosa) or complete (if it penetrates all layers of the uterine wall), causing visceral damage, infection or haemorrhage (Heinemann et al. 2017). Most perforations occur at the time of insertion, with delayed perforation, a process known as IUD migration, being much less common.

The factors that appear to be most closely associated with an increased risk of uterine perforation are: the healthcare provider's experience in inserting devices, cervical stenosis, breastfeeding (which increases the risk sixfold), and insertion within the first 6–9 months after delivery (Heinemann, Reed, Moehner, and Do Minh 2015) (Caliskan et al. 2003) (Harrison-Woolrych et al. 2003) (Kaislasuo et al. 2012) (Andersson et al. 1998) (Heinemann, Reed, Moehner, and Minh 2015) (Heinemann et al. 2017).

However, there does not appear to be any difference in the rate of perforation between the different IUD models analyzed, and it is unclear, according to a Cochrane systematic review, whether armless IUDs are associated with a higher rate of perforation (O'Brien et al. 2008) (O'Brien and Marfleet 2005).

Complications Following Insertion or During Use of the Device

Post-Insertion Bleeding and Menstrual Changes

Most women experience some degree of spotting or genital bleeding immediately after insertion of the Cu-IUD, which may be due to minor cervical trauma during insertion, either from the material used for insertion or from the device itself.

The amount of menstrual bleeding increases in Cu-IUD users by up to 55%. However, in most users there are no significant changes in serum ferritin levels or anemia due to a compensatory increase in the body's absorption of intestinal iron (Milsom et al. 1995) (Black et al. 2016) (Larsson et al. 1993) (Lowe and Prata 2013).

Menstrual changes such as increased menstrual bleeding and longer periods, as well as intermenstrual bleeding, are common side effects during the months following insertion of the copper IUD and decrease over time, especially after the first 6 months of use (Tessa Madden, MD, MPH, n.d.).

Pelvic Pain and Dysmenorrhoea

During the first few days after insertion of an intrauterine device, regardless of the type, women may experience pelvic pain and cramps, which usually subside spontaneously or with commonly used painkillers such as paracetamol or non-steroidal anti-inflammatory drugs (Gillian Dean G, Goldberg AB., n.d.).

However, along with menstrual changes, pelvic pain is the most common reason for discontinuing or abandoning the method (between 4-15% of devices are removed for both reasons during the first year of use) (Grunloh et al. 2013) (Nelson and Massoudi 2016). In turn, the use of copper IUDs may be associated with an increase in dysmenorrhoea, which is more prevalent in nulliparous women, with removal for this reason being more frequent in this group (Caddy et al. 2014).

Pelvic Inflammatory Disease

The main germs involved in the pathogenesis of PID are Chlamydia trachomatis and Neisseria Gonorrhoeae, which are often asymptomatic. Without treatment, up to 30% of these cervical infections will cause ascending pelvic inflammatory disease.

For a long time, it was believed that IUDs increased the risk of pelvic inflammatory disease as a result of certain observational studies that overestimated this risk. However, the available evidence from clinical trials and systematic reviews refutes this relationship. On the one hand, as mentioned above, in the past, IUDs with multifilament threads did seem to promote the ascent of germs into the uterine cavity, causing numerous ascending infections with disastrous results. Once the use of this type of thread was eliminated, various well-designed studies have shown that IUD use is not associated with a substantial increase in the risk of PID, except at the time of insertion and, apparently, in the presence of an undiagnosed STI.

In 1992, Farley et al., members of the WHO's Special Programme of Research and Development in Human Reproduction in Switzerland, published a review study analyzing the risk of PID within a clinical trial conducted by that organization, which analyzed 22,908 IUD insertions with the aim of establishing the incidence and risk of PID during use. The result was 1.6 cases per 1,000 women/years of use, with a higher incidence in the first 20 days of use compared to later stages (9.7 vs. 1.4 per 1,000 women/years, respectively) once adjusted for confounding factors (Farley et al. 1992).

In these first few days after insertion, it appears that manipulation may promote the ascent of pre-existing germs into the endometrial cavity, considering that the risk of PID attributable to the IUD during this period is 1%, with a risk of 0.54% in the first 90 days after insertion (Sufrin and Averbach 2014). Therefore, it would be exposure to sexually transmitted diseases and not the use of the IUD itself that is responsible for PID during the first month of IUD use (Black et al. 2016). For this reason, it is recommended to avoid replacing the IUD before its expiration date, thus avoiding unnecessary removals or insertions, provided that there are no contrainications to continuing its use and the user wishes to continue using it.

A review of recent literature by Jatlaoui et al., which aimed to establish the risk of PID in women with asymptomatic cervicitis or a high risk of acquiring an STI, in women with IUDs compared to women without IUDs, concluded that there was no increase in PID in the group of IUD users and therefore, although scientific evidence is limited, it is not advisable to restrict the use of this contraceptive method in these groups of women (Jatlaoui et al. 2016). Other scientific publications, such as those derived from the CHOICE project carried out in the USA, support this recommendation, obtaining PID rates of less than 1% in women with positive screening for Chlamydia trachomatis and/or Neisseria Gonorrhoeae in IUD users, with no differences compared to users of other contraceptive methods (Birgisson et al. 2015).

Therefore, based on existing evidence, when considering a patient who is a candidate for starting Cu-IUD use, an assessment or screening for sexually transmitted diseases (STDs) should be performed through a proper medical history and pelvic examination prior to the examination. According to the CDC and the United States Preventive Services Task Force (USPSTF), only women at high risk for STDs should undergo laboratory screening for Chlamydia trachomatis and gonorrhoeae, including those ≤ 25 years of age who have not been screened in the previous year, and women with behavioral risk factors, such as previous or current sexually transmitted disease, new or multiple male sexual partners, inconsistent condom use, having sex under the influence of alcohol or drugs, or having sex in exchange for money or drugs (Sufrin and Averbach 2014). In asymptomatic patients who require laboratory screening due to high risk of STIs, insertion would not be delayed; rather, insertion would be performed during the same visit, and in the event of positive results, treatment would be provided as soon as the results were available (Caddy et al. 2014) ('FSRH 2023). However, in accordance with the WHO Medical Eligibility Criteria for Contraceptives, in women in whom physical examination reveals mucopurulent cervicitis or clinical signs of PID, insertion of the device should be delayed until treatment has been completed and laboratory tests have confirmed resolution of the condition, as purulent cervicitis at the time of insertion is a contraindication for insertion (WHO 2015).

On the other hand, a systematic review by the Cochrane Collaboration found no benefit in performing antibiotic prophylaxis prior to IUD insertion, except, as pointed out in the guide "Recommendations on selected practices for contraceptive use" published by the WHO in 2018, in cases where there is a high prevalence of STIs and access to STI screening tests is limited (WHO. 2018) (Grimes and Schulz 2001). In addition, it is currently recommended that in the case of a diagnosis of PID in a woman with an IUD, the device should not be removed if the woman wishes to continue with the IUD, as there is no additional benefit and there is strong evidence that removal could worsen the course of the disease (Tepper et al. 2013). If removal is necessary, it is recommended that it always be done after the start of antibiotic treatment (WHO 2018).

Finally, regarding the risk of vulvovaginal infections, according to the review conducted by the FSRH guidelines in 2023, the Cu IUD has been identified as a possible risk factor for acute and recurrent candidal vulvovaginitis (CVV) (Farr et al. 2021) (Gonçalves et al. 2016) ('FSRH 2023). Apparently, yeasts could adhere to IUDs and produce a biofilm that facilitates recurrent CVV by protecting the yeasts from antifungal agents (Auler et al. 2010). However, there is no consistent evidence that IUDs are associated with an increased incidence of lower genital tract infections. In fact, a recent study analyzing the effects of Cu-IUDs and LNG-IUDs on the vaginal microbiota found no changes in the microbiota after one year of device use, nor did it find any differences in the effects of the two types of IUDs (Bassis et al. 2017). Similarly, there does not appear to be a relationship between the use of the Cu-IUD and an increased risk of bacterial vaginosis (Meirik 2007).

Expulsion and Descent of the IUD

Another possible complication that may arise during IUD use is expulsion. This occurs in 3-6% of cases during the first year of use, and most frequently in the first 3 months (Faculty of Sexual & Reproductive Healthcare 2023) (Curtis et al. 2024).

Traditionally, it was considered that 'properly positioned' IUDs should be located at a maximum distance of 3 cm from the uterine fundus. It was believed that in cases where this distance was greater, there was an increased risk of malposition, expulsion, pain and bleeding. However, these definitions of correct intrauterine position have been questioned as a result of research and knowledge of the migratory patterns of the IUD during the weeks following insertion. It is now known that after insertion, the position of the device within the cavity is fluid, establishing a stable position approximately 3 months after insertion (Evans et al. 2019)..

Currently, for an IUD to be considered correctly positioned in the uterine cavity, it has been established that the distal end of the device must be above the internal cervical os, or in other words, located within the uterine cavity, regardless of the distance to the uterine fundus (Graupera et al. 2012). In this regard, a distinction must be made between expulsion of the device and its descent. In the former case, the IUD leaves the uterine cavity and may even be lost without the wearer noticing when she stops wearing it, thus leading to a situation of absence of contraception and causing unexpected pregnancies. When the IUD descends, it moves distally through the cervix without leaving the cavity completely. This is important because an expelled IUD completely loses its contraceptive capacity, but a descended IUD appears to continue to preserve this capacity to some extent, although it is not very clear how effective it is.

In a review of the literature published in 2015 by Golightly et al, the consequences in terms of efficacy and safety of descent and/or malposition of devices in the uterine cavity were analysed, among other things, concluding that the clinical impact of these findings by ultrasound is often uncertain, with the approach to be followed varying. Given the high frequency of incidental findings of IUD descent and data indicating that devices move within the uterine cavity at different times of the cycle, immediate replacement is not considered necessary, and an individualised approach is recommended for asymptomatic patients in each case. Thus, different options are worth considering, namely: a wait-and-see approach and subsequent re-evaluation with or without additional contraceptive coverage, attempting to modify the position of the device with forceps, replacing the device with a new one while warning the woman that a new descent may occur, or removing the IUD and considering a different contraceptive method. However, in symptomatic women, despite the lack of sufficient evidence to link the symptoms to device descent or malposition, the tendency is to remove the device. Particular caution should be exercised in young women and those with a history of previous device descent, as in these cases the risk of descent and therefore of an unwanted pregnancy appears to be increased (Golightly and Gebbie 2014).

The main risk factors for IUD expulsion appear to be age under 25, insertion after childbirth or second-trimester abortion, and heavy menstrual bleeding or dysmenorrhoea (Madden et al. 2014) (Diedrich et al. 2017) (Patchen and Berggren 2011) (Bayer et al. 2012) (Okusanya et al. 2014) (Zhang et al. 1992).

There is controversy regarding how the type of device influences the risk of expulsion. A Cochrane systematic review published in 2007 found no significant differences between more than 10 types of classic IUDs (with arms or, in English, framed) in terms of expulsion rates. However, another review by the same organisation published in 2005, which compared frameless IUDs with classic IUDs, showed that the former may have a higher expulsion rate in the first year than the latter, which was equal to or better than the classic IUDs after the first year of use, but without significant differences, coinciding in some ways with the results obtained from a randomised clinical trial published in 2009 by Meirik et al., which compared, among other aspects, the efficacy and expulsion rate between the Cu 380A and GyneFix®, where the latter had a higher expulsion and pregnancy rate in the first year of use, but a lower pregnancy rate between the second and eighth years of use. Similarly, and as described in the section on IUD effectiveness and factors that could affect this effectiveness, a subsequent Cochrane study published in 2010, which compared 10 models of IUDs with arms, described a higher expulsion rate with the TCu 380A model, which was also the most effective of all those analysed in the review (O'Brien and Marfleet 2005) (Kulier et al. 2006) (Meirik et al. 2009).

Pregnancy with an IUD

Despite its high effectiveness, as previously described, failures of the method may occur during use of the copper IUD, resulting in unwanted pregnancies, with an approximate frequency of 0.8 pregnancies per 100 users per year of use. Most failures tend to occur during the first year of use of the device, and many of them are a direct consequence of a decrease in effectiveness or inadvertent expulsion of the device.

Intrauterine Pregnancy

Leading scientific institutions and societies (WHO, American College of Obstetricians and Gynaecologists, CDC, FDA, etc.) recommend removing the IUD within the first 12 weeks of pregnancy whenever possible, if the IUD strings are visible through the external cervical os or if the IUD is visible in the cervical canal, as continuing a pregnancy with an IUD in place can increase maternal and foetal risks in up to 60% of cases, compared to 36% in patients who have it removed at the beginning of pregnancy (Ozgu-Erdinc et al. 2014). Although removal of the IUD early in pregnancy reduces the associated risks, it does not eliminate them completely.

The main risks that are increased in pregnancies in the presence of an IUD are as follows:

- Corioamnionitis. Early removal of the IUD appears to reduce the risk, although it does not eliminate it (Kim et al. 2010) (Ganer et al. 2009).
- Increased rates of intra-amniotic infection by Candida spp. A review of the literature published in 2017 analysed 123 published cases of chorioamnionitis caused by Candida spp, of which 26 (21.1%) were related to the presence of an intrauterine device and concomitant pregnancy (Kim et al. 2010) (Maki et al. 2017).
- Abortion, including septic and late abortion (Ozgu-Erdinc et al. 2014) (Kim et al. 2010). Up to 50-60% of pregnancies with IUDs end in spontaneous abortion. This percentage is higher in situations where the IUD remains in place (Inal et al. 2005). Early removal of the IUD appears to be associated with a reduced risk of abortion in the first trimester.
- Preterm birth. Early removal of the IUD also appears to reduce the risk of preterm delivery associated with IUD pregnancy (Ozgu-Erdinc et al. 2014) (Kim et al. 2010) (Ganer et al. 2009).
- Premature detachment of the placenta or abruptio placentae. There appears to be an increased risk in pregnancies with IUDs (Kim et al. 2010).
- Worsening of perinatal outcomes compared to pregnancies without IUDs, resulting from the complications described, including low birth weight (Kim et al. 2010) (Ganer et al. 2009).

If the IUD strings are not visible and the patient wishes to continue with the pregnancy, in addition to informing her of the associated risks, the IUD can be removed under ultrasound guidance using special forceps. Studies have reported an abortion rate of 22% in these cases, which is comparable to the rate associated with device removal when the threads are visible (Schiesser et al. 2004). In fact, different case series have shown remarkably successful results with hysteroscopic removal, with abortion rates much lower than those described with manual removal (Sanders et al. 2016).

If the IUD is not visible on ultrasound during pregnancy or delivery, an abdominal X-ray will be performed after delivery to rule out migration of the device into the abdominal cavity.

Ectopic Pregnancy

The absolute risk of pregnancy, and therefore of ectopic pregnancy, is considerably reduced with the use of the copper IUD compared to non-users of contraception. However, in the event of pregnancy with an IUD, the risk of it being ectopic increases compared to other contraceptive methods. Thus, according to published studies, the rate of ectopic pregnancy in Cu-IUD users is 1.02/1000 women/year for Cu-IUD users compared to 2.6/1000 women/year for non-users of contraception (Franks et al. 1990). Therefore, the IUD does not increase the risk of ectopic pregnancy (EP), but rather its proportion.

Continuation with the Cu IUD as a Contraceptive Method

The copper intrauterine device enjoys high continuation rates among users. According to the results of several published studies focusing on the analysis of this parameter, these continuation rates are around 78-84.5% in the first year of use, 55%-85% in the second year of use, and 32.6-45% in the fifth year of use (Peipert et al. 2011) (Phillips et al. 2017) (Rosenstock et al. 2012) (Jenabi et al. 2006) (Fleming et al. 1998) (Diedrich et al. 2015). This places the Cu IUD among the three reversible contraceptive methods with the highest continuation rates, along with the LNG IUD and the subdermal implant.

It could be that, according to data obtained in different publications, these continuation rates are affected by variables such as the age of users and parity, with lower continuation rates among younger users and nulliparous women. This lower continuation rate seems to be mainly related to poorer tolerance of the method or its possible side effects, making it essential to provide adequate contraceptive counseling to these groups of users, informing them in detail of the possible or expected changes in their menstrual pattern and the appearance of abdominal discomfort or intensification of dysmenorrhea in the first months of use of the device (Jenabi et al. 2006) (Aoun et al. 2014).

Despite this, according to a systematic review conducted by Usinger et al, published in 2016, which studied adherence to the method in women under 25 years of age, it concluded that continuation with the Cu IUD after 12 months of use was higher in this age group compared to other short-term reversible methods (85% Cu IUD -Cu, compared to 39.6% oral contraceptives, 39.8% depo-provera injections, 39.8% patches, 48.9% vaginal rings), finding no statistically significant differences with other LARCs such as the subdermal implant (85.3%) (Usinger et al. 2016). Subsequently, in 2017, Diedrich et al. published a systematic review and meta-analysis to evaluate LARC continuation in the adolescent population in a sample of more than 4,886 women under the age of 25, confirming high continuation rates with IUD -Cu and implants in this population, higher than those of other LARCs (Diedrich et al. 2017).

Return to Fertility

Various studies show that the use of the copper IUD does not reduce fertility after use (Hov et al. 2007) (Skjeldestad and Bratt 1987). According to the literature, pregnancy rates one year after removal of the copper IUD are similar to those after removal or discontinuation of other modern contraceptive methods, such as the subdermal implant, oral contraceptives, the LNG IUD, or barrier methods, with these rates remaining between approximately 70% and 90%, regardless of parity (Mansour et al. 2011) (Stoddard et al. 2015) (Delbarge et al. 2002) (Struthers 1991).

Conclusion

The copper IUD is a long-standing, highly effective method and the most cost-effective of all currently available contraceptive methods. It has high continuation rates, and since it does not contain hormones, it is particularly suitable for users who have contraindications for hormone use and those who do not wish to use hormones.

Its long-lasting contraceptive effect, the possibility of starting immediately after childbirth or abortion, and the possibility of extended use in users aged 40 or older make it an ideal method after childbirth/abortion and especially in the last years of a woman's fertile life, although there are no contraindications for its use due to age or parity.

The risks of insertion and side effects are rare, although not entirely absent. Furthermore, given the absence of hormones in its structure, it has very few contraindications for use, which must be known in order to avoid complications. Given the changes in the menstrual pattern at the beginning of its use, it is crucial to provide potential users with all the relevant information in order to increase adherence and continuation with the method.

References

Advisory Comitee on obstetrics and gynecology. Food and drug administration. 1968. 'Report on Intrauterine Contraceptive Devices'. January.

Al Safty, Ahmed, Abdel Monem Zakaria, and Ahmed Saeed. 2022. 'Efficacy of Immediate Insertion of an Intrauterine Contraceptive Device during Cesarean Section in Comparison with Late Insertion after the Puerperium'. *Al-Azhar International Medical Journal* 0 (0): 0–0. https://doi.org/10.21608/aimj.2023.143720.1982.

Andersson, K., E. Ryde-Blomqvist, K. Lindell, V. Odlind, and I. Milsom. 1998. 'Perforations with Intrauterine Devices. Report from a Swedish Survey'. *Contraception* 57 (4): 251–55.

Anthony, Mary S., Xiaolei Zhou, Juliane Schoendorf, et al. 2022. 'Demographic, Reproductive, and Medical Risk Factors for Intrauterine Device Expulsion'. *Obstetrics & Gynecology* 140 (6): 1017–30. https://doi.org/10.1097/AOG.0000000000005000.

Aoun, Joelle, Virginia A. Dines, Dale W. Stovall, Mihriye Mete, Casey B. Nelson, and Veronica Gomez-Lobo. 2014. 'Effects of Age, Parity, and Device Type on Complications and Discontinuation of Intrauterine Devices'. *Obstetrics and Gynecology* 123 (3): 585–92. https://doi.org/10.1097/AOG.0000000000000144.

Arcangues, Catherine d'. 2007. 'Worldwide Use of Intrauterine Devices for Contraception'. *Contraception* 75 (6 Suppl): S2-7. https://doi.org/10.1016/j.contraception.2006.12.024.

Auler, Marcos E., Debora Morreira, Fabio F. O. Rodrigues, et al. 2010. 'Biofilm Formation on Intrauterine Devices in Patients with Recurrent Vulvovaginal Candidiasis'. *Medical Mycology* 48 (1): 211–16. https://doi.org/10.3109/13693780902856626.

Bassis, Christine M., Jenifer E. Allsworth, Heather N. Wahl, Daniel E. Sack, Vincent B. Young, and Jason D. Bell. 2017. 'Effects of Intrauterine Contraception on the Vaginal Microbiota'. *Contraception* 96 (3): 189–95. https://doi.org/10.1016/j.contraception.2017.05.017.

Bayer, Lisa L., Jeffrey T. Jensen, Hong Li, Mark D. Nichols, and Paula H. Bednarek. 2012. 'Adolescent Experience with Intrauterine Device Insertion and Use: A Retrospective Cohort Study'. *Contraception* 86 (5): 443–51. https://doi.org/10.1016/j.contraception.2012.03.014.

Birgisson, Natalia E., Qiuhong Zhao, Gina M. Secura, Tessa Madden, and Jeffrey F. Peipert. 2015. 'Positive Testing for Neisseria Gonorrhoeae and Chlamydia Trachomatis and the Risk of Pelvic Inflammatory Disease in IUD Users'. *Journal of Women's Health (2002)* 24 (5): 354–59. https://doi.org/10.1089/jwh.2015.5190.

Black, Amanda, Edith Guilbert, Dustin Costescu, et al. 2016. 'Canadian Contraception Consensus (Part 3 of 4): Chapter 7--Intrauterine Contraception'. *Journal of Obstetrics and Gynaecology Canada: JOGC =*

Journal d'obstetrique et Gynecologie Du Canada: JOGC 38 (2): 182–222. https://doi.org/10.1016/j.jogc.2015.12.002.

Boehnke, Tanja, Anja Bauerfeind, Lisa Eggebrecht, et al. 2024. 'Does the Shape of the Copper Intrauterine Device Play a Role in Expulsion? Results from the Ongoing European Active Surveillance Study on LCS12'. *Contraception* 140 (December): 110444. https://doi.org/10.1016/j.contraception.2024.110444.

Caddy, Sheila, Mark H. Yudin, Julie Hakim, Deborah M. Money, Infectious Disease Committee, and Society of Obstetricians and Gynaecologists of Canada. 2014. 'Best Practices to Minimize Risk of Infection with Intrauterine Device Insertion'. *Journal of Obstetrics and Gynaecology Canada: JOGC = Journal d'obstétrique et Gynécologie Du Canada: JOGC* 36 (3): 266–76.

Caliskan, E., N. Oztürk, B. O. Dilbaz, and S. Dilbaz. 2003. 'Analysis of Risk Factors Associated with Uterine Perforation by Intrauterine Devices'. *The European Journal of Contraception & Reproductive Health Care: The Official Journal of the European Society of Contraception* 8 (3): 150–55.

Cheung, Vincent Y. T. 2006. 'GyneFix: A Frameless Intrauterine Device'. *Journal of Minimally Invasive Gynecology* 13 (5): 373–74. https://doi.org/10.1016/j.jmig.2006.03.007.

Chi, I. C. 1991. 'An Evaluation of the Levonorgestrel-Releasing IUD: Its Advantages and Disadvantages When Compared to the Copper-Releasing IUDs'. *Contraception* 44 (6): 573–88.

Chiou, Chiun Fang, James Trussell, Eileen Reyes, et al. 2003. 'Economic Analysis of Contraceptives for Women'. *Contraception* 68 (1): 3–10.

Committee on Practice Bulletins-Gynecology, Long-Acting Reversible Contraception Work Group. 2017. 'Practice Bulletin No. 186: Long-Acting Reversible Contraception: Implants and Intrauterine Devices'. *Obstetrics and Gynecology* 130 (5): e251–69. https://doi.org/10.1097/AOG.0000000000002400.

Cuadros, A., and J. G. Hirsch. 1972. 'Copper on Intrauterine Devices Stimulates Leukocyte Exudation'. *Science (New York, N.Y.)* 175 (4018): 175–76.

Curtis, Kathryn M., Antoinette T. Nguyen, Naomi K. Tepper, et al. 2024. 'U.S. Selected Practice Recommendations for Contraceptive Use, 2024'. *MMWR. Recommendations and Reports: Morbidity and Mortality Weekly Report. Recommendations and Reports* 73 (3): 1–77. https://doi.org/10.15585/mmwr.rr7303a1.

Delbarge, W., I. Bátár, M. Bafort, et al. 2002. 'Return to Fertility in Nulliparous and Parous Women after Removal of the GyneFix Intrauterine Contraceptive System'. *The European Journal of Contraception & Reproductive Health Care: The Official Journal of the European Society of Contraception* 7 (1): 24–30.

Diedrich, Justin T., David A. Klein, and Jeffrey F. Peipert. 2017. 'Long-Acting Reversible Contraception in Adolescents: A Systematic Review and Meta-Analysis'. *American Journal of Obstetrics and Gynecology* 216 (4): 364.e1-364.e12. https://doi.org/10.1016/j.ajog.2016.12.024.

Diedrich, Justin T., Qiuhong Zhao, Tessa Madden, Gina M. Secura, and Jeffrey F. Peipert. 2015. 'Three-Year Continuation of Reversible Contraception'. *American Journal of Obstetrics and Gynecology* 213 (5): 662.e1-8. https://doi.org/10.1016/j.ajog.2015.08.001.

Dueñas, J. L., A. Albert, and F. Carrasco. 1996. 'Intrauterine Contraception in Nulligravid vs Parous Women'. *Contraception* 53 (1): 23–24.

Enjezab, Behnaz, Leila Asadi, and Seyed Abbas Sadat Hosseini. 2023. 'Development of an Informed Consent Form for Intrauterine Device (IUD) Insertion Using the Delphi Method'. *Journal of Midwifery and Reproductive Health*, no. Online First (December). https://doi.org/10.22038/jmrh.2023.68118.1993.

Evans, Adam T., Kam Szlachetka, and Loralei L. Thornburg. 2019. 'Ultrasound Assessment of the Intrauterine Device'. *Obstetrics and Gynecology Clinics of North America* 46 (4): 661–81. https://doi.org/10.1016/j.ogc.2019.07.005.

Faculty of Sexual & Reproductive Healthcare. 2023. 'FSRH Guideline Intrauterine Contraception'. March.

Farley, T. M., M. J. Rosenberg, P. J. Rowe, J. H. Chen, and O. Meirik. 1992. 'Intrauterine Devices and Pelvic Inflammatory Disease: An International Perspective'. *Lancet (London, England)* 339 (8796): 785–88. https://doi.org/10.1016/0140-6736(92)91904-m.

Farr, Alex, Isaak Effendy, Brigitte Frey Tirri, et al. 2021. 'Guideline: Vulvovaginal Candidosis (AWMF 015/072, Level S2k)'. *Mycoses* 64 (6): 583–602. https://doi.org/10.1111/myc.13248.

Fleming, D., J. Davie, and A. Glasier. 1998. 'Continuation Rates of Long-Acting Methods of Contraception. A Comparative Study of Norplant Implants and Intrauterine Devices'. *Contraception* 57 (1): 19–21.

Franks, A. L., V. Beral, W. Cates, and C. J. Hogue. 1990. 'Contraception and Ectopic Pregnancy Risk'. *American Journal of Obstetrics and Gynecology* 163 (4 Pt 1): 1120–23. https://doi.org/10.1016/0002-9378(90)90668-w.

'FSRH Guideline (March 2023) Intrauterine Contraception'. 2023a. *BMJ Sexual & Reproductive Health* 49 (Suppl 1): 1–142. https://doi.org/10.1136/bmjsrh-2023-IUC.

'FSRH Guideline (March 2023) Intrauterine Contraception'. 2023b. *BMJ Sexual & Reproductive Health* 49 (Suppl 1): 1–142. https://doi.org/10.1136/bmjsrh-2023-IUC.

Ganer, Hadas, Amalia Levy, Iris Ohel, and Eyal Sheiner. 2009. 'Pregnancy Outcome in Women with an Intrauterine Contraceptive Device'. *American Journal of Obstetrics and Gynecology* 201 (4): 381.e1-381.e5. https://doi.org/10.1016/j.ajog.2009.06.031.

Gillian Dean G, Goldberg AB. n.d. 'Intrauterine Contraception: Management of Side Effects and Complications. This Topic Last Updated: Jul 14, 2015. In: UpToDate, Basow, DS (Ed), UpToDate, Waltham, MA, 2016.'

Golightly, Ellen, and Ailsa E. Gebbie. 2014. 'Low-Lying or Malpositioned Intrauterine Devices and Systems'. *The Journal of Family Planning and Reproductive Health Care / Faculty of Family Planning & Reproductive Health Care, Royal College of Obstetricians & Gynaecologists* 40 (2): 108–12. https://doi.org/10.1136/jfprhc-2013-100684.

Gonçalves, Bruna, Carina Ferreira, Carlos Tiago Alves, Mariana Henriques, Joana Azeredo, and Sónia Silva. 2016. 'Vulvovaginal Candidiasis: Epidemiology, Microbiology and Risk Factors'. *Critical Reviews in Microbiology* 42 (6): 905–27. https://doi.org/10.3109/1040841X.2015.1091805.

Graupera, Betlem, Lourdes Hereter, M. Angela Pascual, et al. 2012. 'Normal and Abnormal Images of Intrauterine Devices: Role of Three-Dimensional Sonography'. *Journal of Clinical Ultrasound: JCU* 40 (7): 433–38. https://doi.org/10.1002/jcu.21955.

Grimes, D. A., and K. F. Schulz. 2001. 'Antibiotic Prophylaxis for Intrauterine Contraceptive Device Insertion'. *The Cochrane Database of Systematic Reviews*, no. 2: CD001327. https://doi.org/10.1002/14651858.CD001327.

Grunloh, Danielle S., Teya Casner, Gina M. Secura, Jeffrey F. Peipert, and Tessa Madden. 2013. 'Characteristics Associated with Discontinuation of Long-Acting Reversible Contraception within the First 6 Months of Use'. *Obstetrics and Gynecology* 122 (6): 1214–21. https://doi.org/10.1097/01.AOG.0000435452.86108.59.

Hagenfeldt, K. 1972. 'Intrauterine Contraception with the Copper-T Device. Effect on Trace Elements in the Endometrium, Cervical Mucus and Plasma'. *Contraception* 6 (1): 37–54.

Harrison-Woolrych, Mira, Janelle Ashton, and David Coulter. 2003. 'Uterine Perforation on Intrauterine Device Insertion: Is the Incidence Higher than Previously Reported?' *Contraception* 67 (1): 53–56.

Heinemann, Klaas, Clare Barnett, Suzanne Reed, Sabine Möhner, and Thai Do Minh. 2017. 'IUD Use among Parous Women and Risk of Uterine Perforation: A Secondary Analysis'. *Contraception* 95 (6): 605–7. https://doi.org/10.1016/j.contraception.2017.03.007.

Heinemann, Klaas, Suzanne Reed, Sabine Moehner, and Thai Do Minh. 2015. 'Comparative Contraceptive Effectiveness of Levonorgestrel-Releasing and Copper Intrauterine Devices: The European Active Surveillance Study for Intrauterine Devices'. *Contraception* 91 (4): 280–83. https://doi.org/10.1016/j.contraception.2015.01.011.

Heinemann, Klaas, Suzanne Reed, Sabine Moehner, and Thai Do Minh. 2015. 'Risk of Uterine Perforation with Levonorgestrel-Releasing and Copper Intrauterine Devices in the European Active Surveillance Study on Intrauterine Devices'. *Contraception* 91 (4): 274–79. https://doi.org/10.1016/j.contraception.2015.01.007.

Hilgers, T. W. 1974. 'The Intrauterine Device. Contraceptive or Abortifacient?' *Minnesota Medicine* 57 (6): 493-501 p.

Hov, Gunhild Garmo, Finn Egil Skjeldestad, and Torunn Hilstad. 2007. 'Use of IUD and Subsequent Fertility--Follow-up after Participation in a Randomized Clinical Trial'. *Contraception* 75 (2): 88–92. https://doi.org/10.1016/j.contraception.2006.09.010.

Inal, M. M., K. Ertopçu, and I. Ozelmas. 2005. 'The Evaluation of 318 Intrauterine Pregnancy Cases with an Intrauterine Device'. *The European Journal of Contraception & Reproductive Health Care: The Official*

Journal of the European Society of Contraception 10 (4): 266–71. https://doi.org/10.1080/13625180500195340.

Jatlaoui, Tara C., Katharine B. Simmons, and Kathryn M. Curtis. 2016. 'The Safety of Intrauterine Contraception Initiation among Women with Current Asymptomatic Cervical Infections or at Increased Risk of Sexually Transmitted Infections'. *Contraception* 94 (6): 701–12. https://doi.org/10.1016/j.contraception.2016.05.013.

Jenabi, Encieh, Sakine Mohammad Alizade, and Reyhane Ivan Baga. 2006. 'Continuation Rates and Reasons for Discontinuing TCu380A IUD Use in Tabriz, Iran'. *Contraception* 74 (6): 483–86. https://doi.org/10.1016/j.contraception.2006.08.007.

JENNINGS, J.F. 1974. 'Report on Safety and Efficacy of the Dalkon Shield and Other IUDs. Ood and Drug Administration, Washington, DC.'

Johnson, Jo-Ann, Suzanne Tough, and SOGC GENETICS COMMITTEE. 2012. 'Delayed Child-Bearing'. *Journal of Obstetrics and Gynaecology Canada: JOGC = Journal d'obstetrique et Gynecologie Du Canada: JOGC* 34 (1): 80–93. https://doi.org/10.1016/S1701-2163(16)35138-6.

Jonsson, B., B. M. Landgren, and P. Eneroth. 1991. 'Effects of Various IUDs on the Composition of Cervical Mucus'. *Contraception* 43 (5): 447–58.

Kaislasuo, Janina, Satu Suhonen, Mika Gissler, Pekka Lähteenmäki, and Oskari Heikinheimo. 2012. 'Intrauterine Contraception: Incidence and Factors Associated with Uterine Perforation--a Population-Based Study'. *Human Reproduction (Oxford, England)* 27 (9): 2658–63. https://doi.org/10.1093/humrep/des246.

Katherine D Pocius, MD, MPHDeborah A Bartz, MD, MPH. 2025. 'Intrauterine Contraception: Management of Side Effects and Complications'. UpToDate, April.

Kim, Sun Kwon, Roberto Romero, Juan Pedro Kusanovic, et al. 2010. 'The Prognosis of Pregnancy Conceived despite the Presence of an Intrauterine Device (IUD)'. *Journal of Perinatal Medicine* 38 (1). https://doi.org/10.1515/jpm.2009.133.

Kulier, R., F. M. Helmerhorst, P. O'Brien, M. Usher-Patel, and C. d'Arcangues. 2006. 'Copper Containing, Framed Intra-Uterine Devices for Contraception'. *The Cochrane Database of Systematic Reviews*, no. 3: CD005347. https://doi.org/10.1002/14651858.CD005347.pub2.

Larsson, G., I. Milsom, K. Jonasson, G. Lindstedt, and G. Rybo. 1993. 'The Long-Term Effects of Copper Surface Area on Menstrual Blood Loss and Iron Status in Women Fitted with an IUD'. *Contraception* 48 (5): 471–80.

Lee, N. C., G. L. Rubin, H. W. Ory, and R. T. Burkman. 1983. 'Type of Intrauterine Device and the Risk of Pelvic Inflammatory Disease'. *Obstetrics and Gynecology* 62 (1): 1–6.

Lowe, Richard F., and Ndola Prata. 2013. 'Hemoglobin and Serum Ferritin Levels in Women Using Copper-Releasing or Levonorgestrel-Releasing Intrauterine Devices: A Systematic Review'. *Contraception* 87 (4): 486–96. https://doi.org/10.1016/j.contraception.2012.09.025.

Madden, Tessa, Colleen McNicholas, Qiuhong Zhao, Gina M. Secura, David L. Eisenberg, and Jeffrey F. Peipert. 2014. 'Association of Age and Parity With Intrauterine Device Expulsion': *Obstetrics & Gynecology* 124 (4): 718–26. https://doi.org/10.1097/AOG.0000000000000475.

Maki, Yohei, Midori Fujisaki, Yuichiro Sato, and Hiroshi Sameshima. 2017. '*Candida* Chorioamnionitis Leads to Preterm Birth and Adverse Fetal-Neonatal Outcome'. *Infectious Diseases in Obstetrics and Gynecology* 2017: 1–11. https://doi.org/10.1155/2017/9060138.

Mansour, Diana, Kristina Gemzell-Danielsson, Pirjo Inki, and Jeffrey T. Jensen. 2011. 'Fertility after Discontinuation of Contraception: A Comprehensive Review of the Literature'. *Contraception* 84 (5): 465–77. https://doi.org/10.1016/j.contraception.2011.04.002.

Margulies, L. 1975. 'History of Intrauterine Devices'. *Bulletin of the New York Academy of Medicine* 51 (5): 662–67.

Mavranezouli, I. and LARC Guideline Development Group. 2008. 'The Cost-Effectiveness of Long-Acting Reversible Contraceptive Methods in the UK: Analysis Based on a Decision-Analytic Model Developed for a National Institute for Health and Clinical Excellence (NICE) Clinical Practice Guideline'. *Human Reproduction (Oxford, England)* 23 (6): 1338–45. https://doi.org/10.1093/humrep/den091.

McKay, W. J. S. n.d. *The History of Ancient Gynecology*. Tindall and Cox.

'Mechanism of Action, Safety and Efficacy of Intrauterine Devices. Report of a WHO Scientific Group'. 1987. *World Health Organization Technical Report Series* 753: 1–91.

Meirik, Olav. 2007. 'Intrauterine Devices - Upper and Lower Genital Tract Infections'. *Contraception* 75 (6 Suppl): S41-47. https://doi.org/10.1016/j.contraception.2006.12.017.

Meirik, Olav, Patrick J. Rowe, Alexandre Peregoudov, Gilda Piaggio, Max Petzold, and IUD Research Group at the UNDP/UNFPA/WHO/World Bank Special Programme of Research, Development and Research Training in Human Reproduction. 2009. 'The Frameless Copper IUD (GyneFix) and the TCu380A IUD: Results of an 8-Year Multicenter Randomized Comparative Trial'. *Contraception* 80 (2): 133–41. https://doi.org/10.1016/j.contraception.2009.02.006.

Mierzejewska, Anna, Maciej Walędziak, Piotr Merks, and Anna Różańska-Walędziak. 2024. 'Emergency Contraception – A Narrative Review of Literature'. *European Journal of Obstetrics & Gynecology and Reproductive Biology* 299 (August): 188–92. https://doi.org/10.1016/j.ejogrb.2024.06.015.

Milsom, I., K. Andersson, K. Jonasson, G. Lindstedt, and G. Rybo. 1995. 'The Influence of the Gyne-T 380S IUD on Menstrual Blood Loss and Iron Status'. *Contraception* 52 (3): 175–79.

National Institute for Clinical Excellence (NICE). 2014. 'Long Acting Reversible Contraception: The Effective and Appropriate Log-Acting Reversible Contraception.' https://www.nice.org.uk/guidance/cg30.

Nelson, Anita L. 2007. 'Contraindications to IUD and IUS Use'. *Contraception* 75 (6 Suppl): S76-81. https://doi.org/10.1016/j.contraception.2007.01.004.

Nelson, Anita L., and Natasha Massoudi. 2016. 'New Developments in Intrauterine Device Use: Focus on the US'. *Open Access Journal of Contraception* 7: 127–41. https://doi.org/10.2147/OAJC.S85755.

Nguyen, Antoinette T., Kathryn M. Curtis, Naomi K. Tepper, et al. 2024. 'U.S. Medical Eligibility Criteria for Contraceptive Use, 2024'. *MMWR. Recommendations and Reports* 73 (4): 1–126. https://doi.org/10.15585/mmwr.rr7304a1.

O'Brien, P. A., and C. Marfleet. 2005. 'Frameless versus Classical Intrauterine Device for Contraception'. *The Cochrane Database of Systematic Reviews*, no. 1: CD003282. https://doi.org/10.1002/14651858.CD003282.pub2.

O'Brien, Paul A., Regina Kulier, Frans M. Helmerhorst, Margaret Usher-Patel, and Catherine d'Arcangues. 2008. 'Copper-Containing, Framed Intrauterine Devices for Contraception: A Systematic Review of Randomized Controlled Trials'. *Contraception* 77 (5): 318–27. https://doi.org/10.1016/j.contraception.2007.12.011.

Okusanya, Babasola O., Olabisi Oduwole, and Emmanuel E. Effa. 2014. 'Immediate Postabortal Insertion of Intrauterine Devices'. *The Cochrane Database of Systematic Reviews* 7: CD001777. https://doi.org/10.1002/14651858.CD001777.pub4.

Organización Mundial de la Salud. Departamento de Salud Reproductiva e Investigaciones Conexas. 2018. 'Recomendaciones Sobre Prácticas Seleccionadas Para El Uso de Anticonceptivos. Tercera Edición.' http://apps.who.int/iris/bitstream/handle/10665/259814/9789243565408-spa.pdf;jsessionid=CF31E90410F1C5E1C91AF8CA37319DD5?sequence=1.

Ortiz, M. E., and H. B. Croxatto. 1987. 'The Mode of Action of IUDs'. *Contraception* 36 (1): 37–53.

Ortiz, M. E., H. B. Croxatto, and C. W. Bardin. 1996. 'Mechanisms of Action of Intrauterine Devices'. *Obstetrical & Gynecological Survey* 51 (12 Suppl): S42-51.

Ortiz, María Elena, and Horacio B. Croxatto. 2007. 'Copper-T Intrauterine Device and Levonorgestrel Intrauterine System: Biological Bases of Their Mechanism of Action'. *Contraception* 75 (6 Suppl): S16-30. https://doi.org/10.1016/j.contraception.2007.01.020.

Os, W. A. van, M. Thiery, H. van der Pas, et al. 1977. '[Intrauterine contraceptive devices containing copper, the combined multiload copper IUD (MLCu 250)]'. *Nederlands Tijdschrift Voor Geneeskunde* 121 (14): 568–71.

Ozgu-Erdinc, A. Seval, Ufuk Goker Tasdemir, Dilek Uygur, Ayla Aktulay, Nicel Tasdemir, and H. Cavidan Gulerman. 2014. 'Outcome of Intrauterine Pregnancies with Intrauterine Device in Place and Effects of Device Location on Prognosis'. *Contraception* 89 (5): 426–30. https://doi.org/10.1016/j.contraception.2014.01.002.

Parr, E. L., and R. L. Shirley. 1976. 'Embryotoxicity of Leukocyte Extracts and Its Relationship to Intrauterine Contraception in Humans'. *Fertility and Sterility* 27 (9): 1067–77.

Patchen, Loral, and Erica K. Berggren. 2011. 'Use of the Copper T380A Intrauterine Device by Adolescent Mothers: Continuation and Method Failure'. *Journal of Pediatric and Adolescent Gynecology* 24 (2): 71–73. https://doi.org/10.1016/j.jpag.2010.07.010.

Peipert, Jeffrey F., Qiuhong Zhao, Jenifer E. Allsworth, et al. 2011. 'Continuation and Satisfaction of Reversible Contraception.' *Obstetrics and Gynecology* 117 (5): 1105–13. https://doi.org/10.1097/AOG.0b013e31821188ad.

Phillips, Sharon J., Lisa G. Hofler, Anna M. Modest, Lara F. B. Harvey, Lily H. Wu, and Michele R. Hacker. 2017. 'Continuation of Copper and Levonorgestrel Intrauterine Devices: A Retrospective Cohort Study'. *American Journal of Obstetrics and Gynecology* 217 (1): 57.e1-57.e6. https://doi.org/10.1016/j.ajog.2017.03.005.

Pitkin, R. M. 1988. 'The Return of the IUD'. *Obstetrics and Gynecology* 72 (1): 119.

Pust, K. 1923. 'Ein Brauchbarer Frauenschutz.' *Deutsche Medizinische Wochenschrift* 49: 1952–53.

Richter, R. 1909. 'Ein Mittel Zur Verhütung Der Konzeption'. *DEUTSCHE MEDIZINISCHE WOCHENSCHRIFT* 35: 1525–27.

Rosenstock, Jessica R., Jeffrey F. Peipert, Tessa Madden, Qiuhong Zhao, and Gina M. Secura. 2012. 'Continuation of Reversible Contraception in Teenagers and Young Women'. *Obstetrics and Gynecology* 120 (6): 1298–305. http://10.1097/AOG.0b013e31827499bd.

Sallie Craig Huber, M. S. P. H., P. T. Piotrow, PhD., F. 8arbara Orlans, Ph .D., and Geary Kommer, 8. S. N. 1975. 'Population Reports. Intrauterine Devices. Serie B. Num. 2. Department of Medical and Public Affairs.' January.

Sanders, Ari P., Margo R. Fluker, and Barry H. Sanders. 2016. 'Saline Hysteroscopy for Removal of Retained Intrauterine Contraceptive Devices in Early Pregnancy'. *Journal of Obstetrics and Gynaecology Canada: JOGC = Journal d'obstetrique et Gynecologie Du Canada: JOGC* 38 (12): 1114–19. https://doi.org/10.1016/j.jogc.2016.08.013.

Schiesser, M., O. Lapaire, S. Tercanli, and W. Holzgreve. 2004. 'Lost Intrauterine Devices during Pregnancy: Maternal and Fetal Outcome after Ultrasound-Guided Extraction. An Analysis of 82 Cases: Extraction of Lost IUDs'. *Ultrasound in Obstetrics and Gynecology* 23 (5): 486–89. https://doi.org/10.1002/uog.1036.

Scommegna, A., G. N. Pandya, M. Christ, A. W. Lee, and M. R. Cohen. 1970. 'Intrauterine Administration of Progesterone by a Slow Releasing Device'. *Fertility and Sterility* 21 (3): 201–10.

Sivin, I. 1989. 'IUDs Are Contraceptives, Not Abortifacients: A Comment on Research and Belief'. *Studies in Family Planning* 20 (6 Pt 1): 355–59.

Skjeldestad, F. E., and H. Bratt. 1987. 'Return of Fertility after Use of IUDs (Nova-T, MLCu250 and MLCu375)'. *Advances in Contraception: The Official Journal of the Society for the Advancement of Contraception* 3 (2): 139–45.

Sonalkar, Sarita, and Nathalie Kapp. 2015. 'Intrauterine Device Insertion in the Postpartum Period: A Systematic Review'. *The European Journal of Contraception & Reproductive Health Care: The Official Journal of the European Society of Contraception* 20 (1): 4–18. https://doi.org/10.3109/13625187.2014.971454.

Stanford, Joseph B., and Rafael T. Mikolajczyk. 2002. 'Mechanisms of Action of Intrauterine Devices: Update and Estimation of Postfertilization Effects'. *American Journal of Obstetrics and Gynecology* 187 (6): 1699–708.

Stoddard, Amy M., Hanna Xu, Tessa Madden, Jenifer E. Allsworth, and Jeffrey F. Peipert. 2015. 'Fertility after Intrauterine Device Removal: A Pilot Study'. *The European Journal of Contraception & Reproductive Health Care: The Official Journal of the European Society of Contraception* 20 (3): 223–30. https://doi.org/10.3109/13625187.2015.1010639.

Struthers, B. J. 1991. 'Copper IUDs, PID, and Fertility in Nulliparous Women'. *Advances in Contraception: The Official Journal of the Society for the Advancement of Contraception* 7 (2–3): 211–30.

Sufrin, Carolyn B., and Sarah H. Averbach. 2014. 'Testing for Sexually Transmitted Infections at Intrauterine Device Insertion: An Evidence-Based Approach'. *Clinical Obstetrics and Gynecology* 57 (4): 682–93. https://doi.org/10.1097/GRF.0000000000000054.

Tatum, H. J. 1972. 'The First Year of Clinical Experience with the Copper T Intrauterine Contraceptive System in the United States and Canada'. *Contraception* 6 (3): 179–89.

Tepper, Naomi K., Maria W. Steenland, Mary E. Gaffield, Polly A. Marchbanks, and Kathryn M. Curtis. 2013. 'Retention of Intrauterine Devices in Women Who Acquire Pelvic Inflammatory Disease: A Systematic Review'. *Contraception* 87 (5): 655–60. https://doi.org/10.1016/j.contraception.2012.08.011.

Tessa Madden, MD, MPH. n.d. 'Intrauterine Contraception: Background and Device Types - UpToDate'. Accessed 18 May 2025. https://www-uptodate-com.sescam.a17.csinet.es/contents/intrauterine-contraception-background-and-device-types?search=intrauterine%20contraception&source=search_result&selectedTitle=1~150&usage_type=default&display_rank=1.

Thonneau, Patrick F., Thierry Almont, and Thierry E. Almont. 2008. 'Contraceptive Efficacy of Intrauterine Devices'. *American Journal of Obstetrics and Gynecology* 198 (3): 248–53. https://doi.org/10.1016/j.ajog.2007.10.787.

Tietze, C. 1966. 'Contraception with Intrauterine Devices. 1959-1966'. *American Journal of Obstetrics and Gynecology* 96 (7): 1043–54.

Tietze C; Lewit S. 1972. 'Comparison of the Copper-T and Loop D: A Research Report.' *Studies in Family Planning* 3 (11): 277–78.

Trussell, J., J. Koenig, C. Ellertson, and F. Stewart. 1997. 'Preventing Unintended Pregnancy: The Cost-Effectiveness of Three Methods of Emergency Contraception'. *American Journal of Public Health* 87 (6): 932–37.

Trussell, James, Fareen Hassan, Julia Lowin, Amy Law, and Anna Filonenko. 2015. 'Achieving Cost-Neutrality with Long-Acting Reversible Contraceptive Methods'. *Contraception* 91 (1): 49–56. https://doi.org/10.1016/j.contraception.2014.08.011.

Tugrul, Semih, Bekir Yavuzer, Gazi Yildirim, and Arif Kayahan. 2005. 'The Duration of Use, Causes of Discontinuation, and Problems during Removal in Women Admitted for Removal of IUD'. *Contraception* 71 (2): 149–52. https://doi.org/10.1016/j.contraception.2004.08.015.

United Nations. 2024. 'United Nations, Department of Economic and Social Affairs, Population Division (2024). World Contraceptive Use 2024 and Estimates and Projections of Family Planning Indicators 2024. Methodology Report. POP/DB/CP/Rev2024 and POP/DB/FP/Rev2024.'

United Nations, Department of Economic and Social Affairs, Population Division (2022). n.d. 'World Contraceptive Use 2022 and Estimates and Projections of Family Planning Indicators 2022. Methodology Report. POP/DB/CP/Rev2022 and POP/DB/FP/Rev2022'.

US Preventive Services Task Force, Karina W. Davidson, Michael J. Barry, et al. 2021. 'Screening for Chlamydia and Gonorrhea: US Preventive Services Task Force Recommendation Statement'. *JAMA* 326 (10): 949–56. https://doi.org/10.1001/jama.2021.14081.

Usinger, K. M., S. B. Gola, M. Weis, and A. Smaldone. 2016. 'Intrauterine Contraception Continuation in Adolescents and Young Women: A Systematic Review'. *Journal of Pediatric and Adolescent Gynecology* 29 (6): 659–67. https://doi.org/10.1016/j.jpag.2016.06.007.

Wessel, Gary M. 2014. 'Of Camels, Silkworms, and Contraception'. *Molecular Reproduction and Development* 81 (9): Fmi. https://doi.org/10.1002/mrd.22416.

Whiteman, Maura K., Crystal P. Tyler, Suzanne G. Folger, Mary E. Gaffield, and Kathryn M. Curtis. 2013. 'When Can a Woman Have an Intrauterine Device Inserted? A Systematic Review'. *Contraception* 87 (5): 666–73. https://doi.org/10.1016/j.contraception.2012.08.015.

Wiebe, Ellen, and James Trussell. 2016. 'Discontinuation Rates and Acceptability during 1 Year of Using the Intrauterine Ball (the SCu380A)'. *Contraception* 93 (4): 364–66. https://doi.org/10.1016/j.contraception.2015.12.002.

Wildemeersch, D., H. van der Pas, M. Thiery, H. Van Kets, W. Parewijck, and W. Delbarge. 1988. 'The Copper-Fix (Cu-Fix): A New Concept in IUD Technology'. *Advances in Contraception: The Official Journal of the Society for the Advancement of Contraception* 4 (3): 197–205.

Wildemeersch, Dirk, István Batár, Biran Affandi, et al. 2003. 'The "frameless" Intrauterine System for Long-Term, Reversible Contraception: A Review of 15 Years of Clinical Experience'. *The Journal of Obstetrics and Gynaecology Research* 29 (3): 164–73.

Workowski, Kimberly A., Laura H. Bachmann, Philip A. Chan, et al. 2021. 'Sexually Transmitted Infections Treatment Guidelines, 2021'. *MMWR. Recommendations and Reports: Morbidity and Mortality Weekly Report. Recommendations and Reports* 70 (4): 1–187. https://doi.org/10.15585/mmwr.rr7004a1.

World Health Organization, Reproductive Health and Research, and World Health Organization. 2015. *Medical Eligibility Criteria for Contraceptive Use.* http://www.ncbi.nlm.nih.gov/books/NBK321151/.

Wu, Justine P., and Sarah Pickle. 2014. 'Extended Use of the Intrauterine Device: A Literature Review and Recommendations for Clinical Practice'. *Contraception* 89 (6): 495–503. https://doi.org/10.1016/j.contraception.2014.02.011.

Zhang, J., P. J. Feldblum, I. C. Chi, and M. G. Farr. 1992. 'Risk Factors for Copper T IUD Expulsion: An Epidemiologic Analysis'. *Contraception* 46 (5): 427–33.

Zipper, J. A., H. J. Tatum, M. Medel, L. Pastene, and M. Rivera. 1971. 'Contraception through the Use of Intrauterine Metals. I. Copper as an Adjunct to the "T" Device. The Endouterine Copper "T"'. *American Journal of Obstetrics and Gynecology* 109 (5): 771–74.

Zipper, J. A., H. J. Tatum, L. Pastene, M. Medel, and M. Rivera. 1969. 'Metallic Copper as an Intrauterine Contraceptice Adjunct to the "T" Device'. *American Journal of Obstetrics and Gynecology* 105 (8): 1274–78.

Zipper, J., M. Medel, and R. Prager. 1969. 'Suppression of Fertility by Intrauterine Copper and Zinc in Rabbits. A New Approach to Intrauterine Contraception'. *American Journal of Obstetrics and Gynecology* 105 (4): 529–34.

Chapter 10

Female Surgical Contraception

C. García Fernández[1,*], MD
A. Santos Fernández[1], MD
A. García Buendía[1], MD
L. Sales Pérez[2], MD
and J. López Grande[1], MD
[1]Obstetrics and Gynecology Department, University and Hospital of Albacete, Albacete, Spain
[2]Obstetrics and Gynecology Department, Hospital Lluis Alcanyis Xativa, Xativa, Valencia, Spain

Abstract

Definitive female surgical contraception represents a highly effective and permanent option for women who have decided not to have any more children. This chapter provides an in-depth review of the main techniques available, including bilateral salpingectomy, electrocoagulation techniques and mechanical methods, considering their indications, efficacy, reversibility and complications. Essential aspects of prior contraceptive counselling, informed consent and clinical appropriateness criteria are also addressed. In addition, the added value of bilateral salpingectomy as a potential preventive measure against epithelial ovarian cancer is highlighted.

Keywords: woman, sterilisation, surgery, salpingectomy, contraception

Introduction

Surgical contraception or sterilisation is a medical intervention aimed at achieving permanent prevention of pregnancy. It includes procedures performed on both men (vasectomy) and women (tubal sterilisation), the latter being the most common worldwide, with an estimated ratio of 3 women sterilised for every 1 man who has undergone a vasectomy (Moss and Isley 2015).

* Corresponding Author's Email: claragarciafernandez1998@gmail.com

In: Advances in Reproductive Health
Editors: Llanos Belmonte Andujar and Ana Fuentes Rozalen
ISBN: 979-8-90134-038-7

It is estimated that more than 180 million women of reproductive age have chosen sterilisation as a method of contraception, making it one of the most widely used methods globally (Herbert B. Peterson 2008). This choice may be influenced by various demographic, socio-cultural, economic and accessibility factors, as well as individual preference and medical assessment of risk associated with other forms of contraception (Moss and Isley 2015).

Purpose and Characteristics

The main purpose of surgical sterilisation is to provide a permanent and highly effective contraceptive option, especially appropriate for patients with no reproductive desire and a need to avoid user dependent methods. However, its definitive nature requires a thorough counselling process, framed with respect for reproductive autonomy and informed decision-making (Giannakeas et al. 2023; "ACOG Practice Bulletin No. 208: Benefits and Risks of Sterilization" 2019).

Although it is considered a permanent method, its efficacy is not absolute. Occasionally recanalisation occurs, either due to technique failure or at the patient's request. The cumulative 10-year failure rate varies depending on the technique used, with an average of 18.5 pregnancies per 1,000 procedures (Moss and Isley 2015). In addition, in case of failure, there is a high risk of ectopic pregnancy.

Female sterilisation can be performed by different routes: laparoscopic, abdominal via mini laparotomy and hysteroscopic. It can be performed in the immediate postpartum period or outside the obstetric setting.

Techniques used for female sterilisation include mechanical occlusion (clips, rings), coagulation (bipolar or unipolar) and partial or total tubal resection. Among these, bilateral salpingectomy has gained interest for its additional potential to reduce the risk of ovarian cancer. The technique used for male sterilisation is vasectomy.

Despite its high efficacy, sterilisation is not without ethical and personal considerations. Evidence shows that post-procedure regret is more frequent in young women, especially those under 30 years of age, and in those who had no reproductive desire or were under social or medical pressure to undergo these procedures.1 Consequently, current guidelines emphasise the need for comprehensive informed consent, in a context of person-centred, non-coercive contraceptive counselling and ensuring reproductive autonomy (Nguyen et al. 2024).

Indications

Indications for definitive sterilisation may be medical (clinical or psychiatric illnesses, genetic abnormalities or possible obstetric complications) or for contraceptive purposes only. Medical indications include:

- Those situations in which pregnancy entails aggravation of the state of health, or even life threatening: severe heart disease, severe lung disease, severe coagulation disorder, cancer... It is worth mentioning that a scarred uterus, after the third caesarean section, is not currently considered a medical condition. In certain medical conditions, the procedure should be performed in places with experienced surgeons and staff, with adequate anaesthesia equipment and other medical support because of the high risk of surgical and anaesthetic complications, such as in patients with a history of complicated surgery on the uterus (perforation, PID, TB, endometriosis), multiple cardiovascular risk factors, nephropathy, cirrhosis, chronic asthma, emphysema or coagulation disorders. As long as the risks of definitive sterilisation do not outweigh the benefits, otherwise long-term, highly effective contraceptive methods are a valid alternative.

- In case of severe psychiatric disorder, genetic or chromosomal problems, it may be indicated.
- Cases where there is a medical contraindication to the use of reversible methods of contraception ("ACOG Practice Bulletin No. 208: Benefits and Risks of Sterilization" 2019).
- In the case of mental deficiency, the application is made by the legal representatives of the incapable patient, who must give their consent, always with prior judicial authorisation.
- Cancer risk reduction with bilateral salpingectomy, performed during caesarean section or as a stand-alone procedure, has been associated with a reduced risk of epithelial ovarian cancer, which may be an additional consideration for some patients, especially those at increased risk of ovarian cancer: women with a family history of ovarian or breast cancer and women who carry known genetic mutations (with BRCA1 and BRCA2) or a personal history of high-risk gynaecological disease ("ACOG Practice Bulletin No. 208: Benefits and Risks of Sterilisation. 208: Benefits and Risks of Sterilization" 2019; Giannakeas et al. 2023).

Within purely reproductive purposes:

- Women with a desire for permanent contraception who have decided not to have any more children and are looking for a definitive solution ("ACOG Practice Bulletin No. 208: Benefits and Risks of Sterilization" 2019).
- Out of personal preference some patients prefer to avoid user-dependent contraceptive methods during their reproductive years.

Contraindications

There is no medical condition that contraindicates this intervention, although other methods should be considered if the risks outweigh the benefits. If the surgical risk is very high, other long-acting contraceptive methods such as intrauterine devices or implants should also be considered (Nguyen et al. 2024; "ACOG Practice Bulletin No. 208: Benefits and Risks of Sterilization" 2019). Thus, severe hypertension (≥160/100 mm Hg), ischaemic heart disease and peripartum cardiomyopathy with moderate or severely impaired cardiac function, as well as decompensated cirrhosis and malignant liver tumours, are contraindications due to the increased risk of adverse events during the procedure (H. B. Peterson et al. 1983).

- Known allergy or hypersensitivity to the materials used in the procedure. Any known allergy to the materials used in sterilisation should be considered an absolute contraindication.
- Active pelvic infection. The presence of an active pelvic infection is a contraindication to female sterilisation because of the risk of spread of infection and postoperative complications. · Pregnancy. Sterilisation should not be performed in pregnant women. It is essential to confirm the absence of pregnancy before proceeding with surgical contraception.
- Psychological conditions. Patients with severe psychiatric disorders or emotional instability may not be ideal candidates for surgical contraception due to the possibility of impulsive decisions or lack of full understanding of the irreversibility of the procedure.

Patient Counselling

Since surgical contraception is a permanent option, prior clinical counselling should be comprehensive, evidence-based and person-centred, ensuring that the decision is made in an informed manner, free of coercion and aligned with the patient's reproductive values (Vricella, Gawron, and Louis 2019; Zapata et al. 2018).

There is a small percentage of women who may experience regret after sterilisation, so it is essential that patients receive comprehensive counselling on the irreversible nature of these procedures and the alternatives available, such as long-acting reversible contraception (LARC). Permanent contraception does not protect against sexually transmitted infections (STIs), and patients should be counselled on condom use to reduce these risks following sterilisation (Nguyen et al. 2024; "ACOG Practice Bulletin No. 208: Benefits and Risks of Sterilization" 2019).

Assessment of Patient Suitability

Before proceeding with sterilisation, it is essential to assess the patient's medical and personal suitability by performing a correct anamnesis and gynaecological examination. It is necessary to assess whether there are medical conditions that may increase surgical risk, such as severe cardiovascular disease, advanced pulmonary pathology, uncontrolled coagulopathies or liver disease, and social, psychological or personal factors that may interfere with an informed decision (coercion, partner pressure, emotional instability, etc.). A pre-anaesthesia study is also necessary ("ACOG Practice Bulletin No. 208: Benefits and Risks of Sterilization" 2019; Nguyen et al. 2024). It is worth mentioning that there is no evidence of the need for thromboprophylaxis in healthy women without pathology, nor for discontinuation of prior hormonal contraception, whatever the route of approach.

Advice on the Ongoing Nature of the Procedure and Review of Possible Alternatives

Counselling should delve into personal motivations and circumstances, and may require more than one consultation. It is essential that patients understand that this is an irreversible procedure. Although reversal techniques are technically available, recovery of fertility is not guaranteed and often requires complex procedures.

The patients who have the most regrets are those under 30 years of age, who do not have children and who make the decision in crisis contexts (gestational loss, complicated births, etc.). During counselling, a clear and understandable comparison with other methods should be offered, especially long-acting reversible methods (LARCs): hormonal and copper intrauterine devices (IUDs) and subdermal implants. These methods have similar efficacy rates to sterilisation and offer the advantage of reversibility, so they should be considered especially in individuals who express hesitation or ambivalence about staying with the procedure (Zapata et al. 2018; Vricella, Gawron, and Louis 2019).

Information on Risks, Benefits and Surgical Technique

The patient should receive understandable information about the proposed technique, the efficacy of the method (failure is < 1-2% but not 0%), possible surgical complications (bleeding, infection, anaesthesia, technical failure), risk of ectopic pregnancy in case of failure and also about benefits associated with the method, such as its high efficacy, absence of need for user-dependent methods and long-term cost-effectiveness. The patient and her partner should know that vasectomy is a definitive surgical male sterilisation method with a lower failure rate and fewer risks associated with the procedure (Zapata et al. 2018). After receiving this information and understanding it, the patient should sign a clear and explained informed consent form.

Relevant Additional Considerations

In the case of bilateral salpingectomy: it should be reported that this technique, in addition to sterilising, may reduce the risk of epithelial ovarian cancer, and is therefore considered a particularly useful option in women with a personal or family history of gynaecological cancer or risk factors.

The pregnant patient should be informed of the possibility of sterilisation at the same obstetric act, during caesarean section or in the immediate postpartum period.

In those patients who wish to undergo definitive sterilisation outside the puerperal period, which we call interval sterilisation, it is advisable to use a highly effective reversible method beforehand, such as combined hormonal contraceptives or intrauterine devices. In OCP users, it is recommended that treatment be discontinued one week after the operation, and in IUD users, the IUD should be removed no earlier than one week after the operation to avoid unwanted pregnancies in which the blastocyst would have passed the tubal obstruction zone (Grubb and Peterson 1985).

It may be recommended to perform a pregnancy test on the day of the procedure in patients not taking prior contraceptive treatment, although this strategy cannot ignore the possibility of a luteal phase pregnancy. Therefore, if possible, proliferative phase interventions should be scheduled in addition (Lipscomb, Spellman, and Ling 1993).

Procedures

Female sterilisation methods consist of tubal sterilisation by salpingectomy, coagulation techniques or mechanical techniques. It consists of the occlusion, section or removal of one or both segments of the fallopian tubes, preventing the passage of gametes and, therefore, fertilisation. The efficacy of permanent methods of contraception in both men and women is very high, but not absolute. Most failures occur within the first year, but can also occur years later. In case of failure, the risk of ectopic pregnancy is significant, especially with partial occlusion techniques.

Salpingectomy

Salpingectomy is the complete or partial resection of one or both fallopian tubes. The goal is to remove at least the distal third of the tube (including the fimbriae and ampulla), preferably the entire tube, in an attempt to decrease the risk of epithelial ovarian cancer.

There are many surgical techniques that have been used for many years, but their application is based on tradition rather than evidence. The Pomeroy technique is one of the most common forms of tubal sterilisation, especially in the postpartum period and during caesarean section, although it can also be performed laparoscopically. It was originally described as a simple, effective technique with a low complication rate, and has demonstrated comparable efficacy to other tubal methods.

1. Classic procedure, by laparotomy or mini-laparotomy, (Hibbert et al. 1997).
    - The fallopian tube is identified, usually in its proximal isthmic or ampullary portion with an atraumatic forceps and externalised.
    - A ligation is performed with a portion of approximately 3-4 cm of the middle third of the tube. By destroying this length, reversal is made more difficult.
    - This loop is ligated underneath with a fast-absorbing suture such as Poliflactin 910. Rapid absorption reduces the risk of inflammation and fistula formation.
    - The distal portion of the loop is then resected, leaving both ends of the tube separated, and sent to histopathology.
    - The tubes are left in their anatomical position without anastomosis.
2. Modified Pomeroy technique, laparoscopic or microlaparoscopic (Hibbert et al. 1997). The procedure is performed as follows:
    - Laparoscopic access using 2 to 5 mm trocars (microlaparoscopy).
    - A uterine manipulator is used to expose the tube.
    - A ligation with resorbable material is performed on the isthmic segment of the tube.
    - Another ligature is made in the distal third of the ampullary segment of the tube, leaving 3-4cm between the two ligatures.

- The segment between the two ligatures, which remains separated, is severed.
- The tissue is sent to histopathology.

There are other techniques that are currently less commonly used. The Parkland technique consists of accessing an avascular portion of the mesosalpinx and separating the tube and then using it to remove a 2 cm segment of the mid-portion of the tube and ligate both proximal and distal ends. Two even less common and somewhat more difficult procedures are the Irving technique and the Uchida technique.

In the Irving technique, an avascular portion of the mesosalpinx is accessed about 4 cm from the uterotubal junction and the tube is ligated proximally and distally. Subsequently, the intermediate segment is removed and the proximal portion of the tube is inserted into the myometrium through an incision in the posterior uterine wall near the uterotubal junction. The distal portion may be left as is or inserted into the mesosalpinx.

In the Uchida technique, the subserosal layer of the mid-portion of the tube is infiltrated so that an incision can be made. The serosa overlying the proximal segment is then bluntly dissected and the exposed muscular portion is ligated and resected. Finally, the proximal portion is inserted into the mesosalpinx and the distal stump is exteriorised, leaving it open to the peritoneal cavity. Both are very effective and aim to reduce the risk of sterilisation failure due to fistula formation (Wilson 1995; "Käser - Atlas of Gynaecological Surgery | Surgery | Medicine," n. d.).

Regarding the approach, it can be performed by laparoscopy, laparotomy (including postpartum mini laparotomy) or during caesarean section. The morbidity rate in laparoscopy is lower compared to mini laparotomy and, in addition, the surgical time is shorter (Kulier et al. 2004).

Effectiveness

Salpingectomy is considered the most effective method of female sterilisation. In the CREST study, the cumulative 10-year pregnancy rate after partial salpingectomy was 7.5 per 1,000 procedures if performed postpartum and 20.1 per 1,000 in interval surgeries (Lawrie, Kulier, and Nardin 2016; H. B. Peterson et al. 1996). Failures for the classic Pomeroy technique are around 1-1.5% at 10 years (Hibbert et al. 1997). Although there is no such extensive data for total salpingectomy, it is assumed to have superior or equal efficacy, when the tube is completely removed.

Advantages and Disadvantages

The advantages of this technique are that it avoids the use of clips or electrocoagulation, eliminating the risk of mechanical failure or thermal injury, and allows immediate histological documentation and the average operative time is 33 minutes, comparable to standard techniques (Hibbert et al. 1997).

Furthermore, beyond its maximum contraceptive function, as complete removal of the tube reduces failure to a minimum, salpingectomy offers additional benefits such as reducing the risk of ovarian cancer. Multiple studies suggest that high-grade serous carcinoma may originate in the fimbriae of the fallopian tube and that the tube also acts as a conduit for the spread of carcinogens such as endometrial cells or pathogens from ascending infections in cases of endometrioid or clear cell cancer. It is the leading cause of death from gynaecological cancer

(Tone et al. 2012). Bilateral total salpingectomy has been proposed as a primary prevention strategy for this type of cancer, although only for women who are not at high risk of ovarian cancer, such as BRCA mutation carriers or carriers of Lynch syndrome, whose prevention is bilateral adnexectomy from the age of 40-45 years (Narod et al. 2001).

No changes in ovarian reserve have been found following this technique (Findley et al. 2013).

Among the disadvantages are that it is an operator-dependent technique and that if only a small fragment of the tube is resected, spontaneous recanalisation may occur.

Surgical Techniques Using Electrocoagulation

Electrocoagulation has historically been one of the most widely used methods. It consists of applying electric current (unipolar or bipolar) to cause tubal tissue necrosis and subsequent fibrosis.

- *Unipolar* electrocoagulation. This was the first widely used laparoscopic method of tubal occlusion. It consists of carefully identifying the tube and coagulating it about 5cm from the uterus, making a burn of approximately 3-5cm and leaving a safety margin of 2-3cm of healthy tube close to the uterine horn. In this way we avoid uteroperitoneal fistulas caused by activation of the tubal epithelium and increased blood pressure during retrograde menstruation. These fistulas allow sperm access to the peritoneal cavity and the possibility of fertilisation leading to ectopic pregnancy (Shah, Courey, and Cunanan 1977). This technique has a higher risk of generating thermal injury to neighbouring organs, and has therefore been progressively replaced.
- *Bipolar* is safer and more controlled, as it allows energy to be applied to a localised area of the tube, minimising collateral thermal damage (Rioux and Cloutier 1974). The technique consists of coagulating about 3cm of the distal isthmic portion of the tube 3 times, to reduce the likelihood of repermeabilisation and subsequent gestation, leaving a safety margin of 2cm of undamaged tube up to the uterine horn. For this contact electrocoagulation, it would be more appropriate to use the non-modulated mode (cutting mode) with a minimum of 25 watts of power, rather than the modulated mode (coagulation mode) because the latter can produce a superficial carbonisation that prevents obstruction of the deepest layer of the tube. To check if the tube is blocked, we can look at the whitish appearance of the tissue, although this is difficult to check. The long-term probability of pregnancy after tubal sterilisation with bipolar coagulation is lower the more stitches are cauterised, and higher when more than three are performed ("Laparoscopic sterilisation - GLOWM," n. d.).

In both modalities, after coagulation, necrosis and closure of the tube occurs. Subsequently, section of the necrotic segment can be performed for safety, although this is not always essential, as it has been associated with a greater likelihood of fistulae (McCausland 1982).

Efficacy depends on the length of coagulated tube (ideally ≥3 cm), the number of application sites and whether or not the segment is resected after coagulation.

Electrocoagulation shows less postoperative morbidity and less immediate pain than methods such as ring or salpingectomy. The most commonly used approach is the laparoscopic approach.

Effectiveness

According to the CREST study, unipolar electrocoagulation has the lowest cumulative 10-year failure rate, along with postpartum partial salpingectomy, of 7.5/1000 procedures, although it has been abandoned due to the higher complication rate. For bipolar electrocoagulation the 10-year failure rate is 24.8/1000 procedures with bipolar coagulation (2.48%) which decreases to 7.5/1000 in series with resection after coagulation (H. B. Peterson et al. 1996).

Advantages and Disadvantages

The advantages we found are that it is a technique available in most laparoscopic operating theatres, it does not require additional devices (clips, rings) and, if the tube is sectioned, the risk of epithelial ovarian cancer is reduced (Lawrie, Kulier, and Nardin 2016). On the downside, there is a risk of non-visible electrolesion to adjacent organs, it leaves no anatomical specimen to confirm complete disruption, and the possibility of subsequent surgical reversal is low due to extensive thermal damage.

Mechanical Surgical Techniques

Mechanical techniques are based on the physical blocking of the fallopian tube through the application of external devices such as clips or rings.

Tubal clips:

- *Hulka clip:* plastic with metal spring. Covers a small portion of the horn.
- *Filshie clip:* more modern. These are lockable titanium clips coated with a silicone elastomer protection. It is closed by a special clip on the tubal isthmus.

Tubal rings (Yoon or Falope band)

They are placed with the help of an applicator with two hooks with which the mesosalpinx is grasped. With the retraction of the hooks, a silicone elastomer ring is placed around the tubal loop. They can be placed laparoscopically, after a laparotomy or through a vaginal incision. They are associated with more postoperative pain and minor complications compared to other techniques (Oligbo, Revicky, and Udeh 2010; Lawrie, Kulier, and Nardin 2016; Koetsawang, Srisupandit, and Cole 1978).

With mechanical methods, topical local anaesthetics, such as bupivacaine and etidocaine, can be used concomitantly with general or regional anaesthesia on the tubes before and after surgery, as it reduces short-term postoperative pain (Oligbo, Revicky, and Udeh 2010; Harrison, DiNapoli, and Westhoff 2014).

Effectiveness

According to the CREST study, the 10-year cumulative failure rate for Hulka clips is 36.5/1000 procedures, with a rate of 3.65%; Filshie clips improve on these figures with rates close to 1-2%, although without as much long-term data as other techniques. The 10-year efficacy of tubal rings is 17.7/1000 procedures, at 1.77% (Moss and Isley 2015; H. B. Peterson et al. 1996; Lawrie, Kulier, and Nardin 2016).

The immediate postpartum and caesarean section failure and complication rates of Filshie clips are similar to those of the modified Pomeroy technique and are therefore considered a good alternative and quicker to use (Kohaut et al. 2004; Madari, Varma, and Gupta 2011).

Advantages and Disadvantages
The advantages are that these techniques are quick, easy to apply, reproducible and reversible, as they allow greater preservation of the tube and do not generate thermal injury, which favours potential future reversal.

The disadvantages of these techniques are that they require specific instrumentation, they have a risk of failure due to displacement or misplacement of the device, and they leave foreign material in the body.

Time of Realisation

Permanent female sterilisation can be performed after a vaginal delivery, in the course of a caesarean section or outside the puerperal period (interval sterilisation).

- *Puerperal period.*
  - After a vaginal delivery. It is usually performed 24-48 hours postpartum, taking advantage of the fact that the uterine fundus is at the level of the umbilicus and the epidural catheter is in place during labour. It can be performed safely up to 6 days after delivery. Antibiotic and antithrombotic prophylaxis is not necessary in healthy patients without risk factors. The mini laparotomy is the approach of choice. The Pomeroy partial salpingectomy technique is frequently used.
  - During a caesarean section. Partial salpingectomy is performed with the laparotomy already done and with a larger field of view. It has a very high efficacy. The 10-year failure rate of salpingectomy during caesarean section is 7.5/1000 operations, lower than any other sterilisation method and equalled by unipolar electrocoagulation (H. B. Peterson et al. 1996).
  - Interval. This is performed in the non-pregnant woman during the inter-gestational period. It can be performed by mini-laparotomy or laparoscopy, the latter being preferable due to its lower complication rate and shorter surgical time (Kulier et al. 2004). It can also be performed opportunistically, during the course of another gynaecological procedure.

Boarding Routes

The main surgical routes for tubal sterilisation are:

- *Laparoscopic* (more frequent in women in the interval period). Allows the use of clips, rings or coagulation. Minimally invasive and quick recovery.
- *Minilaparotomy* (common in postpartum). It is performed through a suprapubic or mid-infrapubic incision (to access the uterine fundus) of less than 5 cm (Kulier et al.

2004). Once in the abdominal cavity, the uterine fundus is located by extracting the tube through the orifice. In this way we locate the fimbriae to avoid confusing the tube with another adnexal structure such as the broad ligament or the round ligament.

- *Laparotomy* (more during caesarean section). This is an ideal surgical opportunity to perform salpingectomy without increasing morbidity.
- *Transcervical route via hysteroscopy*. It was used with hysteroscopic tubal blocking devices, which has been withdrawn from the market for safety reasons and is no longer possible today ("Revisiting Essure--Toward Safe and Effective Sterilization - PubMed," n. d.).
- *Vaginal route*. Using transluminal endoscopic surgery through natural orifices via the vaginal route or vNOTES. It is a less common technique, but offers superior exposure and access to the pelvic organs, reducing complications associated with trocar placement. It also reduces immediate postoperative pain, leading to earlier discharge from hospital and a better cosmetic outcome for the patient (Yassa et al. 2022). The vaginal route via a 3cm longitudinal or transverse anterior colpotomy through which the cul-de-sac of Douglas is accessed is obsolete. A flap is needed to lift the uterus and the tubes fall into the field. Mechanical methods or salpingectomy can be used. This is a rarely used route. Culdoscopy, with a pneumoperitoneum via a 5mm trocar in the posterior cul-de-sac, is even more rarely used. This access route should not be used for sterilisation (Kulier et al. 2004).

Complications

Surgical contraception, although generally safe and well tolerated, is not without risk. It should be noted that tubal sterilisation techniques have not been associated with menstrual disturbances, adverse hormonal effects, or decreased ovarian reserve since, if performed carefully, ovarian vascularisation is not affected (Gentile et al. 2006; Carmona et al. 2003). Mortality is 2-6 cases per 10000 procedures by any technique (H. B. Peterson et al. 1996), mainly due to complications of general anaesthesia and haemorrhagic complications. The complication rate correlates closely with the laparoscopic procedure (Jamieson et al. 2000). Complications can be divided into immediate, short-term and long-term, and vary according to the technique used and the clinical context.

1. *Immediate and perioperative:*
    - *Haemorrhage*. Both at the point of insertion and intra-abdominal. More frequent in laparoscopic and electrocoagulation techniques.
    - I*njury to adjacent organs*. Injury to bowel, bladder or pelvic vessels, especially during insertion of trocars for laparoscopic forceps. May present clinically for up to 2 weeks in a complicated form with peritonitis and sepsis.
    - *Surgical wound infection or peritonitis* (rare).
    - *Anaesthetic complications*. Nausea, vomiting and other adverse reactions.

2. *Short and long term:*
    - *Post-tubal ligation syndrome*. Described by some women as dysmenorrhoea, menstrual irregularity and/or chronic pelvic pain after sterilisation. Its existence as a separate clinical entity is controversial.
    - *Failure of the procedure*. Although rare, post-sterilisation pregnancies can occur, including ectopic pregnancies. Causes may include poor placement of mechanical methods, ongoing pregnancy on the day of the procedure, or secondary recanalisation. Predisposing factors are the age of the patient, the technique used and the time since the operation (highest failure rate in the first or second year, rarely occurs after 5 years). Pregnancies occurring after tubal sterilisation are usually ectopic and comprise about 33% of pregnancies (H. B. Peterson et al. 1997). The pregnancy rate varies according to the technique used: it is lower with salpingectomy than with clips or rings (H. B. Peterson et al. 1996).
    - *Regret*. Risk factors are: sterilised women under 25 years of age, nulliparous or low parity, in an unstable relationship or in partner conflict, in contexts of socio-economic or personal pressure with insecurity in their decision making, after caesarean section without good decision making, remarriage/change of partner/change in marital status, death of a child and cases of lack of knowledge/limited access to other contraceptive method options. The cumulative probability of regret decreases as the interval between childbirth and sterilisation increases. It also decreases with adequate counselling on the nature of the contraceptive method (Wilcox et al. 1991; Hillis et al. 1999).
3. *Technique-specific complications:*
    - *Electrocoagulation*. Risk of burns to adjacent tissues, less reversibility. Unipolar electrocoagulation was temporarily abandoned when other methods such as clips or bipolar energy appeared, given the high initial complication rate (especially intestinal burns). However, it is likely that there is now a lower rate of complications due to the use of safer electrocoagulators.
    - *Mechanical techniques* (clips, rings). Higher long-term failure rate compared to segmental resection techniques (such as Pomeroy) or salpingectomy.
    - *Salpingectomy*. Slightly higher surgical risk but no increased morbidity compared to other techniques, especially if performed in the context of an already indicated obstetric or gynaecological intervention. The most frequent complications are vascular or visceral injuries during trocar insertion and intestinal burns. Previous abdominal or pelvic surgery, pelvic inflammatory disease, endometriosis and obesity significantly increase the relative risk of complications and the need for laparotomy.

Reversibility

Re-anastomosis of the fallopian tubes after sterilisation may result in high rates of postoperative patency, but may not result in pregnancy or return of fertility.

An advantage of the Pomeroy method over thermal or extensive resection techniques is its potential for surgical reversal, in case total salpingectomy is not performed and a certain length of proximal and distal tube is preserved, which may be more favourable for tubal recanalisation in case of regret (Boeckx et al. 1986). However, like all sterilisation, it should be considered irreversible in clinical practice, and should only be performed in patients who are completely convinced that they do not want future pregnancies. Therefore, the only possibility of conception after this procedure is through assisted reproduction such as in vitro fertilisation (Yossry et al. 2006).

For electrocoagulation techniques, reversibility is limited because extensive coagulation reduces the feasibility of recanalisation, but the risk of ectopic pregnancy is high in case of failure (Prabha, Lunan, and Hill 2003).

Mechanical techniques offer a better prognosis for surgical reversal than coagulation or salpingectomy. Pregnancy rates after recanalisation can reach 40-80% if there is sufficient remaining tube and good microsurgical technique (Boeckx et al. 1986; Prabha, Lunan, and Hill 2003). In addition, both clips and rings may have more technical failures than electrocoagulation or salpingectomy.

Recommendations and Conclusion

Surgical contraception, both female and male, is a safe, effective and definitive option for fertility control. However, because of its permanent nature, it requires a rigorous, ethical and person-centred counselling process. In the light of the scientific evidence and the main clinical guidelines, we conclude the following:

- Prior counselling should be comprehensive and non-coercive, including clear information on the irreversibility of the procedure, failure rates, surgical risks, potential regret - especially in young patients - and available reversible alternatives such as LARC methods.
- The choice of surgical method and technique should be individualised, prioritising the options with the highest efficacy and lowest morbidity. In women, bilateral salpingectomy with the Pomeroy technique is the preferred option when technically possible, given its efficacy and potential oncological benefit.
- The clinical and psychosocial suitability of the patient must be ensured, avoiding hasty decisions in contexts of emotional vulnerability or external pressure. In the case of perinatal sterilisation, consent should be obtained in advance and in a fully informed manner.
- Adequate follow-up and monitoring of complications must be protocolised, ensuring early detection of adverse events such as haematomas, infections, chronic pain or method failure.
- Health care providers must be adequately trained in both surgical techniques and communication skills to promote respectful, evidence-based care focused on the patient's reproductive autonomy.

References

"ACOG Practice Bulletin No. 208: Benefits and Risks of Sterilization." 2019. *Obstetrics & Gynecology* 133 (3): e194-207. https://doi.org/10.1097/AOG.0000000000003111.

Boeckx, W., S. Gordts, K. Buysse, y I. Brosens. 1986. "Reversibility after Female Sterilization." *British Journal of Obstetrics and Gynaecology* 93 (8): 839-42. https://doi.org/10.1111/j.1471-0528.1986.tb07992.x.

Carmona, Francisco, Pilar Cristóbal, Roser Casamitjana, y Juan Balasch. 2003. "Effect of Tubal Sterilization on Ovarian Follicular Reserve and Function." *American Journal of Obstetrics and Gynecology* 189 (2): 447-52. https://doi.org/10.1067/s0002-9378(03)00487-3.

"Esterilización laparoscópica | GLOWM." s. f. Accedido 21 de mayo de 2025. http://www.glowm.com/section-view/heading/Laparoscopic Sterilization/item/402.

Findley, Austin D., Matthew T. Siedhoff, Kumari A. Hobbs, John F. Steege, Erin T. Carey, Christina A. McCall, y Anne Z. Steiner. 2013. "Short-Term Effects of Salpingectomy during Laparoscopic Hysterectomy on Ovarian Reserve: A Pilot Randomized Controlled Trial." *Fertility and Sterility* 100 (6): 1704-8. https://doi.org/10.1016/j.fertnstert.2013.07.1997.

Gentile, Gwen P., Donald W. Helbig, Howard Zacur, Taesung Park, Young Jack Lee, y Carolyn L. Westhoff. 2006. "Hormone Levels before and after Tubal Sterilization." *Contraception* 73 (5): 507-11. https://doi.org/10.1016/j.contraception.2005.12.002.

Giannakeas, Vasily, Ally Murji, Lorraine L. Lipscombe, Steven A. Narod, y Joanne Kotsopoulos. 2023. "Salpingectomy and the Risk of Ovarian Cancer in Ontario." *JAMA Network Open* 6 (8): e2327198. https://doi.org/10.1001/jamanetworkopen.2023.27198.

Grubb, G. S., y H. B. Peterson. 1985. "Luteal Phase Pregnancy and Tubal Sterilization." *Obstetrics and Gynecology* 66 (6): 784-88.

Harrison, Margo S., Marianne N. DiNapoli, y Carolyn L. Westhoff. 2014. "Reducing Postoperative Pain after Tubal Ligation with Rings or Clips: A Systematic Review and Meta-Analysis." *Obstetrics and Gynecology* 124 (1): 68-75. https://doi.org/10.1097/AOG.0000000000000342.

Hibbert, M. L., J. L. Buller, S. D. Seymour, S. E. Poore, y G. D. Davis. 1997. "A Microlaparoscopic Technique for Pomeroy Tubal Ligation." *Obstetrics and Gynecology* 90 (2): 249-51. https://doi.org/10.1016/S0029-7844(97)00234-2.

Hillis, Susan D., Polly A. Marchbanks, Lisa Ratliff Tylor, y Herbert B. Peterson. 1999. "Poststerilization regret: findings from the United States collaborative review of sterilization." *Obstetrics & Gynecology* 93 (6): 889-95. https://doi.org/10.1016/S0029-7844(98)00539-0.

Jamieson, D. J., S. D. Hillis, A. Duerr, P. A. Marchbanks, C. Costello, y H. B. Peterson. 2000. "Complications of Interval Laparoscopic Tubal Sterilization: Findings from the United States Collaborative Review of Sterilization." *Obstetrics and Gynecology* 96 (6): 997-1002. https://doi.org/10.1016/s0029-7844(00)01082-6.

"Käser - Atlas de Cirugía Ginecológica | PDF | Cirugía | Medicina." s. f. Scribd. Accedido 22 de mayo de 2025. https://es.scribd.com/document/384809151/Kaser-Atlas-de-Cirugia-Ginecologica.

Koetsawang, S., S. Srisupandit, y L. P. Cole. 1978. "Laparoscopic Electrocoagulation and Tubal Ring Techniques for Sterilization: A Comparative Study." *International Journal of Gynaecology and Obstetrics: The Official Organ of the International Federation of Gynaecology and Obstetrics* 15 (5): 455-58. https://doi.org/10.1002/j.1879-3479.1977.tb00730.x.

Kohaut, Bettina A., B. Lynn Musselman, Luis Sanchez-Ramos, y Andrew M. Kaunitz. 2004. "Randomized Trial to Compare Perioperative Outcomes of Filshie Clip vs. Pomeroy Technique for Postpartum and Intraoperative Cesarean Tubal Sterilization: A Pilot Study." *Contraception* 69 (4): 267-70. https://doi.org/10.1016/j.contraception.2003.12.007.

Kulier, Regina, Michel Boulvain, Dilys M. Walker, Gabriel De Candolle, y Aldo Campana. 2004. "Minilaparotomy and endoscopic techniques for tubal sterilisation." *The Cochrane Database of Systematic Reviews* 2004 (3): CD001328. https://doi.org/10.1002/14651858.CD001328.pub2.

Lawrie, Theresa A., Regina Kulier, y Juan Manuel Nardin. 2016. "Techniques for the Interruption of Tubal Patency for Female Sterilisation." *The Cochrane Database of Systematic Reviews* 2016 (8): CD003034. https://doi.org/10.1002/14651858.CD003034.pub4.

Lipscomb, G. H., J. R. Spellman, y F. W. Ling. 1993. "The Effect of Same-Day Pregnancy Testing on the Incidence of Luteal Phase Pregnancy." *Obstetrics and Gynecology* 82 (3): 411-13.

Madari, Sheethal, Rajesh Varma, y Janesh Gupta. 2011. "A Comparison of the Modified Pomeroy Tubal Ligation and Filshie Clips for Immediate Postpartum Sterilisation: A Systematic Review." *The European Journal of Contraception & Reproductive Health Care: The Official Journal of the European Society of Contraception* 16 (5): 341-49. https://doi.org/10.3109/13625187.2011.594919.

McCausland, A. 1982. "Endosalpingosis ("endosalpingoblastosis") Following Laparoscopic Tubal Coagulation as an Etiologic Factor of Ectopic Pregnancy." *American Journal of Obstetrics and Gynecology* 143 (1): 12-24. https://doi.org/10.1016/0002-9378(82)90677-9.

Moss, Chailee, y Michelle M. Isley. 2015. "Sterilization." *Obstetrics and Gynecology Clinics of North America* 42 (4): 713-24. https://doi.org/10.1016/j.ogc.2015.07.003.

Narod, S. A., P. Sun, P. Ghadirian, H. Lynch, C. Isaacs, J. Garber, B. Weber, et al. 2001. "Tubal Ligation and Risk of Ovarian Cancer in Carriers of BRCA1 or BRCA2 Mutations: A Case-Control Study." *Lancet (London, England)* 357 (9267): 1467-70. https://doi.org/10.1016/s0140-6736(00)04642-0.

Nguyen, Antoinette T., Kathryn M. Curtis, Naomi K. Tepper, Katherine Kortsmit, Anna W. Brittain, Emily M. Snyder, Megan A. Cohen, et al. 2024. "U.S. Medical Eligibility Criteria for Contraceptive Use, 2024." *MMWR. Recommendations and Reports* 73 (4): 1-126. https://doi.org/10.15585/mmwr.rr7304a1.

Oligbo, Nicholas, Vladimir Revicky, y Rebecca Udeh. 2010. "Pomeroy Technique or Filshie Clips for Postpartum Sterilisation? Retrospective Study on Comparison between Pomeroy Procedure and Filshie Clips for a Tubal Occlusion at the Time of Caesarean Section." *Archives of Gynecology and Obstetrics* 281 (6): 1073-75. https://doi.org/10.1007/s00404-009-1314-7.

Peterson, H. B., F. DeStefano, G. L. Rubin, J. R. Greenspan, N. C. Lee, y H. W. Ory. 1983. "Deaths Attributable to Tubal Sterilization in the United States, 1977 to 1981." *American Journal of Obstetrics and Gynecology* 146 (2): 131-36. https://doi.org/10.1016/0002-9378(83)91040-2.

Peterson, H. B., Z. Xia, J. M. Hughes, L. S. Wilcox, L. R. Tylor, y J. Trussell. 1996. "The Risk of Pregnancy after Tubal Sterilization: Findings from the U.S. Collaborative Review of Sterilization." *American Journal of Obstetrics and Gynecology* 174 (4): 1161-68; discussion 1168-1170. https://doi.org/10.1016/s0002-9378(96)70658-0.

———. 1997. "The Risk of Ectopic Pregnancy after Tubal Sterilization. U.S. Collaborative Review of Sterilization Working Group." *The New England Journal of Medicine* 336 (11): 762-67. https://doi.org/10.1056/NEJM199703133361104.

Peterson, Herbert B. 2008. "Sterilization": *Obstetrics & Gynecology* 111 (1): 189-203. https://doi.org/10.1097/01.AOG.0000298621.98372.62.

Prabha, Sivaraman, C. Burnett Lunan, y Robert Hill. 2003. "Experience of Reversal of Sterilisation at Glasgow Royal Infirmary." *BMJ Sexual & Reproductive Health* 29 (1): 32-33. https://doi.org/10.1783/147118903101196882.

"Revisiting Essure--Toward Safe and Effective Sterilization - PubMed." s. f. Accedido 21 de mayo de 2025. https://pubmed.ncbi.nlm.nih.gov/26397951/.

Rioux, J. E., y D. Cloutier. 1974. "A New Bipolar Instrument for Laparoscopic Tubal Sterilization." *American Journal of Obstetrics and Gynecology* 119 (6): 737-39. https://doi.org/10.1016/0002-9378(74)90084-2.

Shah, A., N. G. Courey, y R. G. Cunanan. 1977. "Pregnancy Following Laparoscopic Tubal Electrocoagulation and Division." *American Journal of Obstetrics and Gynecology* 129 (4): 459-60. https://doi.org/10.1016/0002-9378(77)90597-x.

Tone, Alicia A., Shannon Salvador, Sarah J. Finlayson, Anna V. Tinker, Janice S. Kwon, Cheng-Han Lee, Trevor Cohen, et al. 2012. "The Role of the Fallopian Tube in Ovarian Cancer." *Clinical Advances in Hematology & Oncology: H&O* 10 (5): 296-306.

Vricella, Laura K., Lori M. Gawron, y Judette M. Louis. 2019. "Society for Maternal-Fetal Medicine (SMFM) Consult Series #48: Immediate Postpartum Long-Acting Reversible Contraception for Women at High Risk for Medical Complications." *American Journal of Obstetrics and Gynecology* 220 (5): B2-12. https://doi.org/10.1016/j.ajog.2019.02.011.

Wilcox, L. S., S. Y. Chu, E. D. Eaker, S. L. Zeger, y H. B. Peterson. 1991. "Risk Factors for Regret after Tubal Sterilization: 5 Years of Follow-up in a Prospective Study." *Fertility and Sterility* 55 (5): 927-33.

Wilson, E. W. 1995. "The evolution of methods for female sterilization." *International Journal of Gynecology & Obstetrics*, WHO Consultation on the Development of New Technologies for Female Sterilization, 51 (diciembre): S3-13. https://doi.org/10.1016/0020-7292(95)90363-1.

Yassa, Murat, Cihan Kaya, Erkan Kalafat, Arzu Bilge Tekin, Sema Karakas, Memis Ali Mutlu, Pinar Birol, y Niyazi Tug. 2022. "The Comparison of Transvaginal Natural Orifice Transluminal Endoscopic Surgery and Conventional Laparoscopy in Opportunistic Bilateral Salpingectomy for Permanent Female Sterilization." *Journal of Minimally Invasive Gynecology* 29 (2): 257-264.e1. https://doi.org/10.1016/j.jmig.2021.08.009.

Yossry, M., M. Aboulghar, A. D'Angelo, y W. Gillett. 2006. "In Vitro Fertilisation versus Tubal Reanastomosis (Sterilisation Reversal) for Subfertility after Tubal Sterilisation." *The Cochrane Database of Systematic Reviews* 2006 (3): CD004144. https://doi.org/10.1002/14651858.CD004144.pub2.

Zapata, Lauren B., Karen Pazol, Christine Dehlendorf, Kathryn M. Curtis, Nikita M. Malcolm, Rachel B. Rosmarin, y Brittni N. Frederiksen. 2018. "Contraceptive Counseling in Clinical Settings: An Updated Systematic Review." *American Journal of Preventive Medicine* 55 (5): 677-90. https://doi.org/10.1016/j.amepre.2018.07.006.

Chapter 11

Emergency Contraception

P. Mora Ábalos[1,*], MD
M. Cebrián Marcilla[1], MD
M. Moreno Palmero[1], MD
A. Serrano Sánchez[1], MD
and M. A. Roque Fernández[1,2], PhD
[1]Obstetrics and Gynaecology Department, University and Hospital Complex of Albacete, Spain
[2]Medical Science Department, School of Medicine of Albacete, Universidad de Castilla-La Mancha, Spain

Abstract

Emergency contraception is a key reproductive health intervention aimed at preventing unwanted pregnancies after unprotected sex or contraceptive failure. Since its introduction in the 1960s, it has evolved from high doses of estrogen to safer and more effective methods such as levonorgestrel, ulipristal acetate, and the copper intrauterine device, the latter being considered the most effective method. This chapter reviews the history, indications, mechanisms of action, efficacy, and criteria for choosing among the available methods. Emergency contraception is indicated in cases of contraceptive failure, sexual assault, postpartum, postabortion, and situations of risk of unwanted pregnancy. It should be administered immediately, without prior examinations or diagnostic tests. Oral hormonal methods (levonorgestrel and ulipristal acetate) work by inhibiting or delaying ovulation; the copper intrauterine device also prevents implantation. None of these methods are abortive. Effectiveness depends on the time of the cycle and body mass index: levonorgestrel may be less effective in obese women, unlike ulipristal acetate and the copper intrauterine device. The choice of method should be individualized, considering clinical factors, availability, and the possibility of long-term contraception. Adverse effects are generally mild and transient and do not compromise future fertility. There is a clear need for new options such as the pericoital pill and for strengthening access, education, and public policies to meet the still unmet demand for contraception globally.

Keywords: postcoital contraception, intrauterine devices, levonorgestrel, ulipristal acetate, mifepristone

---

[*] Corresponding Author's Email: pilimora997@gmail.com

In: Advances in Reproductive Health
Editors: Llanos Belmonte Andujar and Ana Fuentes Rozalen
ISBN: 979-8-90134-038-7

Introduction

Research into postcoital contraception began in the 1960s, when methods using high doses of estrogen, such as ethinyl estradiol (steroidal estrogen) and diethylstilbestrol, a non-steroidal estrogen, began to be developed (Ellertson 1994).

In 1974, the first oral emergency contraception (EC) regimen, known as the "Yuzpe method," was introduced, combining estrogen and progestin. This demonstrated that a dose of 100 micrograms of ethinyl estradiol and 0.5 milligrams of levonorgestrel (LNG) (with a second dose repeated 12 hours later) induced changes in the endometrium that prevented the implantation of the fertilized egg (Yuzpe AA, Thurlow HJ, Ramzy I 1974).

In the early 1970s, estrogen-free options were also explored. In South America, research began on the use of LNG (150-400 mcg) as a postcoital contraceptive, administered in a single dose to be taken within three hours of sexual intercourse. However, low doses were ineffective and disrupted the menstrual cycle, prompting the development of more effective LNG-based methods (Kesserü et al. 1974). Beginning in the 1970s, intrauterine devices (IUDs) were also studied as EC.

The most widely used emergency oral contraceptive today is the 1.5 mg LNG pill, which was approved in 1999 and has been available without age restrictions since 2013. In addition, in 2010, the FDA approved a second EC, a pill containing 30 mg of ulipristal acetate (AUP) (Hertzen et al. 2002).

Thus, ECPs have evolved over the decades, offering increasingly accessible and effective options for preventing pregnancy in risky situations, improving the reproductive health of women worldwide.

Indications for Emergency Contraception

Currently, 121 million unwanted pregnancies occur worldwide each year, of which 73.3 million end in abortion, indicating that 61% of these unplanned pregnancies result in termination (Bearak et al. 2020). On the other hand, the probability of a woman having sexual intercourse during her fertile window is 25% (D. Li, Wilcox, and Dunson 2015), which increases the risk of unwanted pregnancy, even with the use of contraceptives. In this sense, EC is presented as a key option for reducing the risk of pregnancy after unprotected sex (UPSI) or insufficient protection, including for victims of sexual assault.

EC is recommended for any woman who does not wish to conceive if there is a potential risk of pregnancy after an episode of UPSI, such as (The Faculty of Sexual & Reproductive Healthcare (FSRH) 2017) (The American College of Obstetricians and Gynecologists (ACOG) 2015) (Salcedo et al. 2023) (Rudzinski et al. 2023):

- *Women who do not use hormonal contraception:* Women who do not use hormonal contraception and have UPSI (including coitus interruptus or errors in calculating the fertile period using natural methods), or if an accident occurs while using a regular contraceptive method, such as condom breakage, retention, or misuse, should resort to EC. This applies to any episode of UPSI that has occurred at any time during the natural menstrual cycle, if they do not wish to conceive.

- *After pregnancy: Women who do not wish to conceive after pregnancy may require EC in the following cases:*
  - After childbirth: If UPSI has occurred since day 21 postpartum (unless the criteria for lactational amenorrhea are met).
  - After an abortion or ectopic pregnancy: If UPSI has occurred since day 5 after a spontaneous abortion, induced abortion, ectopic pregnancy, or uterine evacuation due to gestational trophoblastic disease.
- *Women who use hormonal contraception incorrectly or with method failure:*
  - Recent initiation of hormonal methods without using necessary protection for the required period.
  - Concomitant use of drugs that interact with hormonal contraceptives and may reduce their effectiveness.
  - Detachment of the patch for more than 24 hours or removal of the vaginal ring for more than 3 hours (guidelines such as the FSRH establish a more flexible threshold of up to 48 hours from the detachment of the patch or removal of the vaginal ring to consider it necessary to resort to EC if there has been UPSI or failure of the barrier method during HFI or week 1).
  - Missing two or more active pills of combined contraceptives in week 1, more than 27 hours since the last traditional progestin-only pill (POP) (minipill containing LNG, norethisterone, or linestrenol), or more than 36 hours since the last desogestrel-only pill.
  - More than 14 weeks after the last progestin injection or within the first 7 days after a late injection.
  - Expired implant.
  - IUD removal without immediate replacement, partial or complete expulsion, missing strings, or unknown location of the device.
  - Vomiting that may affect the absorption of the oral contraceptive.
- *Special cases:*
  - Sexual assault in a woman without previous contraception: emergency contraception should be part of the care protocol.
  - Exposure to teratogenic substances in case of UPSI.

Any woman of childbearing age who considers herself at risk of an unwanted pregnancy and is considering using EC should do so, with no age limit (World Health Organization (WHO) 2021). This option is safe for most patients (Krishna K. Upadhya 2019) (ACOG 2015). According to the US Centers for Disease Control and Prevention's Medical Eligibility Criteria for Contraceptive Use (CDC 2024), there are no conditions in which the risks of using EC outweigh the benefits (Kathryn M. Curtis 2010). In addition, it is specifically noted that women with a history of ectopic pregnancy, cardiovascular disease, migraines, liver disease, and those who are breastfeeding can use EC. Therefore, women with contraindications to conventional oral contraceptives can access any EC regimen.

EC should be prescribed immediately, without delays caused by physical examinations or diagnostic tests. It is not necessary to perform a pregnancy test before administering EC (FSRH 2017), as the available tests are not reliable if UPSI occurred in the previous 21 days. The only criterion that contraindicates its use is a confirmed pregnancy, especially in the case of the copper intrauterine device (Cu-IUD). A Cu-IUD can be inserted as EC if all UPSI occurred in the last 5 days, and in the case of a woman with amenorrhea, if all UPSI occurred in the last 21 days and she also has a negative pregnancy test. Finally, if a woman has had UPSI since her last menstrual period and requests EC more than 5 days later, a Cu-IUD can be inserted if it is still within 5 days of the probable date of ovulation.

It is also not necessary to screen for sexually transmitted infections (STIs) before administering EC. In the case of the Cu IUD, routine antibiotic prophylaxis is not recommended before insertion as it does not reduce the risk of pelvic inflammatory disease. However, if women have high risk factors for STIs (detailed in the chapter on Cu IUDs), it is recommended that they be evaluated with specific STI tests at the time of IUD insertion. In any case, insertion should not be delayed while awaiting results in the absence of active mucopurulent discharge, regardless of the patient's personal history of STIs (Salcedo et al. 2023). If an STI is detected later, antibiotic treatment can be started without removing the IUD. It is important to note that insertion is contraindicated in women with purulent cervicitis or a known diagnosis of untreated Chlamydia trachomatis or Neisseria gonorrhoeae infection; in these cases, treatment must be completed before proceeding (ACOG 2017).

If a delay is anticipated before Cu-IUD insertion, it is recommended to offer oral EC at the time of the first consultation, in case the woman does not return for Cu-IUD insertion or if it is not possible to insert it.

Information on all EC methods should be provided, and a referral pathway should be in place to allow women to access their preferred method. Access to these methods is essential to reduce unwanted pregnancies and, consequently, the number of voluntary abortions. Thus, EC offers women the possibility of taking control of their reproductive health, especially when other methods have not been effective or are not available.

Mechanisms of Action of Emergency Contraception

Sperm can remain viable in the female genital tract for approximately 5 days after an episode of UPSI (Wilcox, Weinberg, and Baird 1996) (Ferreira-Poblete 1997). If ovulation occurs within that period, there is a possibility of fertilization, which implies a risk of pregnancy.

It is important to note that EC should not be confused with medical abortion. Medical abortion is used to terminate an established pregnancy, while EC focuses on preventing fertilization or implantation, not on terminating an ongoing pregnancy. EC methods are not abortive, as they do not affect an established pregnancy (WHO 2021).

There are products, both dedicated to EC use and regular contraceptive methods, such as IUDs and combined oral contraceptives (COCs), that can also be used outside their original indication for EC. The available options fall into two main groups: IUD insertion and oral hormonal methods. The latter include LNG, antiprogestogens such as AUP and mifepristone, as well as the Yuzpe method, which consists of a combination of estradiol and LNG. The methods of action of the different types of EC are described below:

Intrauterine Device

The Cu-IUD acts mainly by inhibiting fertilization, through a toxic effect on sperm and eggs. Copper alters sperm motility and viability and also affects egg transport. If fertilization occurs, the inflammatory reaction in the endometrium due to the Cu-IUD prevents implantation (Ortiz and Croxatto 2007) (Stanford and Mikolajczyk 2002). Therefore, the Cu-IUD has both pre- and post-fertilization mechanisms of action (which are detailed in the corresponding chapter of this book). Since implantation usually occurs 6 to 10 days after ovulation, the Cu-IUD can be inserted up to 5 days after ovulation, before the implantation process begins. To ensure this estimation, it is crucial that the date of the last menstrual period (LMP) is accurately known and that the cycles are regular.

Although rare, pregnancies in IUD users have an increase in adverse outcomes. These include miscarriage, premature delivery and septic abortion. Similar considerations apply for patients receiving an IUD as an UA (Brahmi et al. 2012).

Ulipristal Acetate

UPA is a selective modulator of progesterone receptors, with both antagonist and partial agonist effects on these receptors. This action is due to the variable distribution of progesterone receptors in tissues. Structurally similar to mifepristone, UPA is a synthetic steroid derived from 19-norprogesterone, with a half-life of 32 hours. On the hypothalamic-pituitary-gonadal axis, it acts as a progesterone receptor agonist, reducing luteinizing hormone (LH) production and preventing the LH peak, which inhibits ovulation.

UPA can delay ovulation for up to 5 days, which may be enough to close the fertile window if given before ovulation. If ovulation has already occurred it would not be effective, as would LNG. It can reduce LH levels even when it is already rising. Once the LH peak has started and with 18 mm follicles, its therapeutic window is larger than that of LNG depending on the day of the cycle. Ovulation would take place 5 days later, which would be enough to close the fertile window since the sperm have entered the female genital tract.

At doses used for EC, it does not affect gamete transport or fertilization (Gemzell-Danielsson, Berger, and Lalitkumar 2013). The effects on the fallopian tubes are unclear: some studies suggest that it could inhibit ciliary movement due to its agonist action on progesterone receptors, while others point out that its antagonist effect could reduce such movement (Rosato, Farris, and Bastianelli 2016). Regarding the endometrium and implantation, most studies indicate that low doses of UPA do not significantly affect endometrial thickness or embryo attachment. However, in vitro studies suggest that UPA may interfere with implantation, showing alterations in markers of endometrial receptivity and a decrease in trophoblast spheroid adhesion.

Levonorgestrel

LNG is a progestogen with progesterone receptor agonist action. Its half-life is 43 hours. LNG in EC inhibits ovulation for up to five days by delaying follicular rupture and inducing luteal phase dysfunction. It acts on the hypothalamic-pituitary-gonadal axis by reducing LH secretion through negative feedback, thereby preventing the preovulatory LH surge and subsequent ovulation (Ortiz and Croxatto, 2007). Unlike UPA, LNG is ineffective once LH levels have begun to rise. Unlike UPA, it does not act once the LH elevation has begun.

LNG is effective before ovulation, but not after ovulation, as it does not prevent implantation (Novikova et al. 2007). Likewise, LNG does not affect the endometrium or embryo receptivity, nor does it significantly alter sperm motility. Furthermore, it does not interfere with an established pregnancy (Zhang et al. 2009).

Mifepristone

Mifepristone or RU 486 is a synthetic steroid with antiprogestational activity, originally developed and approved in high doses for the pharmacological induction of abortion. Its mechanism of action varies depending on the phase of the menstrual cycle: it can inhibit ovulation if administered during the follicular phase and may impair endometrial receptivity if given in the early luteal phase. Low doses (e.g., 10 mg) have shown no significant effect on the endometrium (Gemzell-Danielsson, Berger, and Lalitkumar 2013).

The Yuzpe Method

The Yuzpe method is an effective EC option when COCs containing 100 micrograms of ethinyl estradiol and 0.5 milligrams of LNG are available. A second dose is administered 12 hours after the first to ensure efficacy. The current regimen consists of 0.2 mg of ethinyl estradiol and 1 mg of LNG, given in two doses 12 hours apart, and within 72 hours of UPSI. Although no specific commercial formulation exists for this indication, commercially available COCs can be adapted to achieve the necessary dosage. Individuals who correctly combine the pills to reach the appropriate dose of ethinyl estradiol and LNG can effectively reduce the risk of pregnancy following UPSI. The mechanism of action is thought to involve delayed ovulation due to the effect of progestins, as well as alterations in the endometrium.

Danazol

Danazol is a synthetic steroid that interferes with the development of the dominant follicle at the ovarian level and exerts antiprogestational effects on the endometrium, leading to endometrial atrophy. For EC, the recommended dose of danazol is 600 mg every 12 hours, for a total of two doses.

Effectiveness of Currently Available Emergency Contraceptive Methods

The ideal method of EC would combine safety, high acceptability, and ease of use, and could be administered up to 120 hours after UPSI. This time frame is critical, as sperm can remain viable in the female reproductive tract for up to five days. In addition, an optimal EC method would be effective throughout the entire fertile window of the menstrual cycle, even after fertilization. Ideally, it would also provide a dual mechanism of action, targeting multiple steps in the reproductive process to prevent pregnancy. However, despite advances in EC, no current method meets all of these ideal criteria.

The efficacy of currently available EC methods varies significantly depending on the type of method used and the timing of administration. These methods must be used within a specific window to achieve maximum effectiveness. The available methods are listed below in decreasing order of efficacy:

Cu-IUD

The Cu-IUD is recognized as the most effective method of EC and is recommended as the first-line option for all women seeking protection after UPSI. This recommendation is supported by a systematic review that evaluated 7,034 Cu-IUD insertions performed between 1979 and 2011 across six countries. The overall pregnancy rate was only 0.09%, meaning that fewer than 1 in 1,000 women became pregnant when the Cu-IUD was inserted within 120 hours (5 days) after UPSI. This represents an efficacy of 99.9%, significantly higher than that of oral emergency contraceptives (Cleland et al. 2012).

In a more recent study, an even larger cohort was analyzed, yielding similar findings with a pregnancy rate of 0.1%, further supporting the high efficacy of the Cu-IUD. Importantly, this study also demonstrated that efficacy does not decline in women with a high body mass index (body mass index (BMI) >30), in contrast to some oral EC methods such as LNG, which may be less effective in overweight or obese women (Kaiser et al. 2023).

Notably, a 2021 study by Bakenra et al. examined late Cu-IUD insertion, between 6 and 14 days after UPSI. Among 1,200 cases, no pregnancies were reported during follow-up, suggesting that the protective effect of the Cu-IUD may extend beyond the conventionally accepted 5-day window. This has important clinical implications, offering a wider window for effective intervention in women who present late.

Finally, the Cu-IUD provides both economic and clinical benefits as a long-term contraceptive following its use for EC (Praditpan et al. 2017). Once inserted, it offers up to 10 years of continuous protection, reducing the need for repeated interventions, lowering healthcare costs, and improving adherence. The annual cost of protection with the Cu-IUD has been estimated to be up to 80% lower than that of hormonal methods or repeated use of oral EC.

DIU-LNG

While the Cu-IUD has historically been the preferred intrauterine method for EC, recent research has explored the feasibility of the 52 mg LNG-IUD as an alternative. A randomized noninferiority clinical trial demonstrated that, when inserted within five days of UPSI, the LNG-IUD offers comparable efficacy to the Cu-IUD, with pregnancy rates of 0.3% and 0.0%, respectively (Turok et al. 2021).

Both devices have shown similar safety profiles, with no significant differences in the incidence of adverse events or discontinuation rates after one year of follow-up. One pregnancy was reported in each group at one year (Kaiser et al. 2023). LNG-IUDs are approved for contraceptive use for up to eight years (Bayer HealthCare Pharmaceuticals Inc., 2008), making them an effective long-acting alternative.

In addition to high efficacy, LNG-IUDs offer clinical benefits such as reduced menstrual bleeding and cramping, which may make them more acceptable to some users compared to the Cu-IUD. Like copper devices, LNG-IUDs can be retained after EC use as a long-acting reversible contraceptive (LARC) method.

However, despite these advantages, the use of the LNG-IUD for EC is not currently recommended in clinical guidelines. The primary limitation is the limited body of evidence regarding its specific effectiveness in the EC setting, particularly beyond five days after UPSI. Furthermore, barriers remain in terms of provider knowledge, clinical training, and public health policy, which hinder its systematic adoption.

Therefore, although preliminary findings are promising, larger and more methodologically rigorous studies are needed to confirm its efficacy in emergency contexts. If validated, the LNG-IUD could not only broaden the range of available EC options but also promote wider adoption of LARC methods among individuals seeking contraception after UPSI.

Ulipristal Acetate

UPA is considered the most effective oral emergency contraceptive pill (Sprem Goldstajn et al. 2014). UPA, administered in a single 30 mg dose, is effective for up to 120 hours (five days) after UPSI, with no significant decline in efficacy observed throughout this interval (Moreau and Trussell 2012). This feature clearly distinguishes it from LNG, whose effectiveness is limited to the early stages of the fertile window and decreases progressively with time after UPSI.

Unlike LNG, which delays ovulation only when administered before the LH surge, UPA remains effective even after the LH surge has begun. However, its efficacy diminishes as the periovulatory period progresses, becoming ineffective once the LH peak is reached. At this point, its primary action may shift to the endometrium, where it induces less morphological change than it does at the follicular level (Mozzanega et al. 2014).

Several studies have shown that UPA is more effective than LNG for EC, with lower reported pregnancy rates (1.2% vs. 1.2–2.1%) (Shen et al. 2017). It is estimated to prevent 60–80% of expected pregnancies after UPSI (Li et al. 2016).

A clinically relevant advantage of UPA is its ability to delay ovulation even when it is imminent, making it the preferred option for women in the later phases of the menstrual cycle. However, because ovulation can be significantly delayed following UPA administration, the risk of pregnancy increases if further UPSI occurs within the same cycle (Brache et al. 2013). Therefore, it is essential to advise patients to use a reliable contraceptive method for the remainder of the cycle.

Additionally, it is important to note that hormonal contraceptives containing progestins should not be initiated within five days after UPA administration, as they may antagonize its mechanism of action.

Mifepristone

Mifepristone is currently available as a prescription-only method of EC in a limited number of countries, including Armenia, Russia, Ukraine, China, and Vietnam (European Consortium for Emergency Contraception (ECEC) 2023). Depending on the phase of the menstrual cycle, different post-coital regimens have been utilized. These include two doses of 100 mg administered between days 4 and 7 after the basal body temperature rise; daily doses of 100 to 200 mg for four days between days 23 and 27 of the cycle; or a single dose of 400 to 600 mg on the estimated day of menstruation.

At lower doses (between 10 and 25 mg), mifepristone has been shown to be effective for up to 120 hours (five days) after UPSI (Gemzell-Danielsson, Berger, and Lalitkumar 2013). Increasing evidence suggests that mifepristone is more effective than the Yuzpe method and likely superior to LNG at low to moderate doses (25 to 50 mg) (Shen et al. 2017). A clinical trial conducted in Cuba compared 5 mg and 10 mg doses of mifepristone administered within six days of UPSI. Both groups exhibited a pregnancy rate of only 1.2%, corresponding to an efficacy rate of 98.8% in preventing unintended pregnancies. The authors concluded that both doses are equally effective and safe for use as EC (Mirás, Adriana, and Sánchez 2014).

Levonorgestrel

LNG, when used as EC after a single episode of UPSI, has been associated with pregnancy rates ranging from 1.7% to 2.6% per cycle (Hang et al. 2023). It is officially approved for use within 72 hours following UPSI, although some studies suggest it may retain limited efficacy up to 96 hours. However, evidence between 96 and 120 hours post-UPSI is insufficient to confirm its effectiveness (Hertzen et al. 2002). The WHO supports potential use up to 96 hours, but acknowledges that this recommendation is based on low-quality evidence (Piaggio, Kapp, and Hertzen 2011). Consequently, use beyond 72 hours is not supported by product labeling and is not currently recommended. It is also well-established that LNG becomes ineffective if administered after ovulation has occurred (Li et al. 2016).

In an effort to enhance its effectiveness, the combination of LNG with piroxicam (a single 40 mg oral dose) has been investigated. A recent randomized clinical trial found that this combination significantly reduced pregnancy rates compared to LNG plus placebo (Hang et al. 2023). However, these findings should be interpreted with caution, as the study was limited to women with a single UPSI episode and an average BMI of 21 kg/m^2, limiting generalizability to populations with higher BMI. Nevertheless, when piroxicam is available over the counter and there are no contraindications, this combination may be a viable option.

Finally, it is crucial to advise patients that LNG does not provide contraceptive protection for subsequent UPSI during the same menstrual cycle. To avoid the risk of pregnancy, a reliable ongoing contraceptive method should be initiated immediately following LNG administration.

Effect of Body Weight on Emergency Contraception

The Cu-IUD and the 52 mg LNG-IUD maintain high efficacy regardless of body weight or BMI, making them the most reliable EC options for all patients (Cleland et al. 2012; Turok et al. 2021). In contrast, some studies suggest that oral EC with LNG or UPA may be less effective in overweight or obese women, particularly with LNG (Jatlaoui and Curtis 2016). However, the European Medicines Agency (EMA) concluded in 2014 that the available evidence was insufficient to definitively confirm reduced efficacy in individuals with higher BMI (European Medicines Agency 2014).

Several clinical studies have reported diminished efficacy of LNG in women with obesity, a phenomenon attributed to pharmacokinetic changes. Increased BMI has been associated with lower plasma concentrations of LNG, as demonstrated in comparative studies involving women with normal BMI, obesity, and extreme obesity (Natavio et al. 2019). Although doubling the LNG dose to 3 mg can restore serum levels comparable to those in individuals of normal weight, this approach has not been shown to improve clinical outcomes such as ovulation delay or suppression (Edelman et al. 2022).

By contrast, UPA appears to maintain consistent pharmacokinetics irrespective of BMI. A crossover study involving 32 women found no significant differences in serum UPA levels between individuals with normal BMI and those with obesity, and no dose adjustment based on weight is required (Praditpan et al. 2017). Additionally, a recent trial comparing standard-dose UPA with single and double dose LNG regimens found no statistically significant differences in pregnancy rates, although methodological limitations prevent definitive conclusions (Jensen et al. 2016).

For patients who have undergone bariatric surgery involving a malabsorptive component, the absorption of oral LNG may be significantly impaired, thereby compromising its efficacy as EC. Currently, there is no conclusive evidence on the pharmacokinetics of UPA in this population. In such clinical scenarios, the Cu-IUD remains the most effective and potentially the only reliable option for EC.

Medical Criteria for Choice

The choice of EC method should be individualized according to the patient's preferences, taking into account efficacy, availability, accessibility, and the possibility of initiating long-term contraception. The decision must balance these clinical and personal factors.

Cu-IUD

All women requiring EC should be offered a Cu-IUD whenever possible, as it is the most effective method available. However, its insertion requires face-to-face medical care, which may delay access and pose an economic barrier for individuals without health coverage. Ideally, the Cu-IUD should be inserted at the earliest opportunity. If immediate insertion is not feasible at the point of care, an alternative oral EC method should be provided, and Cu-IUD insertion scheduled as soon as possible. Some patients may decline the Cu-IUD due to personal reasons or prior unfavorable experiences, and this preference should be respected.

The primary advantage of the Cu-IUD lies in its dual function: besides serving as EC, it provides highly effective LARC. Its efficacy is independent of the timing within the menstrual cycle relative to the exposure risk. Current guidelines also recommend offering the Cu-IUD to adolescents at risk of unintended pregnancy (Krishna K. Upadhya 2019).

From a clinical perspective, contraindications for the use of the Cu-IUD in the context of EC coincide with those established for its routine use (see corresponding chapter) (WHO 2021) (UKMEC 2016) (World Health Organization 2021; UK Medical Eligibility Criteria 2016). Nulliparity, young age, history of ectopic pregnancy, and STI risk are not absolute contraindications, though STI risk should be assessed individually.

There are conditions in which the use of the Cu-IUD is absolutely contraindicated, classified as Category 4 (CDC 2024; WHO 2021), due to an unacceptable risk to health; and others classified as Category 3, where the risks may outweigh the benefits, requiring an individualized clinical assessment. These situations are detailed earlier in the corresponding chapter.

Oral Emergency Contraception

There is no medical eligibility category that restricts the use of pharmacological EC, except for Category 4, which applies to known pregnancy. However, if EC is inadvertently taken by a woman who is already pregnant, it will not terminate an established pregnancy nor will it harm the developing embryo (WHO 2021; ACOG 2015).

Ulipristal Acetate

UPA is currently considered the most effective form of oral EC. There are no specific contraindications for the use of UPA as EC (CDC 2024; UKMEC 2016), although its label advises against use in women with severe asthma controlled by oral glucocorticoids, due to its anti-glucocorticoid effect. It also warns that, in the absence of conclusive safety data, use should be avoided in women with hepatic impairment. However, it is important to note that pregnancy poses a significant clinical risk in women with severe hepatic insufficiency, and expert opinion supports the administration of a single 30 mg dose of UPA in these cases, always under medical supervision (FSRH 2017). Additionally, UPA contains lactose, which may be relevant for patients with lactose intolerance or malabsorption.

Levonorgestrel

Although less effective than UPA, LNG is an oral EC option available without prescription in the United States and in several European countries, including Spain, France, Finland, the Netherlands, Norway, Slovakia, Sweden, and the United Kingdom. This accessibility makes it a widely used alternative.

There are no specific contraindications for the use of LNG as EC (UKMEC 2016). However, its product label indicates that it is not recommended for use in patients with severe hepatic dysfunction (Bayer Plc 2021). Nonetheless, given that pregnancy may pose a significant clinical risk in such cases, expert opinion supports the use of a single 1.5 mg dose of LNG under medical supervision (FSRH 2017).

It should also be noted that commercially available 1.5 mg LNG products contain lactose, which is relevant for women with lactose intolerance.

Side Effects of Emergency Contraception

In general, EC methods are extremely safe and do not pose long-term risks to fertility (Lee and Schwarz 2017).

The Cu-IUD is a safe EC method when insertion is performed by trained clinicians. The risk of uterine perforation is low, approximately 1 in 1,000 insertions. In women at high risk for infection, prophylactic administration of antibiotics targeting prevalent sexually transmitted infections may be considered (FSRH 2017).

The most common side effects are similar to those seen with regular use of the IUD: insertion-related pain, increased menstrual bleeding, and longer menstrual cycles, symptoms that generally decrease over time (Cleland et al. 2012).

Oral EC with either LNG or UPA is considered safe for all women, including adolescents. These methods can be used throughout the reproductive lifespan, from menarche until menopause. Perimenopausal women may continue to ovulate despite irregular menstruation, and thus should consider EC after UPSI, particularly in cases of incorrect hormonal contraceptive use. EC is generally not necessary for women over 50 years of age who have experienced one year of natural amenorrhea. However, it may still be required for women under 50 with fewer than two years of amenorrhea, particularly those under age 45, as ovulation may still occur. Hormone replacement therapy (HRT) is not a contraceptive and, when combined with contraceptive methods or EC, may reduce the efficacy of UPA (FSRH 2017).

Adverse effects associated with EC are rare in healthy women (Jatlaoui, Riley, and Curtis 2016). To date, there have been no reported deaths or serious complications linked to the use of EC. Moreover, its use has not been shown to negatively affect future fertility (FSRH 2017).

Both LNG and UPA have favorable safety profiles. In cases of accidental administration during pregnancy, no significant teratogenic risk has been identified (Berger et al. 2015). Furthermore, no increased risk of venous thromboembolism or cancer has been documented among EC users. The most commonly reported side effects include headache, nausea, and dysmenorrhea, each affecting approximately 10% of users (Glasier et al. 2010).

Vomiting

The Yuzpe regimen is associated with the highest incidence of nausea and vomiting among EC methods. Approximately 50% of users experience nausea, and 20% report vomiting (Shen et al. 2017).

If vomiting occurs within two hours of taking LNG or within three hours of taking other oral EC methods, the dose should be repeated, or the insertion of a Cu-IUD should be considered. Routine use of antiemetics is not recommended (WHO 2021).

Ectopic Pregnancy

Although available evidence is not entirely conclusive, EC does not appear to increase the risk of ectopic pregnancy. A systematic review concluded that the rate of ectopic pregnancy following EC failure with LNG or mifepristone did not exceed that of the general population (Cleland et al. 2010). UPA also does not appear to increase this risk (Glasier 2014).

The Cu-IUD does not raise the absolute risk of ectopic pregnancy, as it prevents the vast majority of pregnancies. However, in the rare instance that pregnancy occurs with an IUD in place, the likelihood of it being ectopic is higher compared to pregnancies in women not using an IUD (ACOG 2017).

Menstrual Cycle Alterations

Menstrual irregularities are common following EC use. Patients should be informed about the possibility of changes in cycle length or intermenstrual bleeding. If menstruation is delayed by more than seven days, a pregnancy test should be conducted (FSRH 2017).

In phase III studies of UPA, 75% of women menstruated on schedule or within seven days of the expected date. Around 20% experienced delays of more than seven days, and 4% reported delays exceeding 20 days (Moreau and Trussell 2012). Fewer than 10% reported intermenstrual bleeding.

For LNG, most users menstruated within seven days of the expected date. Delays of more than one week occurred in fewer than 10% of cases (Bayer Plc 2021).

Abdominal Pain

Lower abdominal pain is more frequently reported among users of the Cu-IUD and the Yuzpe regimen compared to those who use mifepristone. Nonetheless, the Cu-IUD is associated with an overall lower incidence of side effects than hormonal EC methods such as LNG or moderate-to high-dose mifepristone (Shen et al. 2017). Between 5–6% of LNG and UPA users report abdominal pain (Glasier et al. 2010).

In summary, EC methods such as LNG, UPA, and the Cu-IUD are highly safe and effective at preventing unintended pregnancy. While side effects may occur, they are generally mild and transient. There is no evidence of serious complications or long-term effects on fertility. It is essential that healthcare professionals provide patients with clear information on potential adverse effects and guidance on how to manage them.

Emergency Contraception in Women with Previous Hormonal Treatment

Cu-IUD Insertion After Misuse of Combined Hormonal Contraceptives (CHC)

When CHC methods, such as the pill, patch, or vaginal ring) are used incorrectly during the first week of the cycle, or when the HFI is extended, there may be a risk of ovulation. A systematic review reported that ovulation may occur as early as 8 days after the last correctly taken pill. Another study observed ovulation 13 days after an extended HFI in vaginal ring users. However, no equivalent data are available for the contraceptive patch (Zapata et al. 2013).

Based on this evidence, it is recommended that a Cu-IUD may be inserted for EC up to 13 days after the beginning of an extended HFI, provided that CHC was used correctly beforehand. This approach aims to ensure that the Cu-IUD is inserted before implantation occurs, even in the unlikely event of ovulation occurring 8 days after CHC discontinuation.

Cu-IUD Insertion After Misuse of POP

A recent clinical trial observed that ovulation may occur as early as 9 days after discontinuation of desogestrel, following two months of correct use (Duijkers et al. 2015). However, data on the precise timing of ovulation after missed doses of POP remain limited. As a result, the Guideline Development Group (GDG) does not issue a definitive recommendation on this matter.

Nevertheless, since cervical mucus remains a barrier to sperm migration if POP has been used correctly, the Cu-IUD may be inserted for EC up to 5 days after the first episode of UPSI following a missed pill. This applies to both desogestrel-containing and traditional POP formulations.

Cu-IUD Insertion for Emergency Contraception After Recent Expiration of Depot Medroxyprogesterone Acetate (DMPA)

A systematic review concluded that the return of ovulation after the last injection of DMPA is highly variable, ranging from 15 to 49 weeks (Paulen and Curtis 2009). Therefore, the insertion of a Cu-IUD as EC is only recommended within 5 days after the first episode of UPSI occurring more than 14 weeks after the last DMPA dose.

Cu-IUD Insertion for Emergency Contraception After Recent Implant Removal

Ovulation may resume rapidly following the removal of a contraceptive implant, although precise data on the timing of ovulation are limited. The GDG recommends that a Cu-IUD can be inserted within 5 days of the first UPSI following implant removal.

Cu-IUD Insertion for Emergency Contraception After Recent LNG-IUD Removal

Ovulation may occur at any time before or after the removal of a LNG-IUD. Since the contraceptive effect ends shortly after removal, it is essential to evaluate pregnancy risk based on the timing of UPSI:

- If no UPSI occurred in the 5 days prior to IUD removal, a Cu-IUD may be inserted within 5 days of the first UPSI that occurs after removal.

- If UPSI occurred within the 5 days prior to IUD removal, a Cu-IUD must be inserted within 5 days of that UPSI. In either case, if no UPSI occurred before removal, the Cu-IUD can still be placed within 5 days following the next UPSI.

Oral Emergency Contraception

When EC is needed due to incorrect use of a hormonal method, it is important to consider that residual progestogen may reduce the efficacy of UPA. In these situations, the clinician may opt for LNG and initiate an appropriate contraceptive method immediately. If UPA is chosen, initiation or resumption of hormonal contraception should be delayed for at least 5 days.

Exceptionally, if COCs are restarted after an extended HFI and pills are missed during the first week, LNG should be preferred. If UPA is used in this scenario, the COCs should still be restarted immediately (Munyaneza et al. 2009).

Recently Expired LNG-IUD or Implant

The risk of pregnancy remains extremely low during the fourth year of contraceptive implant use and the sixth year of the 52 mg LNG-IUD (Ali et al. 2016). In these cases, EC is generally not required. However, LNG may be considered, along with the immediate initiation of an appropriate hormonal contraceptive method. The efficacy of UPA in the presence of residual progestogen from an expired LNG-IUD or implant is uncertain. If UPA is administered, hormonal contraception should not be initiated for 5 days afterward.

Emergency Contraception During Lactation

All EC methods are considered acceptable during lactation (CDC 2024). In women who are exclusively breastfeeding and remain amenorrheic, contraception (including EC) is not required during the first six months postpartum. However, it becomes necessary if any of the following occurs: exclusive breastfeeding is discontinued, menstruation resumes, or six months have elapsed postpartum, whichever occurs first. Women who do not meet the criteria for lactational amenorrhea should initiate contraception from day 21 postpartum (FSRH 2020).

IUD

The use of any type of IUD is permitted during lactation. However, Cu-IUD insertion is relatively contraindicated between 48 hours and 28 days postpartum due to the increased risk of uterine perforation and expulsion (FSRH 2020). Although this is a relative contraindication, the absolute risk remains low. It is estimated that the rate of uterine perforation in breastfeeding women less than 36 weeks postpartum is approximately 6 per 1,000 insertions (Heinemann et al. 2015).

Oral EC

UPA is excreted into breast milk and can be detected for up to five days after ingestion. Therefore, it is recommended to avoid breastfeeding for seven days following administration, during which time milk should be expressed and discarded.

In the case of LNG, it is recommended to avoid breastfeeding for at least eight hours after intake (Bayer Plc 2021). However, available evidence has not shown adverse effects in infants or significant impact on milk production (Jatlaoui, Riley, and Curtis 2016). The GDG considers it safe to continue breastfeeding after LNG administration. LNG is excreted in breast milk in minimal amounts and is not contraindicated during lactation.

Can Emergency Contraception Be Taken More Than Once in a Cycle?

If a woman has used UPA or LNG in one cycle, she can receive the same treatment again after a new UPSI in that cycle. It is important to inform about the increased risk of pregnancy with additional UPSI and the need to continue with effective contraceptive methods. UPA is well tolerated and can delay ovulation, which reduces the likelihood of ovulation at the time of UPSI. If UPA is taken, LNG should not be administered within 5 days, and vice versa, if LNG is taken, UPA may be less effective within 7 days. In both cases, use of a Cu-IUD is a recommended alternative, or repeat UA treatment (Halpern, Raymond, and Lopez 2014).

The dose of LNG as a UA is lower than that of regular birth control pills and does not present a risk of overdose. Repeated use of LNG is not associated with serious health risks beyond cycle alterations. No minimum interval between treatments has been established, but if new risky intercourse occurs within 12 hours of taking LNG, no retreatment is required (Brache et al. 2013).

Looking to the Future

Despite growing support for reproductive autonomy and efforts to ensure universal access to sexual and reproductive health, progress in meeting contraceptive needs remains slow. Currently, 218 million women in low- and middle-income countries have an unmet need for modern contraception (Sully et al. 2020). Although this need has remained steady, the reasons for nonuse of contraceptives have shifted. Today, many women do not use contraception because available methods do not meet their needs, rather than due to lack of knowledge or access (Sedgh, Ashford, and Hussain 2016).

One recent innovation in contraception is the development of on-demand pills, such as the "pericoital pill," which can be taken close to the time of UPSI, offering a flexible option for women who have infrequent sex or prefer not to use contraception continuously. The specific active ingredient of the pericoital pill is still under investigation, and it is anticipated that this method would be used regularly but not continuously, unlike EC, which is intended for unexpected situations. This method could benefit those who prefer not to rely on daily or long-term contraception and may help reduce side effects experienced with continuous methods (Odwe et al. 2022).

A recent analysis demonstrates high interest in this type of contraceptive, particularly among women engaging in casual or spontaneous sex (Bell et al. 2024). Furthermore, discreet use of the pericoital pill has shown promise in contexts where reproductive autonomy is limited. The development of methods such as the pericoital pill could help satisfy the unmet demand of women dissatisfied with current options by providing greater control over their reproductive health.

Therefore, it is essential to support research and development of these products with the objective of bringing them to market and expanding contraceptive options tailored to the needs and realities of all people.

Conclusion

EC represents an essential tool in the prevention of unintended pregnancy, offering a safe, effective, and accessible solution in situations of reproductive risk. Its historical evolution has facilitated the development of more tolerable methods, characterized by lower side effect profiles and higher efficacy rates, such as the Cu-IUD and UPA.

The choice of method should be individualized, taking into account clinical factors, availability, body weight, menstrual cycle timing, and personal preferences. This underscores the importance of comprehensive sexual and reproductive health education, as well as timely and informed access to these methods, particularly among vulnerable populations.

Despite notable progress, challenges remain regarding barriers to access, widespread misinformation, and inequalities in care, highlighting the urgent need for public policies that ensure universal access to emergency contraception.

In summary, emergency contraception not only fulfills a critical clinical role but also plays a fundamental role in supporting women's autonomy and their right to make informed decisions about their reproductive health.

References

Ali, Moazzam, Ayse Akin, Luis Bahamondes, Vivian Brache, Ndema Habib, Sihem Landoulsi, and David Hubacher. 2016. "Extended Use up to 5 Years of the Etonogestrel-Releasing Subdermal Contraceptive Implant: Comparison to Levonorgestrel-Releasing Subdermal Implant." *Human Reproduction* 31 (11): 2491–98. https://doi.org/10.1093/humrep/dew222.

American College of Obstetricians and Gynecologists. 2015. "Practice Bulletin No. 152: Emergency Contraception." *Obstetrics & Gynecology* 126 (3): e1–11. https://doi.org/10.1097/aog.0000000000001047.

Bakenra, Abena, Alexandra Gero, Jessica Sanders, Rebecca Simmons, Kathryn Fay, and David K. Turok. 2021. "Pregnancy Risk by Frequency and Timing of Unprotected Intercourse Before Intrauterine Device Placement for Emergency Contraception." *Obstetrics and Gynecology* 138 (1): 79–84. https://doi.org/10.1097/AOG.0000000000004433.

Bayer HealthCare Pharmaceuticals. 2008. *Mirena® (levonorgestrel-releasing intrauterine system). Patient Information.* https://www.accessdata.fda.gov/drugsatfda_docs/label/2008/021225s019lbl.pdf. Accessed June 11, 2025.

Bearak, Jonathan, Anna Popinchalk, Bela Ganatra, Ann-Beth Moller, Özge Tunçalp, Cynthia Beavin, Lorraine Kwok, and Leontine Alkema. 2020. "Unintended Pregnancy and Abortion by Income, Region, and the Legal Status of Abortion: Estimates from a Comprehensive Model for 1990–2019." *The Lancet Global Health* 8 (9): 1–10. https://doi.org/10.1016/S2214-109X(20)30315-6.

Bell, Stephen, Susannah Gibbs, Abigail Winskell, Xaviera Villarino, Halle Gill, and Kristen Little. 2024. "Acceptability of an On-Demand Pericoital Oral Contraceptive Pill: A Systematic Scoping Review." *Reproductive Health* 21 (1): 1–15. https://doi.org/10.1186/s12978-024-01829-7.

Berger, C., N. R. Boggavarapu, J. Menezes, P. G.L. Lalitkumar, and K. Gemzell-Danielsson. 2015. "Effects of Ulipristal Acetate on Human Embryo Attachment and Endometrial Cell Gene Expression in an in Vitro Co-Culture System." *Human Reproduction* 30 (4): 800–811. https://doi.org/10.1093/humrep/dev030.

Brache, Vivian, Leila Cochon, Maëva Deniaud, and Horacio B Croxatto. 2013. "Ulipristal Acetate Prevents Ovulation More Effectively than Levonorgestrel: Analysis of Pooled Data from Three Randomized Trials of Emergency Contraception Regimens ☆." *Contraception* 88 (5): 611–18. https://doi.org/10.1016/j.contraception.2013.05.010.

Cleland, Kelly, Elizabeth Raymond, James Trussell, Linan Cheng, and Haoping Zhu. 2010. "Ectopic Pregnancy and Emergency Contraceptive Pills: A Systematic Review." *Obstetrics and Gynecology* 115 (6): 1263–66. https://doi.org/10.1097/AOG.0b013e3181dd22ef.

Cleland, Kelly, Haoping Zhu, Norman Goldstuck, Linan Cheng, and James Trussell. 2012. "The Efficacy of Intrauterine Devices for Emergency Contraception: A Systematic Review of 35 Years of Experience." *Human Reproduction* 27 (7): 1994–2000. https://doi.org/10.1093/humrep/des140.

Centers for Disease Control and Prevention. 2024. *U.S. Medical Eligibility Criteria for Contraceptive Use, 2024*. Vol. 73. Atlanta: U.S. Department of Health and Human Services.

Duijkers, Ingrid J. M., Doris Heger-Mahn, Dominique Drouin, and Sven Skouby. 2015. "A Randomised Study Comparing the Effect on Ovarian Activity of a Progestogen-Only Pill (POP) Containing Desogestrel and a New POP Containing Drospirenone in a 24/4 Regimen." *European Journal of Contraception and Reproductive Health Care* 20 (6): 419–27. https://doi.org/10.3109/13625187.2015.1044082.

Edelman, Alison B., Jon D. Hennebold, Kise Bond, Jeong Y. Lim, Ganesh Cherala, David F. Archer, and Jeffrey T. Jensen. 2022. "Double Dosing Levonorgestrel-Based Emergency Contraception for Individuals With Obesity." *Obstetrics & Gynecology* 140 (1): 48–54. https://doi.org/10.1097/AOG.0000000000004717.

Ellertson, Charlotte. 1996. "History and Efficacy of Emergency Contraception: Beyond Coca-Cola." *International Family Planning Perspectives* 22 (2): 52–56. https://www.jstor.org/stable/i348657.

European Medicines Agency. 2014. "Levonorgestrel and Ulipristal Remain Suitable Emergency Contraceptives for All Women, Regardless of Bodyweight." Published July 24, 2014. https://www.ema.europa.eu/en/news/levonorgestrel-ulipristal-remain-suitable-emergency-contraceptives-all-women-regardless-bodyweight.

Ferreira-Poblete, A. 1997. "The Probability of Conception on Different Days of the Cycle with Respect to Ovulation: An Overview." *Advances in Contraception* 13 (2–3): 83–95. https://doi.org/10.1023/A:1006527232605.

Faculty of Sexual & Reproductive Healthcare. 2017. *FSRH Guideline: Emergency Contraception*. March 2017, 1–68. https://www.communitypharmacy.scot.nhs.uk/media/3132/fsrh-guideline-ec-dec-17.pdf

FSRH Clinical Effectiveness Unit. 2017. *FSRH Guideline: Contraception for Women Aged Over 40 Years*. Agosto 2017. https://www.fsrh.org/Common/Uploaded%20files/documents/fsrh-guideline-contraception-for-women-aged-over-40-years-august-2017-amended-july-2023-.pdf

Faculty of Sexual & Reproductive Healthcare. 2020. *Contraception After Pregnancy: Detail of Changes to Original Guidance. BMJ Sexual & Reproductive Health* 27 (supplement 2): 1–96. https://www.fsrh.org/Common/Uploaded%20files/documents/contraception-after-pregnancy-guideline-oct2020.pdf.

Faculty of Sexual and Reproductive Healthcare. 2016. *UK Medical Eligibility Criteria for Contraceptive Use (UKMEC 2016)*. London: Faculty of Sexual and Reproductive Healthcare. https://www.fsrh.org/standards-and-guidance/documents/ukmec-2016/.

Gemzell-Danielsson, Kristina, Cecilia Berger, and P. G.L. Lalitkumar. 2013. "Emergency Contraception - Mechanisms of Action." *Contraception* 87 (3): 300–308. https://doi.org/10.1016/j.contraception.2012.08.021.

Glasier, Anna, Sharon T. Cameron, Diana Blithe, Bruno Scherrer, Henri Mathe, Delphine Levy, Erin Gainer, and Andre Ulmann. 2011. "Can We Identify Women at Risk of Pregnancy despite Using Emergency Contraception? Data from Randomized Trials of Ulipristal Acetate and Levonorgestrel." *Contraception* 84 (4): 363–67. https://doi.org/10.1016/j.contraception.2011.02.009.

Glasier, Anna F., Sharon T. Cameron, Paul M. Fine, Susan J.S. Logan, William Casale, Jennifer Van Horn, Laszlo Sogor, et al. 2010. "Ulipristal Acetate versus Levonorgestrel for Emergency Contraception: A

Randomised Non-Inferiority Trial and Meta-Analysis." *The Lancet* 375 (9714): 555–62. https://doi.org/10.1016/S0140-6736(10)60101-8.

Halpern, Vera, Elizabeth G. Raymond, and Laureen M. Lopez. 2014. "Repeated Use of Pre- and Postcoital Hormonal Contraception for Prevention of Pregnancy." *Cochrane Database of Systematic Reviews* 2014 (9). https://doi.org/10.1002/14651858.CD007595.pub3.

Hang, Raymond, Wun Li, Sue Seen, Tsing Lo, Kristina Gemzell-Danielsson, Carol Ho, Yi Fong, Pak Chung Ho, Ernest Hung, and Yu Ng. 2023. "Oral Emergency Contraception with Levonorgestrel plus Piroxicam: A Randomised Double-Blind Placebo-Controlled Trial." *The Lancet* 402 (10405): 851–58. https://doi.org/10.1016/S0140-6736(23)01240-0.

Heinemann, Klaas, Suzanne Reed, Sabine Moehner, and Thai Do Minh. 2015. "Risk of Uterine Perforation with Levonorgestrel-Releasing and Copper Intrauterine Devices in the European Active Surveillance Study on Intrauterine Devices." *Contraception* 91 (4): 274–79. https://doi.org/10.1016/j.contraception.2015.01.007.

Hertzen, Helena Von, Gilda Piaggio, Juhong Ding, Junling Chen, Si Song, György Bártfai, and Ernest Ng. 2002. "Low Dose Mifepristone and Two Regimens of Levonorgestrel for Emergency Contraception: A WHO Multicentre Randomised Trial." *The Lancet* 360 (1803): 1803–10.

Jatlaoui, Tara C., Halley Riley, and Kathryn M. Curtis. 2016. "Safety Data for Levonorgestrel, Ulipristal Acetate and Yuzpe Regimens for Emergency Contraception." *Contraception* 93 (2): 93–112. https://doi.org/10.1016/j.contraception.2015.11.001.

Jatlaoui, Tara C., and Kathryn M. Curtis. 2016. "Represent the Official Position of the US Centers for Disease Control and Prevention." *Contraception*. https://doi.org/10.1016/j.contraception.2016.05.002.

Jensen, Jeffrey T., Alison Edelman, Carolyn L. Westhoff, Courtney A. Schreiber, David F. Archer, Stephanie Teal, Michael Thomas, Jill Brown, and Diana L. Blithe. 2016. "Use of Serum Evaluation of Contraceptive and Ovarian Hormones to Assess Reduced Risk of Pregnancy among Women Presenting for Emergency Contraception in a Multicenter Clinical Trial." *Contraception* 137: 110475. https://doi.org/10.1016/j.contraception.2024.110475.

Kaiser, Jennifer E., David K. Turok, Alexandra Gero, Lori M. Gawron, Rebecca G. Simmons, and Jessica N. Sanders. 2023. "One-Year Pregnancy and Continuation Rates after Placement of Levonorgestrel or Copper Intrauterine Devices for Emergency Contraception: A Randomized Controlled Trial." *American Journal of Obstetrics and Gynecology* 228 (4): 438.e1-438.e10. https://doi.org/10.1016/j.ajog.2022.11.1296.

Curtis, Kathryn M., PhD. 2010. "U.S. Medical Eligibility Criteria for Contraceptive Use, 2010: Adapted from the World Health Organization Medical Eligibility Criteria for Contraceptive Use, 4th Edition." *MMWR. Recommendations and Reports: Morbidity and Mortality Weekly Report. Recommendations and Reports /Centers for Disease Control* 59 (RR-4): 1–86. http://ovidsp.ovid.com/ovidweb.cgi?T=JS&PAGE=reference&D=emed9&NEWS=N&AN=20559203.

Kesserü, E., F. Garmendia, N. Westphal, and J. Parada. 1974. "The Hormonal and Peripheral Effects of D-Norgestrel in Postcoital Contraception." *Contraception* 10 (4): 411–24. https://doi.org/10.1016/0010-7824(74)90041-9.

Upadhya, Krishna K., MD. 2019. "Emergency Contraception." *Pediatrics* 144 (6). https://doi.org/10.1542/peds.2019-3149.

Lee, Jessica K., and Eleanor Bimla Schwarz. 2017. "The Safety of Available and Emerging Options for Emergency Contraception." *Expert Opinion on Drug Safety* 16 (10): 1163–71. https://doi.org/10.1080/14740338.2017.1354985.

Levonelle 1500 Microgram Tablet. 2021. *Summary of Product Characteristics*. Bayer plc. Updated July 28, 2021. https://www.medicines.org.uk/emc/product/6085/smpc.

Li, Daniel, Allen J. Wilcox, and David B. Dunson. 2015. "Benchmark Pregnancy Rates and the Assessment of Post-Coital Contraceptives: An Update." *Contraception* 91 (4): 344–49. https://doi.org/10.1016/j.contraception.2015.01.002.

Li, H. W. R., S. S. T. Lo, E. H. Y. Ng, and P. C. Ho. 2016. "Efficacy of Ulipristal Acetate for Emergency Contraception and Its Effect on the Subsequent Bleeding Pattern When Administered before or after Ovulation." *Human Reproduction* 31 (6): 1200–1207. https://doi.org/10.1093/humrep/dew055.

Sprem Goldstajn, M., D. Piljac, I. Grabnar, B. Peterlin, and M. Gužvić. 2014. "Ulipristal Acetate for Emergency Contraception." *Collegium Antropologicum* 38: 379–384. https://doi.org/10.1345/aph.1P704.

Moreau, Caroline, and James Trussell. 2012. "Results from Pooled Phase III Studies of Ulipristal Acetate for Emergency Contraception." *Contraception* 86 (6): 673–80. https://doi.org/10.1016/j.contraception.2012.05.012.

Mozzanega, Bruno, Salvatore Gizzo, Stefania Di Gangi, Erich Cosmi, and Giovanni Battista Nardelli. 2014. "Ulipristal Acetate: Critical Review About." *Reproductive Sciences* (January). https://doi.org/10.1177/1933719113519178.

Munyaneza, Charles, Emmanuel Nteziryayo, Celestin Ugirashebuja, and Hugo Keith. 2009. "Judgment As Approved by the Court." *Communications* 770 (December 2008): 1–5.

Natavio, Melissa, Frank Z. Stanczyk, Emilie A. G. Molins, Anita Nelson, and William J. Jusko. 2019. "Pharmacokinetics of the 1.5 mg Levonorgestrel Emergency Contraceptive in Women with Normal, Obese and Extremely Obese Body Mass Index." *Contraception* 99 (5): 306–11. https://doi.org/10.1016/j.contraception.2019.01.003.

Novikova, Natalia, Edith Weisberg, Frank Z. Stanczyk, Horacio B. Croxatto, and Ian S. Fraser. 2007. "Effectiveness of Levonorgestrel Emergency Contraception Given before or after Ovulation – A Pilot Study." *Contraception* 75 (2): 112–18. https://doi.org/10.1016/j.contraception.2006.08.015.

Odwe, George, Brent McCann, Wilson Liambila, Jessica Vandermark, Daniel Mwanga, Edna Anab, Moses Wanami, and Saumya Ramarao. 2022. "Feasibility of E-Commerce Pharmacy Provision and Acceptability of Levonorgestrel 1.5 mg for Pericoital Use in Urban and Peri-Urban Settings in Kenya: A Prospective Cohort Study." *BMJ Sexual and Reproductive Health* 49 (1): 35–42. https://doi.org/10.1136/bmjsrh-2022-201653.

Ortiz, María Elena, and Horacio B. Croxatto. 2007. "Copper-T Intrauterine Device and Levonorgestrel Intrauterine System: Biological Bases of Their Mechanism of Action." *Contraception* 75, no. 6 (Supplement): 16–30. https://doi.org/10.1016/j.contraception.2007.01.020..

Paulen, Melissa E., and Kathryn M. Curtis. 2009. "When Can a Woman Have Repeat Progestogen-Only Injectables—Depot Medroxyprogesterone Acetate or Norethisterone Enantate?" *Contraception* 80, no. 4: 391–408. https://doi.org/10.1016/j.contraception.2009.03.023.

Piaggio, Gilda, Nathalie Kapp, and Helena Von Hertzen. 2011. "Effect on Pregnancy Rates of the Delay in the Administration of Levonorgestrel for Emergency Contraception: A Combined Analysis of Four WHO Trials." *Contraception* 84, no. 1: 35–39. https://doi.org/10.1016/j.contraception.2010.11.010.

Praditpan, Piyapa, Angie Hamouie, Cale N. Basaraba, Renu Nandakumar, Serge Cremers, Anne R. Davis, and Carolyn L. Westhoff. 2017. "Pharmacokinetics of Levonorgestrel and Ulipristal Acetate Emergency Contraception in Women with Normal and Obese Body Mass Index." *Contraception* 95, no. 5: 464–69. https://doi.org/10.1016/j.contraception.2017.01.004.

Rosato, Elena, Manuela Farris, and Carlo Bastianelli. 2016. "Mechanism of Action of Ulipristal Acetate for Emergency Contraception: A Systematic Review." *Frontiers in Pharmacology* 6 (January). https://doi.org/10.3389/fphar.2015.00315.

Rudzinski, Patryk, Inga Lopuszynska, Dorota Pazik, Dominik Adamowicz, Anna Jargielo, Aleksandra Cieslik, Karolina Kosieradzka, Justyna Stanczyk, Astrik Meliksetian, and Alicja Wosinska. 2023. "Emergency Contraception – A Review." *European Journal of Obstetrics and Gynecology and Reproductive Biology* 291 (November): 213–18. https://doi.org/10.1016/j.ejogrb.2023.10.035.

Sedgh, Gilda, Lori S. Ashford, and Rubina Hussain. 2016. "Unmet Need for Contraception in Developing Countries: Examining Women's Reasons for Not Using a Method." Guttmacher Institute, June, 1–93. https://www.guttmacher.org/sites/default/files/report_pdf/unmet-need-for-contraception-in-developing-countries-report.pdf.

Shen, J., Y. Che, E. Showell, K. Chen, and L. Cheng. 2017. "Interventions for Emergency Contraception (Review)." Cochrane Database of Systematic Reviews, no. 8. https://doi.org/10.1002/14651858.CD001324.pub5.

Stanford, Joseph B., and Rafael T. Mikolajczyk. 2002. "Mechanisms of Action of Intrauterine Devices: Update and Estimation of Postfertilization Effects." *American Journal of Obstetrics and Gynecology* 187 (6): 1699–1708. https://doi.org/10.1067/mob.2002.128091.

Sully, E. A., A. Biddlecom, J. Darroch, T. Riley, L. Ashford, and N. Lince-Deroche. 2020. "Investing in Sexual and Reproductive Health." Guttmacher Institute, October.

Turok, David K., Alexandra Gero, Rebecca G. Simmons, Jennifer E. Kaiser, Gregory J. Stoddard, Corinne D. Sexsmith, Lori M. Gawron, and Jessica N. Sanders. 2021. "Levonorgestrel vs. Copper Intrauterine Devices for Emergency Contraception." *New England Journal of Medicine* 384 (4): 335–44. https://doi.org/10.1056/nejmoa2022141.

Vol. Federal Register, and No. Tuesday. 1997. "Federal Register / Vol. 62, No. 37 / Tuesday, February 25, 1997 / Notices." *Federal Register* 62 (37): 8610–12.

Wilcox, Allen J., Clarice R. Weinberg, and Donna D. Baird. 1996. "Timing of Sexual Intercourse in Relation to Ovulation." *Obstetrical & Gynecological Survey* 51 (6): 357–58. https://doi.org/10.1097/00006254-199606000-00016.

Yuzpe, A. A., H. J. Thurlow, I. Ramzy, and J. I. Leyshon. 1974. "Post Coital Contraception—A Pilot Study." *Journal of Reproductive Medicine*, 53–58.

Zapata, Lauren B., Maria W. Steenland, Dalia Brahmi, Polly A. Marchbanks, and Kathryn M. Curtis. 2013. "Effect of Missed Combined Hormonal Contraceptives on Contraceptive Effectiveness: A Systematic Review." *Contraception* 87 (5): 685–700. https://doi.org/10.1016/j.contraception.2012.08.035.

Zhang, Lin, Junling Chen, Yasun Wang, Fangming Ren, Wen Yu, and Linan Cheng. 2009. "Pregnancy Outcome after Levonorgestrel-Only Emergency Contraception Failure: A Prospective Cohort Study." *Human Reproduction* 24 (7): 1605–11. https://doi.org/10.1093/humrep/dep076.

Chapter 12

Male Surgical Contraception

A. Serrano Sánchez[1,*], MD
M. P. Mora Ábalos[1], MD
M. Cebrián Marcilla[1], MD
M. M. Castillo García[1], MD
and M. A. Roque Fernández[1,2], PhD
[1]Obstetrics and Gynecology Department, University and Hospital of Albacete, Albacete, Spain
[2]Medical Science Department, School of Medicine of Albacete, Universidad de Castilla-La Mancha, Spain

Abstract

Vasectomy is one of the mainstays of male contraception. It is a relatively simple surgical procedure with few complications, although it is not without them. This technique, which is inexpensive compared to other methods, is highly effective with a low pregnancy rate. The evolution of the surgical technique has led to an improvement in the results, resulting in a decrease in post-surgical complications. Although its reversal is described as achieving adequate subsequent pregnancy rates, it is important to remember that it is considered a permanent method and should be presented as such.

Keywords: vasectomy, vas deferens, male contraception

Introduction

Vasectomy is one of the surgical methods, along with tubal ligation or salpingectomy, used as a permanent method of contraception, reserved for individuals who desire permanent sterilisation. It is one of the most widely used contraceptive methods among the male population, although a decrease in the trend of its use has been found. In the United States in the 2000s, vasectomy was estimated to be the contraceptive method of choice for approximately 5% of the population, being the fourth most used method behind condoms, tubal ligation and oral hormonal contraceptives (Martinez et al. 2006). Although it is a contraceptive method used

* Corresponding Author's Email: alexcvii16@gmail.com

In: Advances in Reproductive Health
Editors: Llanos Belmonte Andujar and Ana Fuentes Rozalen
ISBN: 979-8-90134-038-7

by a large part of the population, it shows a decline in its use in 2015 in the US population, in which only around 527,000 vasectomies were performed, with a greater trend in the 35-45 age group (Ostrowski et al. 2018).

The mechanism of action of vasectomy is the interruption of the passage of spermatozoa in the vas deferens. This is achieved by occluding or sectioning the vas deferens using various surgical techniques.

With a very high efficacy, vasectomy is one of the cheapest contraceptive methods, along with the copper IUD and the Levonorgestrel IUD. Compared to tubal ligation, vasectomy is four times cheaper than tubal ligation as a method of definitive sterilisation (Trussell et al. 2009).

Effectiveness

The post-vasectomy pregnancy rate is extremely low, less than 1% (Schwingl and Guess 2000; Jamieson et al. 2004), although this percentage may vary depending on the technique used. Although it is a safe method of contraception, a minimal risk of pregnancy remains, and patients should be informed accordingly. The technique is considered effective when azoospermia or severe oligospermia is achieved. The use of another method of contraception is recommended until azoospermia is confirmed by a seminal sample after surgery. Even if vasectomy is confirmed to be effective, it has a minimal risk of failure of 0.05%, with the risk of post-vasectomy pregnancy being 1 in 2000 (Sharlip et al. 2012). Despite the reversibility of the technique, vasectomy should be offered as a definitive sterilisation method for men who do not wish to have any more offspring.

Indications and Contraindications

The main indication is permanent male contraception. Vasectomy is usually requested by adult males with fulfilled reproductive desires.

The only contraindication to vasectomy is the presence of an acute event affecting the male genitalia, such as epididymitis or scrotal haematoma. After resolution of the process, vasectomy can be performed.

There are other relative contraindications, where it is considered that there may be greater post-realisation regret, such as being under 30-35 years of age and not having offspring (Anderson et al. 2022). Other contraindications that may be considered are: suffering from a serious illness, not being in a relationship at the time the intervention is requested, being coerced, or being in a time of conflict in life.

Contraceptive Counselling

As previously mentioned, and despite the possibility of reversal, vasectomy is considered a definitive method of contraception and should be offered as such. The patient should be aware of this fact and should be adequately informed about the technique and complications, as well as about other alternatives.

Adequate contraceptive counselling should be provided prior to vasectomy, explaining clearly that this method is definitive, and if there are doubts about performing vasectomy, alternative methods should be offered. It is important to emphasise that vasectomy does not prevent the risk of contracting sexually transmitted diseases, so condom use would be recommended in patients who do not have a regular partner.

Finally, the need to use alternative methods should be explained for a period of time, until it is clear that vasectomy has been effective.

Surgical Anatomy

It is necessary to know the anatomy in order to understand the vasectomy surgical procedure. Within the male genital tract, we will focus mainly on the two structures that are affected during the procedure: the scrotum and the spermatic cord.

The scrotum is the layer of skin covering the testes and their associated structures. It is innervated by fibres of the ilioinguinal nerve and by the genital branch of the genitofemoral nerve. Below this we find the spermatic cord.

Thus, we find the following layers from the outside to the inside:

- Scrotal skin.
- Dartos muscle and its fascia.
- External spermatic fascia.
- Cremaster muscle and its fascia.
- Internal spermatic fascia.

Inside the spermatic cord are the deferens artery and the pampiniform plexus, which are responsible for the irrigation and drainage of the area. The branch of the genitofemoral nerve is also found here.

Surgical Procedure

The vasectomy procedure is a surgical procedure that can be performed on an outpatient basis under local anaesthesia and is well accepted by the men who undergo it (Vienot et al. 2023).

The different techniques have the same objective: to isolate and expose the vas deferens (through one or more incisions of varying length) and section it to interrupt the flow of sperm. In turn, different variants can be used to isolate the vas deferens and to increase effectiveness

Ligation of the sperm ducts with resorbable sutures or clips is one of the least effective alternatives. The use of end ligation as a sole method should be avoided as it has been associated with an increased incidence of failure of the technique (Denniston 1985). The isolated use of clips is also controversial as it has a higher failure rate. This is reflected in a study published in 2002 comparing the use of clips and excision of a section of the deferens with cauterisation of the deferens and fascial interposition, showing a higher failure rate of the technique in the clip-only group (Labrecque et al. 2002).

Excision of a more or less long section of the vas deferens is a less effective measure compared to other techniques. It was suggested that the longer the length of vas deferens removed, the lower the rate of recanalisation and failure of the technique. A case-control study aimed at assessing the association between the length of the severed vas and the risk of recanalisation found no association between the two. No significant differences were found between three length intervals (less than 10 millimetres, between 10 and 14 millimetres, and more than 15 millimetres), with a similar recanalisation rate (Labrecque, Hoang, and Turcot 2003).

The techniques that have proven most effective are fascial interposition and vas deferens cauterisation.

Fascial interposition consists of separating both ends of the severed vas deferens into distinct strata by a layer of fascia from the vas deferens. Several studies have demonstrated its usefulness in reducing the failure of the technique and improving its effectiveness. For example, a randomised study compared vasectomy without fascial interposition with vasectomy plus fascial interposition. This study showed that men in the fascial interposition group took less time to achieve azoospermia in subsequent controls compared to the control group, in turn reducing the failure rate by half (12% vs. 6%) (David Sokal et al. 2004). Another advantage of the fascial interposition technique is that it has a lower post-technique failure rate (Lynley A. Cook et al. 2014).

Cauterisation involves applying electrical energy to fulgurate the ends of the vas deferens. If combined with fascial interposition, the failure rate of the technique is greatly reduced. This is concluded in a study by Schmidt in which a single surgeon performed 6248 vasectomies in combination with fascial interposition and electrocautery. In this study the author reports no post-vasectomy pregnancies (Schmidt 1995).

From the point of view of incision and access to the vas deferens, there are two variants: conventional or classic and minimally invasive. The less invasive variant has been associated with fewer complications such as post-surgical pain or scrotal haematoma (L. A. Cook et al. 2007), and the contraceptive efficacy of both variants is practically the same, with no differences between them (D. Sokal et al. 1999). This makes minimally invasive vasectomy the technique of choice for many practitioners (Sharlip et al. 2012).

The specific procedure for each technique is described below.

- Conventional technique: This technique can be performed through two bilateral incisions on each side of the scrotal raphe or through a single incision, as long as it allows access to both vasa deferens.

First, local disinfection is performed with povidone iodine or chlorhexidine or another antiseptic, the vas deferens is located and fixed in the surgeon's fingers. After fixation, local anaesthesia is administered in order to form a skin wheal. Once effective anaesthesia has been achieved, an incision is made over the described area and the different layers are dissected until the fibrous layer of the vas deferens is reached.

Once the vas deferens is located, it is clamped with a clamp (usually Allis or Adson) and sectioned.

In the event of section or injury to the deferential artery, the artery must be ligated at both ends to avoid the formation of a large haematoma.

Once the process has been performed on both vas deferens, the technique is considered complete. The ducts are buried back into the scrotum and the Dartos muscle and the incision must be closed with a resorbable suture.

- Minimally invasive technique or percutaneous vasectomy: Initially described by Li in 1974 (Li et al. 1991), this technique was described with the aim of increasing the acceptability of vasectomy by decreasing the fear caused by the scalpel incision. As previously mentioned, it has fewer complications compared to the conventional technique (Labrecque et al. 2004).

In order to perform this technique, a circular forceps is needed to grasp the deferens, and a sharp dissector to pierce the skin and reach the deferens.

The vas deferens is located and fixed using three fingers: one finger is placed below the vas deferens; the other two fingers are placed above the skin and the vas deferens, fixing it and bringing it to the scrotal midline.

The local anaesthetic is injected, producing a wheal. Then, the vas deferens and the skin surrounding it are fixed with the circular forceps described above. Subsequently, with the help of the dissector, the skin of the scrotum is incised until the duct is reached, and with the help of the dissector it is located and extracted to expose it. The vasectomy continues as normal, with the vas deferens being sectioned.

In this technique it is not necessary to suture the skin, as the wound closes and heals correctly with the contraction of the cremaster muscle.

The postoperative period is usually painful and swollen. It is recommended that the patient wear tight-fitting underwear for one or two days. Ice may also be recommended to reduce swelling. Pain is usually adequately controlled with non-steroidal anti-inflammatory drugs.

Sexual abstinence should be maintained for at least one week ('Vasectomy Guideline - American Urological Association', n. d.). Rest is recommended for the next 24 hours after the procedure; normal activity is usually restored within a week.

Confirmation of Sterility

The effectiveness of vasectomy should be evidenced by semen analysis after surgery. Semen analysis should be obtained after at least 12 weeks (Hancock et al. 2016). It is therefore recommended to be performed at around 12-16 weeks.

In addition to the minimum time required, it is recommended that at least 20 ejaculations have occurred in this time, as with these characteristics it is estimated that 80% of patients achieve azoospermia (Griffin et al. 2005).

Semen analysis should be performed in a laboratory according to World Health Organization recommendations, without the need for centrifugation ('FSRH Service Standards for Vasectomy (April 2024)', n. d.).

After the analysis we can find ourselves in three situations:

- Azoospermia: The technique is effective and no other contraceptive method or follow-up is necessary.
- Presence of motile sperm: this finding must be confirmed with a subsequent control. If it persists, the technique is considered to have failed.
- Presence of immotile sperm: a rare finding, another semen control may be recommended, although it may be considered as a rare way to achieve sterility, so that the use of other contraceptive methods would not be necessary (Sharlip et al. 2012).

Complications

Despite being a relatively safe procedure, vasectomy, like any other surgical intervention, is not without complications. These include:

- *Haematoma:* usually caused by involvement of the pampiniform plexus or injury of the deferential artery, and is one of the most common complications associated with vasectomy (Yang et al. 2021). It rarely requires reoperation and drainage. It is usually self-limiting, reabsorbing on its own over time.
- *Infection*: with the haematoma, this is one of the most frequent complications, being more frequent in the conventional technique compared to the minimally invasive one. As they are mild and self-limiting, they usually subside with antibiotic treatment.
- *Sperm granuloma*: Granulomas are produced by the inflammatory effect generated by the spermatozoa when they exit through the sectioned duct, causing their aggregation and the body's reaction. They are usually asymptomatic.
- *Epididymitis*: due to traumatic epididymal congestion, usually not infectious in nature.
- *Post-vasectomy pain syndrome*: this is due to chronic epididymitis due to the constant outflow of sperm and discharge. This can lead to chronic inflammation affecting the patient's quality of life, although it has a low incidence (Manikandan et al. 2004). The first step of treatment includes anti-inflammatory drugs and warm baths, rarely requiring re-intervention.
- *Recanalisation of the vas deferens*:
  - *Early recanalisation*: that which occurs in the first few months post-surgery, where motile spermatozoa are visible in control tests.
  - *Late or spontaneous recanalisation of the vas*: a very rare complication with an incidence of less than 1% (Awsare et al. 2005), defined as the presence of spermatozoa after a control sample with azoospermia criteria.

One of the comorbidities associated and studied after vasectomy is the possible association with the development of prostate cancer. Observational studies have observed that there may be a relationship between these processes (Siddiqui et al. 2014; Bernal-Delgado et al. 1998), but no causal relationship has been demonstrated to explain this association.

A 2018 meta-analysis involving nearly 700,000 patients from Canada, Australia and the UK suggests there is no association with prostate cancer. The patient pool was divided into two groups: the first of 9700 men who underwent vasectomy reversal, the second larger group of almost 684,600 patients with vasectomy but without reversal. The analysis showed that vasectomy reversal did not act as a protective effect for prostate cancer compared to the non-reversed vasectomy group (Randall et al. 2018). These data suggest that there is no risk associated with developing this cancer.

Another cancer that may be related to vasectomy is testicular cancer, although cohort studies have shown no increased risk compared to the non-vasectomised population (Møller, Knudsen, and Lynge 1994).

It was thought that post-vasectomised men might in turn be more likely to be at increased risk of a cardiovascular event, due to the theory that vasectomy increases the incidence of atherosclerosis. This theory was disproved in a cohort study that followed a group of 3900 post-vasectomised patients for 9 years and demonstrated no association between vasectomy and atherosclerosis (Coady et al. 2002).

Reversal

Although vasectomy is considered to be a definitive method of contraception, and should be offered as such, it is true that in some patients who have undergone this type of intervention, a new genital desire may be awakened. This, although infrequent, often occurs in men who have found a new partner (Hendry 1994), or especially in young patients who opted for vasectomy as a contraceptive method around the age of 20 (Potts et al. 1999).

In the event of this desire, a reversal can be offered by vasovasostomy, a technique that consists of an anastomosis of the vas deferens using microsurgery. The main factor influencing the outcome of the reversal and the possibility of subsequent pregnancy is the time that has elapsed between the vasectomy and the reversal. In a study of the pregnancy rate after vasectomy reversal involving around 1469 patients, the pregnancy rate was found to be higher the shorter the time between the two surgeries. If the interval was less than 3 years, the pregnancy rate after reversal was 76%, which decreased drastically the more years elapsed (Belker et al. 1991).

Another technique that can be used if vasovasostomy is not possible is vasoepididymostomy, which involves anastomosing the epididymis to the vas deferens.

Although not considered a reversal technique, in vitro fertilisation (IVF) or in vitro fertilisation with intracytoplasmic sperm injection (ICSI) with sperm obtained from a testicular biopsy can be considered as an alternative in case the patient does not want to undergo this surgery.

The efficacy of in vitro fertilisation compared to vasectomy reversal appears that it may have similar results in terms of pregnancy ratc. This is reflected in a retrospective study comparing the efficacy between these techniques in men with post-vasectomy reproductive desire. The first group of 99 men underwent reversal by reanastomosis, performed by a single surgeon. The second group of 64 couples underwent direct assisted reproductive techniques (IVF-ICSI). There were no statistically significant differences between the two groups in terms of live birth rate, but there was a shorter time to pregnancy in the IVF-ICSI group (Uvin et al. 2018). Other studies also show that both options are valid in terms of efficacy, with reanastomosis being cheaper (Dubin et al. 2021).

Conclusion

Vasectomy is a highly effective, safe and cost-effective method of contraception, with low pregnancy rates. Minimally invasive vasectomy is the technique of choice as it has been associated with fewer post-surgical complications.

Adequate contraceptive counselling should be provided prior to the procedure, offering alternative methods.

Although reversal is possible, and different possibilities of achieving a new pregnancy have been described, vasectomy should be offered as a definitive contraceptive method.

References

Anderson, Danyon J., Morgan Lucero, Stephen Vining, Charles Daniel, Jamal Hasoon, Omar Viswanath, Alan D. Kaye, y Ivan Urits. 2022. "Vasectomy Regret or Lack Thereof." *Health Psychology Research* 10 (3): 38241. https://doi.org/10.52965/001c.38241.

Awsare, Ninaad S., Jai Krishnan, Greg B. Boustead, Damian C. Hanbury, y Thomas A. McNicholas. 2005. "Complications of Vasectomy." *Annals of the Royal College of Surgeons of England* 87 (6): 406-10. https://doi.org/10.1308/003588405X71054.

Belker, A. M., A. J. Thomas, E. F. Fuchs, J. W. Konnak, y I. D. Sharlip. 1991. "Results of 1,469 Microsurgical Vasectomy Reversals by the Vasovasostomy Study Group." *The Journal of Urology* 145 (3): 505-11. https://doi.org/10.1016/s0022-5347(17)38381-7.

Bernal-Delgado, E., J. Latour-Pérez, F. Pradas-Arnal, y L. I. Gómez-López. 1998. "The Association between Vasectomy and Prostate Cancer: A Systematic Review of the Literature." *Fertility and Sterility* 70 (2): 191-200. https://doi.org/10.1016/s0015-0282(98)00142-3.

Coady, Sean A., A. Richey Sharrett, Zhi-Jie Zheng, Gregory W. Evans, y Gerardo Heiss. 2002. "Vasectomy, Inflammation, Atherosclerosis and Long-Term Follow up for cardiovascular diseases: No Associations in the Atherosclerosis Risk in Communities Study." *The Journal of Urology* 167 (1): 204-7.

Cook, L. A., A. Pun, H. van Vliet, M. F. Gallo, y L. M. Lopez. 2007. "Scalpel versus No-Scalpel Incision for Vasectomy." *The Cochrane Database of Systematic Reviews*, n.º 2 (abril), CD004112. https://doi.org/10.1002/14651858.CD004112.pub3.

Cook, Lynley A., Huib A. A. M. Van Vliet, Laureen M. Lopez, Asha Pun, y Maria F. Gallo. 2014. "Vasectomy Occlusion Techniques for Male Sterilization." *The Cochrane Database of Systematic Reviews* 2014 (3): CD003991. https://doi.org/10.1002/14651858.CD003991.pub4.

Denniston, G. C. 1985. "Vasectomy by Electrocautery: Outcomes in a Series of 2,500 Patients." *The Journal of Family Practice* 21 (1): 35-40.

Dubin, Justin M., Joshua White, Jesse Ory, y Ranjith Ramasamy. 2021. "Vasectomy Reversal vs. Sperm Retrieval with in Vitro Fertilization: A Contemporary, Comparative Analysis." *Fertility and Sterility* 115 (6): 1377-83. https://doi.org/10.1016/j.fertnstert.2021.03.050.

"FSRH Service Standards for Vasectomy (April 2024) "s. f. Accessed May 3, 2025. https://www.fsrh.org/Public/Public/Documents/fsrh-service-standards-for-vasectomy-april-2024.aspx.

Griffin, Tabatha, Rebecca Tooher, Kris Nowakowski, Mark Lloyd, y Guy Maddern. 2005. "How Little Is Enough? The Evidence for Post-Vasectomy Testing." *The Journal of Urology* 174 (1): 29-36. https://doi.org/10.1097/01.ju.0000161595.82642.fc.

Hancock, P., B. J. Woodward, A. Muneer, y J. C. Kirkman-Brown. 2016. "2016 Laboratory Guidelines for Postvasectomy Semen Analysis: Association of Biomedical Andrologists, the British Andrology Society and the British Association of Urological Surgeons." *Journal of Clinical Pathology* 69 (7): 655-60. https://doi.org/10.1136/jclinpath-2016-203731.

Hendry, W. F. 1994. "Vasectomy and Vasectomy Reversal." *British Journal of Urology* 73 (4): 337-44. https://doi.org/10.1111/j.1464-410x.1994.tb07592.x.

Jamieson, Denise J., Caroline Costello, James Trussell, Susan D. Hillis, Polly A. Marchbanks, Herbert B. Peterson, y US Collaborative Review of Sterilization Working Group. 2004. "The Risk of Pregnancy after Vasectomy." *Obstetrics and Gynecology* 103 (5 Pt 1): 848-50. https://doi.org/10.1097/01.AOG.0000123246.11511.e4.

Labrecque, Michel, Caroline Dufresne, Mark A. Barone, y Karine St-Hilaire. 2004. "Vasectomy Surgical Techniques: A Systematic Review." *BMC Medicine* 2 (mayo):21. https://doi.org/10.1186/1741-7015-2-21.

Labrecque, Michel, Diem-Quan Hoang, y Lucile Turcot. 2003. "Association between the Length of the Vas Deferens Excised during Vasectomy and the Risk of Postvasectomy Recanalization." *Fertility and Sterility* 79 (4): 1003-7. https://doi.org/10.1016/s0015-0282(02)04924-5.

Labrecque, Michel, Hanif Nazerali, Myrto Mondor, Vincent Fortin, y Marlina Nasution. 2002. "Effectiveness and Complications Associated with 2 Vasectomy Occlusion Techniques." *The Journal of Urology* 168 (6): 2495-98; discussion 2498. https://doi.org/10.1016/S0022-5347(05)64176-6.

Li, S. Q., M. Goldstein, J. Zhu, y D. Huber. 1991. "The No-Scalpel Vasectomy." *The Journal of Urology* 145 (2): 341-44. https://doi.org/10.1016/s0022-5347(17)38334-9.

Manikandan, R., S. J. Srirangam, E. Pearson, y G. N. Collins. 2004. "Early and Late Morbidity after Vasectomy: A Comparison of Chronic Scrotal Pain at 1 and 10 Years." *BJU International* 93 (4): 571-74. https://doi.org/10.1111/j.1464-410x.2003.04663.x.

Martinez, Gladys M., Anjani Chandra, Joyce C. Abma, Jo Jones, y William D. Mosher. 2006. "Fertility, Contraception, and Fatherhood: Data on Men and Women from Cycle 6 (2002) of the 2002 National Survey of Family Growth." *Vital and Health Statistics. Series 23, Data from the National Survey of Family Growth*, n.º 26 (mayo), 1-142.

Møller, H., L. B. Knudsen, y E. Lynge. 1994. "Risk of Testicular Cancer after Vasectomy: Cohort Study of over 73,000 Men." *BMJ (Clinical Research Ed.)* 309 (6950): 295-99. https://doi.org/10.1136/bmj.309.6950.295.

Ostrowski, Kevin A., Sarah K. Holt, Brandon Haynes, Benjamin J. Davies, Eugene F. Fuchs, y Thomas J. Walsh. 2018. "Evaluation of Vasectomy Trends in the United States." *Urology* 118 (agosto):76-79. https://doi.org/10.1016/j.urology.2018.03.016.

Potts, J. M., F. F. Pasqualotto, D. Nelson, A. J. Thomas, y A. Agarwal. 1999. "Patient Characteristics Associated with Vasectomy Reversal." *The Journal of Urology* 161 (6): 1835-39.

Randall, Sean, James Boyd, Emma Fuller, Caroline Brooks, Carole Morris, Craig C. Earle, Anna Ferrante, Rachael Moorin, James Semmens, y C. D'Arcy J. Holman. 2018. "The Effect of Vasectomy Reversal on Prostate Cancer Risk: International Meta-Analysis of 684,660 Vasectomized Men." *The Journal of Urology* 200 (1): 121-25. https://doi.org/10.1016/j.juro.2018.03.005.

Schmidt, S. S. 1995. "Vasectomy by Section, Luminal Fulguration and Fascial Interposition: Results from 6248 Cases." *British Journal of Urology* 76 (3): 373-74; discussion 375.

Schwingl, P. J., y H. A. Guess. 2000. "Safety and Effectiveness of Vasectomy." *Fertility and Sterility* 73 (5): 923-36. https://doi.org/10.1016/s0015-0282(00)00482-9.

Sharlip, Ira D., Arnold M. Belker, Stanton Honig, Michel Labrecque, Joel L. Marmar, Lawrence S. Ross, Jay I. Sandlow, David C. Sokal, y American Urological Association. 2012. "Vasectomy: AUA Guideline." *The Journal of Urology* 188 (6 Suppl): 2482-91. https://doi.org/10.1016/j.juro.2012.09.080.

Siddiqui, Mohummad Minhaj, Kathryn M. Wilson, Mara M. Epstein, Jennifer R. Rider, Neil E. Martin, Meir J. Stampfer, Edward L. Giovannucci, y Lorelei A. Mucci. 2014. "Vasectomy and Risk of Aggressive Prostate Cancer: A 24-Year Follow-up Study." *Journal of Clinical Oncology: Official Journal of the American Society of Clinical Oncology* 32 (27): 3033-38. https://doi.org/10.1200/JCO.2013.54.8446.

Sokal, D., S. McMullen, D. Gates, y R. Dominik. 1999. "A Comparative Study of the No Scalpel and Standard Incision Approaches to Vasectomy in 5 Countries. The Male Sterilization Investigator Team." *The Journal of Urology* 162 (5): 1621-25.

Sokal, David, Belinda Irsula, Melissa Hays, Mario Chen-Mok, Mark A. Barone, y Investigator Study Group. 2004. "Vasectomy by Ligation and Excision, with or without Fascial Interposition: A Randomized Controlled Trial [ISRCTN77781689]." *BMC Medicine* 2 (marzo):6. https://doi.org/10.1186/1741-7015-2-6.

Trussell, James, Anjana M. Lalla, Quan V. Doan, Eileen Reyes, Lionel Pinto, y Joseph Gricar. 2009. "Cost Effectiveness of Contraceptives in the United States." *Contraception* 79 (1): 5-14. https://doi.org/10.1016/j.contraception.2008.08.003.

Uvin, Valerie, S. De Brucker, M. De Brucker, V. Vloeberghs, P. Drakopoulos, S. Santos-Ribeiro, y H. Tournaye. 2018. "Pregnancy after Vasectomy: Surgical Reversal or Assisted Reproduction? " *Human Reproduction (Oxford, England)* 33 (7): 1218-27. https://doi.org/10.1093/humrep/dey101.

"Vasectomy Guideline - American Urological Association." s. f. Accessed April 26, 2025. https://www.auanet.org/guidelines-and-quality/guidelines/vasectomy-guideline.

Vienot, S., O. Skowron, C. Valignat, V. Xardel, L. Ngo, y V. Arnoux. 2023. " [Vasectomy under local anesthesia, retrospective evaluation of patient satisfaction in CH Annecy Genevois] ". *Progres En Urologie: Journal De l'Association Francaise D'urologie Et De La Societe Francaise D'urologie* 33 (15-16): 1002-7. https://doi.org/10.1016/j.purol.2023.09.008.

Yang, Fang, Junjun Li, Liang Dong, Kun Tan, Xiaopeng Huang, Peihai Zhang, Xiaozhang Liu, Degui Chang, y Xujun Yu. 2021. "Review of Vasectomy Complications and Safety Concerns." *The World Journal of Men's Health* 39 (3): 406-18. https://doi.org/10.5534/wjmh.200073.

Chapter 13

Drug Interactions with Hormonal Contraceptives

C. Aparicio Martínez[1,*], MD
G. Serrano García[2], MD
S. Rico Cardenal[3], MD
M. M. Haro Pérez[2], MD
and L. Gómez Muñoz[1], MD

[1]Obstetrics and Gynaecology Department, Hospital of Tomelloso, Tomelloso, Ciudad Real, Spain
[2]Obstetrics and Gynaecology Department, Albacete University Hospital Complex, Albacete, Spain
[3]Obstetrics and Gynaecology Department, Hospital of Villarrobledo, Villarrobledo, Albacete, Spain

Abstract

Hormonal contraceptives are the second most used contraceptive method. They are medications for long-term continuous use, so secondary drug interactions are one of the major problems we face. These interactions can have repercussions on the effect and safety of both the oral contraceptive and the patient's other regular medication.

These interactions are known through the study of the pharmacodynamics and pharmacokinetics of the drugs, with those that influence pharmacokinetics being more frequent and predictable.

Drug-drug interactions with contraceptives are more frequent in the absorption of the drugs and, above all, in their metabolism. At this point, the influence of Cytochrome P450 must be taken into account, which acts as an enzyme inducer and inhibitor when certain drugs are combined with contraceptives, thus varying their bioavailability and thus their adverse effects and contraceptive effectiveness. The most common drug interactions with contraceptives are antibiotics, antiepileptics, antiretrovirals and to a lesser extent benzodiazepines. The duration of treatment must also be taken into account to ensure the contraceptive effect and another effective contraceptive method must be considered if the contraceptive effect cannot be ensured or if adverse effects occur.

These interactions have to be taken into account in the different routes of administration of the contraceptive, with the peculiarities of each one, including emergency contraception.

Keywords: pharmacokinetics, pharmacodynamics, drug interactions, absorption, metabolism

---

* Corresponding Author's Email: claraapa@hotmail.com

In: Advances in Reproductive Health
Editors: Llanos Belmonte Andujar and Ana Fuentes Rozalen
ISBN: 979-8-90134-038-7

Introduction

Medications for long-term continuous use, such as hormonal contraceptives, may have drug-drug interactions secondary to biochemical, physiological and pharmacological factors.

These interactions can affect the efficacy and safety of both the oral contraceptive and the patient's other regular medications by increasing or decreasing their concentration, although the main cause of contraceptive failure is still a dosing failure. For this reason, it is a priority to know the metabolism of drugs to prevent unwanted interactions.

In the specific case of oral contraceptives, the metabolism of ethinylestradiol is taken as a model, since it is the most widely used oestrogen. This chapter discusses possible interactions during its metabolism, the most frequent being during absorption and hepatic metabolism, with liver isoenzymes, in particular cytochrome P450, being of great importance.

Alternative routes of administration and possible interactions with non-oral contraceptives are also discussed.

In recent years, new formulations with natural oestrogens have been introduced, showing no differences in the interactions described in the literature with ethinylestradiol.

Types of Drug Interactions: Pharmacokinetics and Pharmacodynamics

Pharmacokinetics refers to the series of processes that a drug undergoes in the body. Pharmacodynamics, on the other hand, corresponds to the relationship between the plasma concentration and its effect.

A change in the behaviour of the drug in the body would affect its pharmacokinetics, either during absorption, distribution, metabolism or excretion, thereby increasing or decreasing its plasma concentration and bioavailability. Pharmacokinetic interactions are the most common and therefore widely studied, as well as being the most predictable.

Pharmacodynamic interactions, however, are less predictable as they result from the combination of the hormonal contraceptive and a drug that may cause an increase or decrease in its action when used together. The alterations caused in this case cannot be explained pathophysiologically.

Pharmacokinetic Cycle and Hormone Metabolism

The pharmacokinetics of most medicines are based on the following steps:

- The drug is ingested (orally or parenterally) and absorbed.
- It gives rise to active metabolites through metabolism.
- It is distributed through the body. It may be bound to transporter proteins.
- Binding to target organs
- Excretion

In all these steps, the drug is exposed to possible interferences, especially in absorption and metabolism.

In the specific case of oral contraceptives, the metabolism of ethinylestradiol is taken as a model, since it is the most widely used oestrogen and the sequence is well known (Stanczyk, Archer, y Bhavnani 2013).

In this metabolism, the role of phase I enzymes, responsible for oxidation, reduction and hydrolysis, and phase II enzymes, responsible for glycation, sulphation and acetylation, should be highlighted. These include cytochrome P-450, specifically the CYP3A4 subtype, which is responsible for the hydroxylation of oestrogens, maintaining their hormonal capacity but allowing them to be eliminated more quickly. This enzyme is also a key point in the metabolism of other drugs, so it is one of the main points to be taken into account when detecting possible drug interactions.

Ethinylestradiol Metabolism

Ethinyl estradiol (EE) is first ingested orally and absorbed in the small intestine. After that, a small part is first metabolised by cytochrome P450 in the intestine to ethinyl estradiol sulphate. Most of the ethinylestradiol absorbed in the intestine passes into the portal circulation, initiating the so-called first-pass hepatic metabolism. Of this percentage, a small part of it enters the systemic circulation (bioavailable fraction) and the other part is hydroxylated in the liver by cytochrome P450, yielding catecholestrogen metabolites. Sixty per cent of these metabolites are conjugated in the liver with glucuronic acid and give rise to ethinylestradiol glucuronate, while the remainder is excreted in the urine.

The second hepatic step follows the action of intestinal bacteria in the colon. These bacteria hydroxylate ethinyl estradiol sulphate from the intestine and ethinyl estradiol glucuronate from the bile. This releases ethinylestradiol back into the porto-hepatic circulation. Ethinyl estradiol is then distributed to its target organs, mostly bound to albumin (97%).

Vaginal or transdermic administration of oestrogens has the same pharmacokinetic cycle as the oral one, so there are no differences in metabolic interactions. The only drug to drug interactions that are not affected by transdermal or vaginal administration are the absorption interactions, because first-pass hepatic metabolism is only present in oral administration.

As for progestins, many of them are ingested in inactive forms, so they do not pass through the enterohepatic circulation and are metabolised in the liver. They then reach the target organs mostly bound to the transporter protein sex hormone binding globulin (SHGB). Other transporter proteins are also present, such as corticoisteroid-binding globulin (CBG) and albumin. Since their metabolism has less well-established steps than that of ethinyl estradiol, the interactions of oral progestogen-only contraceptives are more unknown than in combination (Bick et al. 2021).

Once the metabolic cycle of the hormones involved in contraceptives is understood, pharmacokinetic interactions are largely predictable. Such interactions can occur at all the steps described above, but are most frequent during absorption and, above all, metabolism. This leads to an increase or decrease in the bioavailability of the hormone in serum and thus to alterations in its effect.

Absorption Interactions

- Alterations in gastric pH, altering hormone absorption: antacids and gastric pH modifiers (antacids, proton pump inhibitors).

- Motility modifiers
  - Increase gastric motility, decreasing the absorption of the contraceptive and thus its effect: metoclopramide, domperidone.
  - Decrease gastric motility, increasing the absorption and bioavailability of the hormone, and thus its side effects: anticholinergics, atropine, hyoscine.
- Alteration of the intestinal flora: some antibiotics (tetracyclines, erythromycin, beta-lactams, sulphonamides, neomycin, quinolones) alter the intestinal flora and thus decrease the absorption of the antibiotic, although there is no evidence of a decrease in the effect at the clinical level.
- At the colon level, there are drugs that decrease the reabsorption of oestrogen in the colon by the bile, decreasing the second hepatic step and increasing its excretion in the faeces: Laxatives and fibre. They decrease absorption by 20-30%, although they have not been shown to decrease contraceptive efficacy at the clinical level. This group also includes activated charcoal, which has not shown any alteration at the clinical level if administered 3 hours before or 12 hours after the contraceptive (World Health Organization 2015).
- There are drugs (paracetamol, ascorbic acid and fluconazole) that interfere with the sulphation of oestrogens, increasing their concentration and thus their absorption, which in high doses can lead to side effects of combined oral contraceptives (COCs)

Interactions in Metabolism

The hydroxylation that occurs in the liver metabolism process is the critical point for drug-drug interferences. At this level, isoenzymes present in the mitochondria and endoplasmic reticulum of the liver, in particular those present in cytochrome P450, can be altered and thus change the bioavailability of the contraceptive.

Cytochrome P450 contains at least forty enzymes, of which CYP 3A4 is the most important for hormone metabolism. This enzyme, when induced, increases metabolism, thus decreasing the bioavailability and thus the effect of the contraceptive. Within contraceptives, the only routes that would not be affected by this phenomenon would be the injectable and the intrauterine device (IUD). In the opposite case, inhibition would increase the likelihood of side effects by increasing the bioavailability of the hormone ("FSRH CEU Guidance: Drug Interactions with Hormonal Contraception (May 2022) ", s. f.).

The following table (Table 1) summarises the enzyme inducing/inhibiting drugs known to date (Wilbur y Ensom 2000; Simmons et al. 2018; Zhanel et al. 1999; Crawford et al. 1990):

In patients chronically taking any of these drugs, it is recommended to avoid their use and change for contraceptives that do not interfere with Cytochrome P450 such as levonorgestrel-releasing intrauterine system (LNG-IUS), copper intrauterine device (Cu-IUD) or Medroxyprogesterone depot). If the combination of the contraceptive with any of the drugs in the table is less than two months, it is recommended to continue using both drugs and to use barrier methods during this period of time and the month after taking the contraceptive.

Table 1. Enzyme inducing/inhibiting drugs

Enzyme inducers	Antibiotics	Rifampicin Rifabutin
	Antiepileptics	Phenytoin, Primidone, Carbamazepine, Slicarbamazepine, Oxcarbazepine, Topiramate Felbamate, Ethosuximide Rufinamide, Lamotrigine (monotherapy)
	Antiretrovirals	- Protease inhibitors (Ritonavir, Saquinavir, Atazanavir, Tripanavir) - Efavirenz - Non-nucleoside reverse transcriptase inhibitors (Efavirenz, Nevirapine)
	Benzodiazepines	Clordiazepoxide, Diazepam, Nitrozepam, Alprazolam, Flurazepam, Bromazepam, Medazepam
	Others	Ethanol, St John's wort, Bosetan, Modafinil, Aprepitant
Enzyme inhibitors	Antifungals	Fluconazole, Itraconazole, Ketoconazole, Voriconazole
	Immunosuppressant	Tracholimus
	Anti-inflammatory	Etoricoxib
	Antibacterial	Erythromycin
	Antiretroviral	Atazanavir not boosted
	Statins	Atorvastatin, Rosuvastatin
	Benzodiazepines	Lorazepam, Oxazepam, Temazepam, Triazolam
	Vasodilatador	Sitaxentan sodium

The risk of interactions of contraceptive methods with enzyme inducers is summarised in Table 2.

Table 2. Risk of interactions of contraceptive methods with enzyme inducers

METHOD	Recommendations	Additional information
COCs (oral, transdermic, vaginal)	- Contraception is reduced - Recommend use barrier methods while the treatment with enzyme-inducer longs and 28 days after - If the enzyme inducer treatment lasts more than two months, recommend another contraception method	- If the patient does not want to change oral COCs to another method, they could use two EE monophasic combined oral contraceptive pills together (a total of 50 µg) in continuous regimen (or only 4 days free-hormone interval). Patients should be advised that this is not as effective as change for another method and that there is an increased risk of thrombosis. - Do not use two patches or two vaginal rings together
POP (progestogen only pill)	The same as COCs	Do not take two pills together
ENG - IMP	The same as COCs	Do not use two implants together
DMPA Progestogen-only injectable: depot medroxyprogesterone acetate	Contraception is not reduced Effective method while enzyme-induce treatments longs	
LNG-IUS	Contraception is not reduced Effective method while enzyme-induce treatments longs	
Cu-IUD	Contraception is not reduced Effective method while enzyme-induce treatments longs	

If emergency contraception is needed, a cu IUD is the most effective method of emergency contraception. Alternatively, a double dose of oral levonorgestrel (30mg) or a single dose of ulipristal acetate can be offered, but patients should be advised that effectiveness in this situation is unknown.

Alterations in Excretion

There are different drugs that can alter the excretion of sex hormones at the renal, hepatic or intestinal level.

The use of diuretic drugs can accelerate their renal excretion; however, if they are combined with calcium blockers, the opposite effect is achieved.

Cholestyramine or colestipol modify biliary excretion, as does chitin. In addition to increasing the excretion of bile products, chitin decreases intestinal absorption and increases the excretion of oral hormonal contraceptives in which the first hepatic step is significantly present.

Non-Oral Routes of Administration

The main non-oral routes available are parenteral, vaginal and transdermal.

Both the LNG Diu and the injectable route have been shown to be used in conjunction with enzyme inhibitors without affecting their contraceptive capacity.

As for the other routes, more and more studies are being conducted to assess the interactions of the non-oral routes. Two studies conclude that oral amoxicillin and doxycycline, like vaginal miconazole, do not affect the contraceptive efficacy of the ring (Lazorwitz et al. 2017; Leticee et al. 2012).

However, as a general rule, when using both the vaginal route (contraceptive ring) and the transdermal route (transdermal patch), it is important to know that, although there are differences with the oral route in terms of pharmacokinetics, they undergo hepatic metabolism. This fact should lead us to recommend the same contraceptive protection measures when using them together with drugs with significant enzyme induction.

Natural Oestrogens

When using COCs with Estradiol or Estradiol Valerate, it is important to know that they have a greater effect on protein synthesis in the liver.

Despite this, the recommendations do not differ from those for other COCs *("FSRH CEU Guidance: Drug Interactions with Hormonal Contraception (May 2022) ", s. f.).*

Conclusion

An understanding of drug pharmacokinetics and pharmacodynamics is essential to identify drug-drug interactions. Most interactions occur in the absorption and metabolism of contraceptives, in particular when they are inhibited or induced by isoenzymes present in hepatic metabolism, the most important being cytochrome P450.

These interactions change the bioavailability of the drugs and thus their contraceptive capacity and side effects. It is therefore important to know the possible drug-drug interactions of contraceptives according to the route of administration and to advise the patient on the contraceptive best suited to her situation. DMPA, LNG IUS and cu-IUD have the least metabolic interactions and are the most effective in the case of regular use of Cytochrome P450 inducers or inhibitors. In addition, in the case of emergency contraception, the cu-IUD has been shown to be the most effective in these situations.

It is essential to inform the patient of this situation and to advise them on the contraceptive method, taking into account their preferences.

References

Bick, Alexis J., Renate Louw-du Toit, Salndave B. Skosana, Donita Africander, y Janet P. Hapgood. 2021. "Pharmacokinetics, metabolism and serum concentrations of progestins used in contraception." *Pharmacology & Therapeutics* 222 (junio):107789. https://doi.org/10.1016/j.pharmthera.2020.107789.

Crawford, P, D J Chadwick, C Martin, J Tjia, D J Back, y M Orme. 1990. "The interaction of phenytoin and carbamazepine with combined oral contraceptive steroids. " *British Journal of Clinical Pharmacology* 30 (6): 892-96. https://doi.org/10.1111/j.1365-2125.1990.tb05457.x.

"FSRH CEU Guidance: Drug Interactions with Hormonal Contraception (May 2022) ". s. f. https://www.fsrh.org/Public/Public/Documents/ceu-clinical-guidance-drug-interactions-with-hormonal.aspx.

Lazorwitz, Aaron, Anne Davis, Maryke Swartz, y Maryam Guiahi. 2017. "The Effect of Carbamazepine on Etonogestrel Concentrations in Contraceptive Implant Users." *Contraception* 95 (6): 571-77. https://doi.org/10.1016/j.contraception.2017.03.004.

Leticee, Nadia, Jean-Paul Viard, Amina Yamgnane, Marina Karmochkine, y Alexandra Benachi. 2012. "Contraceptive Failure of Etonogestrel Implant in Patients Treated with Antiretrovirals Including Efavirenz." *Contraception* 85 (4): 425-27. https://doi.org/10.1016/j.contraception.2011.09.005.

Simmons, KB, LB Haddad, K Nanda, y KM Curtis. 2018. "Drug interactions between rifamycin antibiotics and hormonal contraception: a systematic review." *BJOG: an international journal of obstetrics and gynaecology* 125 (7): 804-11. https://doi.org/10.1111/1471-0528.15027.

Stanczyk, Frank Z., David F. Archer, y Bhagu R. Bhavnani. 2013. "Ethinyl estradiol and 17β-estradiol in combined oral contraceptives: pharmacokinetics, pharmacodynamics and risk assessment." *Contraception* 87 (6): 706-27. https://doi.org/10.1016/j.contraception.2012.12.011.

Wilbur, Kerry, y Mary H. H. Ensom. 2000. "Pharmacokinetic Drug Interactions Between Oral Contraceptives and Second-Generation Anticonvulsants." *Clinical Pharmacokinetics* 38 (4): 355-65. https://doi.org/10.2165/00003088-200038040-00004.

World Health Organization. 2015. *Medical Eligibility Criteria for Contraceptive Use*. 5th ed. Geneva: World Health Organization. https://iris.who.int/handle/10665/181468.

Zhanel, George G, Shannon Siemens, Kathryn Slayter, y Lionell Mandell. 1999. "Antibiotic and oral contraceptive drug interactions: Is there a need for concern? " *The Canadian Journal of Infectious Diseases* 10 (6): 429-33. https://doi.org/10.1155/1999/539376.

Chapter 14

Non-Contraceptive Benefits of Contraceptives

S. Rico Cardenal[1,*], MD
C. Aparicio Martínez[2], MD
L. M. Gómez Muñoz[2], MD
G. Serrano García[3], MD
and M. M. Pérez Haro[3,4], MD
[1]Obstetrics and Gynaecology Department, Hospital of Villarrobledo, Villarrobledo, Albacete, Spain
[2]Obstetrics and Gynaecology Department, Hospital of Tomelloso, Tomelloso, Ciudad Real, Spain
[3]Obstetrics and Gynecology Department, University and Hospital of Albacete, Albacete, Spain
[4]Instituto Bernabeu of Alicante, Spain

Abstract

Pregnancy planning is the main indication for the use of contraceptives, thus avoiding unwanted pregnancies and abortions. However, the different hormonal preparations exert effects on ovulation, endometrial growth and uterine contractility and this has led them to offer a profile of beneficial and non-contraceptive side effects that has led to their use for purposes other than purely contraceptive. These purposes include the control of cycle-related symptoms and the treatment of diseases such as endometriosis and endometrial hyperplasia, among others.

Keywords: contraception, oral contraception, oral contraceptives, combined oral hormone contraception, combined oral contraceptive, combined oral contraception, progestins, progestogens, levonorgestrel-releasing intrauterine system, subdermal implantable contraceptives, non-contraceptive benefits, dysmenorrhea, endometriosis, abnormal uterine bleeding, heavy menstrual bleeding, uterine fibroids, endometrial hyperplasia, ovarian cysts, ectopic pregnancy, PCOS, polycystic ovary syndrome, pelvic inflammatory disease, human papillomavirus, anemia, iron deficiency, bone mineral density

---

* Corresponding Author's Email: src4393@gmaill.com

In: Advances in Reproductive Health
Editors: Llanos Belmonte Andujar and Ana Fuentes Rozalen
ISBN: 979-8-90134-038-7

Introduction

Contraceptives have numerous beneficial effects aside from those derived from the prevention of unwanted pregnancies. These advantages have led gynecology specialists to use them for the management of episodes of uterine bleeding, pelvic pain related or unrelated to the menstrual cycle, control of diseases such as endometriosis, and even for the treatment of other premalignant diseases such as endometrial hyperplasia. On the other hand, contraceptives have also proven useful in the prevention of sexually transmitted diseases, in the management of symptoms associated with premenstrual syndrome, in the improvement of anemia parameters, as well as in many other areas.

Benefits in Pelvic Pain: Dysmenorrhea, Chronic Pelvic Pain, Pain Related to Endometriosis, Ovulatory Pain (Mittelschmerz) and Premenstrual Syndrome

Primary Dysmenorrhea

Dysmenorrhea is a colicky and recurrent abdominal pain that occurs during menstruation. It is a very common disorder in women of childbearing age and has a great social, functional, occupational, sexual, physical and social impact. Primary dysmenorrhea is a condition in which there is no demonstrable cause or disease that explains these symptoms, so its diagnosis is a diagnosis of exclusion. Secondary dysmenorrhea, on the other hand, has the same symptoms but there are identifiable underlying causative disorders (e.g., adenomyosis, endometriosis, myomas) (O'Hara, Shan, & Yau, 2024). In addition, in secondary dysmenorrhea there are other signs and symptoms (dyspareunia, enlarged uterus...) that help differentiate it from primary dysmenorrhea.

The goal of dysmenorrhea treatment is to provide symptomatic pain relief so that patients can perform most of their daily activities while maintaining their usual productivity (Schoep et al. 2019). First-line treatment includes nonsteroidal anti-inflammatory drugs, hormonal contraceptives, or a combination of both. In the case of nonsteroidal anti-inflammatory drugs, treatment is started just before menstruation and continued for two to three days depending on the duration of menstruation. This helps to relieve pain and quality of life during this period.

Hormonal contraceptives are one of the main treatments for primary dysmenorrhea (Schroll, Black, Farquhar, and Chen, 2023), as they reduce endometrial thickness and maturation. A thinner endometrium contains less arachidonic acid (less prostaglandin synthesis) and results in less menstrual flow. Thus, the ultimate effect is lighter menstruation, less uterine inflammation and contractility, and ultimately reduced pain (Dawood 2006).

A meta-analysis showed that combined oral contraceptives produce an improvement in dysmenorrhea superior to placebo with no differences between the various oral formulations (Wong et al. 2009. Estrogen dose also has no influence on pain relief. However, continuous regimens seem to achieve better symptomatic control compared to cyclic regimens (Machado et al. 2010). Regarding the vaginal ring, no differences in dysmenorrhea control have been found with respect to combined pills (Roumen 2007). On the other hand, the contraceptive patch offers poorer control of dysmenorrhea (Audet et al. 2001).

Regarding methods based solely on progestogens, we found that, in a meta-analysis of 11 studies involving 1200 patients (Imai et al. 2014), the Levonorgestrel IUD was shown to have similar efficacy to combined oral contraceptives in relieving dysmenorrhea due to a reduction in menstrual flow or even due to amenorrhea caused in some patients. The same is not true for the copper IUD which has been shown to increase dysmenorrhea. On the other hand, progesterone-only pills reduce secondary dysmenorrhea related to endometriosis but their effect on primary dysmenorrhea is not as well demonstrated (Al-Jefout et al. 2016).

Pain Related to Endometriosis

Endometriosis is an estrogen-dependent inflammatory disease characterized by the presence of endometrial tissue outside the uterine cavity (Beker et al. 2022). Being hormone-dependent, it mainly affects women of reproductive age although its clinical consequences may persist until menopause. The 2022 ESRHE guideline (Becker et al. 2022) recommends offering hormonal treatment to women with endometriosis to reduce the pain associated with this disease and advises using combined hormonal contraceptives or those based solely on progestogens as the first-choice treatment. Due to their adverse effect profile, GnRH agonists or antagonists would be reserved as a second therapeutic line when the former fail. For pain refractory to previous medical or surgical therapies, this guideline recommends using aromatase inhibitors alone or in combination with previous treatments.

A systematic review (Vercellini et al. 2016) that included randomized clinical trials and observational studies of relevance evaluated the efficacy and safety of combined hormonal contraceptives and progestogen-only contraceptives in the treatment of endometriosis. By inhibiting ovulation, inducing endometrial atrophy of eutopic and ectopic tissue, and decreasing menstrual bleeding, contraceptives improve dysmenorrhea, non-cyclic pelvic pain, and quality of life in two-thirds of patients. This review also highlights the anti-inflammatory properties of contraceptives and their similar effect regardless of the type of progesterone used and the route of administration of the contraceptive. Furthermore, it recommends using the combined hormonal contraceptive regimen with the lowest possible estrogen dose to optimize the suppression of endometrial growth and avoid thrombotic events. On the other hand, it is also worth highlighting the role of contraceptives based only on progestogens because, in addition to not increasing the risk of thrombosis, they are the indicated treatment in those women with dyspareunia and deep endometriosis who do not tolerate or have contraindications to estrogens. For all these reasons, hormonal contraceptives are the first-line treatment in this type of patient, without any differences between them in terms of pain reduction (Practice Committee of the American Society for Reproductive Medicine).

Focusing on progestogens, a systematic review (Allen et al. 2025) of 21 randomized clinical trials (19 related to endometriosis and two related to fibroids) involving a total of 2745 participants (1317 treated with progesterone and 1428 treated with placebo, danazol or GnRH analogues) showed that progestins produced a statistically significant reduction in endometriosis-related pain with spotting/irregular bleeding being the main adverse effect, whereas in the comparison group it was hot flushes.

As for the etonogestrel implant (Grandi et al. 2019), there is little evidence for its use in endometriosis although it does appear to produce a reduction in pain. For its part, the Levonorgestrel IUD improves dysmenorrhea but is less effective in the management of chronic pelvic pain and dyspareunia and has also not been shown to reduce disease recurrences. Thus, the ESHRE guideline (Beker et al. 2022) considers postoperative insertion of a Levonorgestrel IUD (or combined hormonal contraceptive) for at least 18 to 24 months for secondary prevention of endometriosis-associated dysmenorrhea to be appropriate.

Regarding combined oral contraceptives, several studies (Zorbas, Economopoulos, and Vlahos 2015; Muzii et al. 2016) have shown that, compared to conventional regimens (regimens of 21 tablets plus 7 placebo tablets), continuous regimens or regimens have been able to achieve a better reduction in pain, quality of life and sexual function; therefore, the continuous regimen could constitute a more effective therapeutic option for women with pelvic pain associated with endometriosis.

In addition, hormonal treatment with a monophasic regimen at low doses of ethinylestradiol has been shown to significantly reduce the volume of endometriomas and dysmenorrhea compared to the placebo group without adding serious adverse effects (Harada et al. 2008).

Finally, a systematic review (Grandi et al. 2019) evaluated the efficacy of different contraceptives in the control of postsurgical disease recurrences and in the treatment of endometriosis-associated pain (dysmenorrhea, pelvic pain, and dyspareunia). Both combined contraceptives and progestogen-only methods improved quality of life and significantly reduced dysmenorrhea, noncyclic pelvic pain, and dyspareunia; however, only combined contraceptives were shown to decrease the risk of postsurgical disease recurrence. However, a subsequent meta-analysis (Muzii et al. 2023) compared dienogest with GnRH analogs and demonstrated that post-surgical treatment with this progestogen is as effective as GnRH analogs in reducing the recurrence rate of endometriotic cysts, both being significantly superior to placebo. In addition, dienogest produces a significant reduction in pain but with a better tolerated side effect profile than GnRH analogues.

Chronic Pelvic Pain

In chronic pelvic pain, there is a hormonal imbalance that favors pelvic vasoconstriction and the occurrence of pain. In this context progestogens, with their vasodilator action, can improve the pain associated with such pelvic congestion (Gavrilov and Turischeva, 2017). In fact, a randomized clinical trial involving 47 patients with pure pelvic congestion showed improvement of pelvic congestion, pain and other symptoms after six months of treatment with goserelin or medroxyprogesterone acetate (Soysal et al., 2001).

Ovulatory Pain (Mittelschmerz).

Some women experience intense pain mid-cycle related to ovulation. This pain can also be caused by endometriosis or the formation of hemorrhagic follicles. The best way to prevent it is the use of combined hormonal contraceptives or progestogen-only contraceptives that prevent ovulation or follicular rupture, and therefore the peritoneal irritation associated with it (Jensen and Speroff 2000).

Premenstrual Syndrome

Premenstrual syndrome is a set of physical and psychological symptoms that occur recurrently in the luteal phase of the menstrual cycle and interfere with a woman's normal activities. The γ-aminobutyric acid (GABA) pathway is responsible for mood changes related to the menstrual cycle. This pathway is sensitive to changes in the levels of progesterone and its metabolites. Allopregnanolone is a neurosteroid with anxiolytic and anticonvulsant effects and its levels fluctuate during a menstrual cycle with progesterone levels. Progestins exert diverse effects on allopregnanolone depending mainly on their androgenic activity (Fruzzetti and Fidecicchi 2020).

Drospirenone is a common progestogen in the management of premenstrual syndrome. A Cochrane meta-analysis (Lopez et al. 2012) analyzed 6 randomized clinical trials and compared the combination of ethinylestradiol with drospirenone against placebo and other hormonal contraceptives combined with gestagens other than drospirenone. Their results showed that preparations with drospirenone could be more effective in the management of premenstrual syndrome, which could be attributed to its antimineralocorticoid and antiandrogenic properties that give it a more favorable profile in terms of fluid retention, irritability and emotional changes.

On the other hand, regimens with a shorter hormone-free interval (24 days of estrogen plus drospirenone followed by 4 days of rest) produce less hormone fluctuation and have been postulated as a good strategy to achieve greater control of PMS symptoms (Bustillos-Alamilla et al. 2010).

However, the role of drospirenone in menstrual syndrome is less clear from a more current Cochrane meta-analysis (Ma and Song 2023) that included five randomized clinical trials looking at 858 women diagnosed with premenstrual dysphoric disorder (severe form of premenstrual syndrome) who were treated for at least three months with: placebo, combined oral contraceptives with drospirenone, or combined oral contraceptives containing a different progestogen. The quality of evidence was very low-moderate with significant heterogeneity. The conclusions were that contraceptives with drospirenone can reduce premenstrual symptoms and improve quality of life during the first 3 months; however, placebo was also shown to have a relevant effect with a lower rate of adverse effects. In fact, contraceptives with drospirenone were associated with a higher incidence of nausea, intermenstrual bleeding, mastalgia and a higher dropout rate due to these adverse effects. Finally, this meta-analysis also highlights the lack of knowledge as to whether drospirenone-based regimens work in women with less severe symptoms, whether they work after three months of use, or whether they are superior to other oral contraceptives combined with a different progestogen.

Currently, two phase 3 clinical trials have been published that provide more recent data. The first (Bitzer et al. 2024) included 1553 women from Europe and Russia and the second (Bouchard et al. 2025) included 1864 patients from the United States and Canada. Participants were treated with 15 mg stetrol + 3 mg drospirenone for up to 13 cycles. These trials observed that those patients who initiated treatment showed significant improvement on the Menstrual Distress Questionnaire. The Bitzer trial showed significant improvements in the areas of menstrual and premenstrual pain, water retention and negative affect for women taking stetrol + drospirenone for the first time. While the Bouchard trial showed that, in this group of women, menstrual pain, premenstrual and menstrual fluid retention and premenstrual negative affect were significantly reduced. This study also observed an improvement in over 40% of patients in general muscle pain, headache, cramps, mastalgia, irritability, etc. However, both studies showed that patients who had previously used another contraceptive method had hardly any significant changes in the parameters evaluated by the Menstrual Distress Questionnaire.

Benefits in Heavy Menstrual Bleeding

Hypermenorrhea or Heavy Menstrual Bleeding

Heavy menstrual bleeding (Bofill Rodriguez et al. 2019) is defined as a loss of menstrual blood perceived by patients as excessive and which affects their health and interferes with their quality of life. The first-line treatment for habitual hypermenorrhea is the 52 mg levonorgestrel IUD, because the atrophy it produces at the endometrial level translates into a decrease in the volume of menstrual bleeding. This is reflected in a clinical trial (Creinin et al. 2023) in which it was shown that the Levonorgestrel IUD was able to reduce menstrual volume by more than 90% over a period of 6 months, regardless of the woman's BMI or parity, and without serious adverse effects. This makes patients prefer it over other treatments, since, in addition, about 60% of them remain amenorrheic (Davies and Kadir 2017).

As a second line of treatment, after the levonorgestrel IUD, come combined hormonal contraceptives. A meta-analysis including 8 randomized clinical trials and a total of 805 women (Lethaby et al. 2019) showed that combined oral contraceptives (estradiol valerate + dienogest) normalized bleeding by reducing menstrual volume significantly (12-77% success rate with combined oral contraceptives vs 3% with placebo). However, when compared to Levonorgestrel IUD, the latter was significantly more effective in reducing bleeding. The comparison of combined oral contraceptives with other routes of administration such as the vaginal ring is still inconclusive. Finally, it should be noted that continuous or extended-cycle therapies reduce the number of days of menstrual bleeding per year; however, they are associated with a higher number of unscheduled bleeding episodes.

Regarding cyclic progestogens, a review (Bofill Rodriguez et al. 2019) of 15 randomized controlled trials with a total of 1071 concluded that they are not as effective as other treatments in reducing bleeding, so they should be considered a third line therapy behind Levonorgestrel IUD and other treatments.

In this sense, and returning to methods based on progestogens alone, the etonogestrel implant could also constitute an alternative, although not as effective as the levonorgestrel IUD, since it manages to maintain amenorrhea in 30-40 % of patients one year after its insertion (Power et al. 2007).

Abnormal and Severe Uterine Bleeding

We define acute abnormal uterine bleeding as bleeding of uterine origin, unrelated to pregnancy, that is excessively heavy in quantity or duration requiring urgent intervention (Pravata-Rezende et al. 2025). It can take place with ovulation or occur in an anovulatory cycle (Munro et al. 2013).

Management in the context of hemodynamically unstable patients is beyond the scope of our book. However, as a summary, we could say that initially we would perform resuscitative measures with fluids and blood products, together with uterine tamponade with a Foley catheter, and then move on to therapeutic measures: uterine curettage (of choice) or intravenous estrogens at high doses. Intravenous estrogens (25 mg every 4 - 6 hours for 24 hours) are an alternative in patients in whom we can wait at least three to five hours and manage to stop bleeding in 72 % in 5 h (Munro et al. 2013). Finally, if with these measures we cannot control uterine bleeding, we will move on to measures such as uterine artery embolization, endometrial ablation or hysterectomy (Pravata-Rezende et al. 2025).

On the other hand, in the management of hemodynamically stable patients, we can perform an initial evaluation before starting treatment. Thus, in those patients with denuded endometrium (ultrasonographically thin) and in whom we can wait 48 hours without further complications, we will use combined oral hormonal contraceptives at high doses, because in most patients they cause cessation of bleeding in this period of time (Munro et al. 2013).

Various high-dose regimens of combined oral contraceptives have been studied (Pravata-Rezende et al. 2024). One example would be to take a tablet every 6-8 hours until bleeding stops (maintaining the dose for at least two days) followed by maintenance of one tablet per day for three to six weeks. Another pattern would be one tablet every 8 hours for two to seven days, followed by one tablet every 12 hours for two to seven days, and then one tablet a day for at least four weeks. Other studies recommend using other dosages. Munro's review (Munro et al. 2013) uses 3-4 pills a day for a few days and then tapering off progressively. Another example (James et al. 2011) would be to use a high-dose ethinylestradiol contraceptive with the following dosage: 5 pills on the first day, 4 pills on the second day, 3 pills on the third day, 2 pills on the fourth day and one pill on the fifth day; after the bleeding subsides, again, a maintenance of one to three weeks with one pill a day is proposed and then discontinued to allow withdrawal bleeding. After all this, a monthly or extended regimen of contraception at normal doses can be restarted to prevent further episodes of acute bleeding. It should be noted that for this indication, dose adjustments cannot be made with patches or vaginal rings, as opposed to combined hormonal contraceptives via oral contraceptives.

An alternative to combined oral contraceptives would be the use of oral estrogen at high doses. We would treat with 2.5 mg of conjugated equine estrogen every six hours, which would be equivalent to between 8-40 mg of ethinylestradiol. When the bleeding disappears or is very little, we can reduce the dose to 2.5 mg every 12 hours (Speroff and Fritz 2005). The duration of treatment is 21 to 25 days. With this treatment, bleeding is likely to stop within 10 hours, making it a faster treatment than high-dose combined oral contraceptives. Estrogens promote rapid regeneration of the denuded endometrium and this leads to cessation of bleeding. After discontinuation it is necessary to administer a progestogen for 10 days.

Finally, the role of gestagens in severe hemorrhage would be relegated to those anovulatory bleedings in stable patients in whom ultrasound shows a hypertrophic endometrium. Progesterone inhibits endometrial growth and supports and organizes the endometrium previously sensitized by estrogens, allowing its effective detachment after hormonal deprivation. Various progestogens and doses can be used; an example would be to use 10 mg medroxyprogesterone acetate 2 or 3 times daily for 5-10 days (Munro et al. 2013); (James et al. 2011).

Benefits Related to Benign and Premalignant Gynecological Pathology: Endometriosis, Adenomyosis, Myomas, Endometrial Hyperplasia, Adnexal Cysts, Ectopic Pregnancy, Hyperandrogenism (PCOS, Hirsutism and Acne) and Benign Breast Pathology

Endometriosis

See the section on "pain related to endometriosis."

Adenomyosis

In adenomyosis we find endometrial tissue in the muscular thickness of the uterine wall, which produces uterine enlargement, abnormal bleeding and dysmenorrhea. A narrative review (Etrusco et al. 2023) found that, in the first 3-6 months, the Levonorgestrel IUD reduces the symptoms associated with adenomyosis: dysmenorrhea, menstrual bleeding volume and in some cases even uterine size. Progestogen-only contraceptives such as Dienogest are anti-inflammatory and cause atrophy of the endometrium, bringing benefits to this pathology, especially in terms of improvement of dysmenorrhea, although there is less evidence.

A prospective study (Carrillo Torres et al. 2023) conducted a follow-up of up to 24 months in women with adenomyosis and endometriosis who received treatment with dienogest plus ethinylestradiol. This study observed an improvement in dysmenorrhea, dyspareunia, chronic pelvic pain, myometrial asymmetry and MUSA characteristics by ultrasound, which led the author to suggest a possible reduction of adenomyosis after two years of treatment. However, current reviews (Muzii et al. 2023b; Etrusco et al. 2023) state that combined contraceptives may be an option although less effective for symptom control than methods based on gestagens alone.).

Myomas

Leiomyomas, fibroids or myomas are the most frequent benign gynecological neoplasm in women. Patients with submucosal fibroids accessible to hysteroscopy are subsidiaries of resection of the same by this approach. In those patients with myomas that do not deform the cavity and have heavy menstrual bleeding, the Levonorgestrel IUD can be used as a treatment, achieving a significant reduction in their bleeding, improving their quality of life and having a beneficial effect on ferritin and hemoglobin levels (Vannuccini et al. 2024). Levonorgestrel

IUD insertion in myomas that deform the cavity may be more difficult and this condition is associated with a higher rate of expulsion of the IUD.

A Cochrane review (Sangkomkamhang et al. 2020) sought to determine the effectiveness of gestagens and the Levonorgestrel IUD in the treatment of uterine fibroids in premenopausal women. For this purpose, it analyzed four randomized clinical trials involving 221 women, but the evidence of the analysis was of very low quality due to imprecise information in the included studies. For this reason, this review could not conclude with certainty whether the levonorgestrel IUD reduces the size of fibroids. Nor was it able to determine whether oral gestagens reduce abnormal uterine bleeding in the same way as goserelin acetate, although women did report fewer adverse events such as hot flashes.

Subsequently, another systematic review (Allen et al. 2025) that included randomized clinical trials related to fibroids found that progestins produce significant reductions in pain although there were no statistically significant differences compared to the control group (placebo, danazol or GnRH analogues). The most frequent adverse effect of progestins was spotting/irregular bleeding, while in the comparison group it was hot flushes.

Combined oral contraceptives are frequently used as first-line treatment in women with abnormal uterine bleeding associated with myomas, especially when the myomas are small and subserosal or intramural and do not deform the endometrial cavity. They are less effective than other options such as Levonorgestrel IUD and GnRH agonists/antagonists in controlling bleeding in myomatous uteri. Their efficacy is limited when myomas distort the endometrial cavity and they also do not reduce myoma size (Vannuccini et al. 2024).

Therefore, to date, we could conclude that hormonal contraceptive treatment could contribute to the control of bleeding and dysmenorrhea but with no additional benefit for this pathology.

Endometrial Hyperplasia

Endometrial hyperplasia is an endometrial glandular growth that presents a risk of progression to endometrial cancer. For those women with a desire of pregnancy or in whom hysterectomy is not a possibility, gestagens are a therapeutic option due to their antiproliferative effect at the endometrial level.

A meta-analysis of seven randomized clinical trials involving 766 women (Abu Hashimet al. 2015) compared the efficacy of Levonorgestrel IUD versus oral progestogens in the treatment of hyperplasia without atypia. That meta-analysis evidenced higher therapeutic or histologic regression rates and lower hysterectomy rates in the Levonorgestrel IUD intervention group. These results were significant for both simple hyperplasia and complex hyperplasia without atypia and were observed throughout follow-up at 3, 6, 12 and 24 months. Therefore, in the treatment of endometrial hyperplasia without atypia, we should consider the Levonorgestrel IUD as a preferential treatment over other forms of progestogens.

Along the same lines, another meta-analysis (Elassall et al. 2022) compared the efficacy of the Levonorgestrel IUD with oral or injectable gestagens to evaluate the resolution of endometrial hyperplasia (with and without atypia), treatment failure rates and the need for hysterectomy. After analyzing 5 randomized clinical trials and 7 observational studies, this meta-analysis concludes that the Levonorgestrel IUD significantly achieves a higher regression rate, lower treatment failure and lower need for hysterectomy with respect to the control group in endometrial hyperplasia in general. The evidence for cases of complex endometrial hyperplasia is less robust, but in these cases, it appears that the efficacy of the levonorgestrel IUD and systemic gestagens is similar.

Focusing on hyperplasia with atypia, a prospective study including 105 women with endometrial hyperplasia with and without atypia (Varma et al. 2008), showed a histological regression of almost 70% in the group of patients with endometrial hyperplasia with atypia treated with Levonorgestrel IUD (and 92% in cases of hyperplasia without atypia treated with Levonorgestrel IUD) at two years of follow-up. A more recent review (Fernandez-Montoli et al. 2025) compared the efficacy and safety of different conservative treatments in women with atypical endometrial hyperplasia and stage IA grade 1 endometrioid cancer. In this review, the Levonorgestrel IUD had a higher rate of regression of hyperplasia with atypia than the group treated with oral progestogens. However, the difference was not statistically significant. However, the evidence from this meta-analysis is inconclusive as only a single trial of those included in the analysis dealt with hyperplasia with atypia and this had a low sample size.

Therefore, we could conclude that the Levonorgestrel IUD is significantly superior to oral progestogens for the conservative treatment of hyperplasia without atypia. In the case of hyperplasia with atypia, it could also be more effective but further research is needed to confirm this superiority.

Functional Ovarian Cysts

Combined oral contraceptives protect against the appearance of functional ovarian cysts and hemorrhagic follicles, although they do not improve the resolution of existing ones (Grimes et al. 2014). This effect would be due to the fact that progesterone inhibits LH secretion and ovulation, while estrogen inhibits FSH secretion and the formation of the dominant follicle (Bahamondes et al. 2015).

Ectopic Pregnancy

Pregnancy prevention is the main mechanism for reducing the risk of ectopic gestation by contraceptives (combined or gestagen-only). However, the very reduction in the incidence of Pelvic Inflammatory Disease (PID) may also contribute to a reduction in ectopic pregnancy rates (Raine-Bennett et al. 2022; Kopp-Kallner et al. 2022).

Hyperandrogenism: Polycystic Ovary Syndrome, Hirsutism and Acne

Polycystic ovary syndrome (PCOS) affects 10% of women of reproductive age and is a syndrome characterized by anovulation, oligomenorrhea / amenorrhea, hirsutism, acne, obesity and even alopecia (Helena J. Teede et al. 2023). In this condition, anovulation leads to a state of hyperandrogenism whose cutaneous manifestations would be hirsutism and acne, since the excess of androgens increases the production of sebum and the growth of the pilosebaceous gland (Nissa et al. 2023). On the other hand, this syndrome also associates metabolic alterations such as insulin resistance, diabetes, metabolic syndrome, increased risk of cardiovascular disease, etc. (Stańczak et al. 2024).

Contraceptives provide advantages in this picture (Teede et al. 2018) because they reduce androgen production by inhibiting the release of gonadotropins. In addition, estrogens increase the production of SHBG (Sex Hormone Binding Globulin) which transports more androgens thus decreasing their free fraction in blood. Progestogens in general, but especially those with anti-androgenic action such as dienogest and drospirenone, inhibit 5 alpha reductase, which is the enzyme in charge of transforming testosterone into dihydrotestosterone (the most potent metabolite), thus also reducing circulating androgens and those present in the hair follicle. Furthermore, gestagens exert a protective effect in situations of chronic anovulation, where the endometrium is chronically exposed to estrogenic stimulus without receiving gestagenic compensation to reduce the risk of endometrial hyperplasia.

The objective is to reduce the production of androgens, circulating androgens and to limit their action on the pilosebaceous units. The most commonly used combined oral contraceptives will be those with the most anti-androgenic progestogens: cyproterone acetate, chlormadinone acetate, dienogest and drospirenone (Requena and Llombart 2020). These have been shown to improve the aesthetic condition of patients by reducing alopecia in 86% of patients, acne in up to 70% and hirsutism in 36% of users (Barrionuevo et al. 2018).

In summary, both estrogens and progestogens improve the androgen profile and acne. Given the beneficial effect of estrogens, combined hormonal contraceptives are preferred as the first line of treatment. In addition, combined contraceptives allow better cycle control. Therefore, the ESHRE guideline on polycystic ovary syndrome (Helena J. Teede et al. 2023) recommends combined oral contraceptives with anti-androgen progestogens (drospirenone, cyproterone, dienogest) as the first line of treatment for polycystic ovary syndrome, especially if there are symptoms of hyperandrogenism.

Benign Breast Pathology

Combined oral contraceptives, by decreasing cyclic hormonal stimulation, may reduce the incidence of benign breast disease such as fibrocystic mastopathy (Caserta et al. 2014).

A retrospective study (Johansson et al. 2021) analyzed 61,617 Swedish women aged 40-69 years and evaluated the association between different benign breast diseases and their relationship with age, hormonal factors, and family history of breast cancer. This study found that the use of combined oral contraceptives for a period of time longer than 8 years was associated with a significant reduction in the occurrence of fibroadenomas in premenopausal women. Therefore, it appears that hormonal contraceptives reduce the risk of proliferative disease without histological atypia and this reduction is greater the longer they are used.

Benefits on Infectious Diseases: Prevention of Sexually Transmitted Diseases and Pelvic Inflammatory Disease

Sexually transmitted diseases are highly prevalent in society with a significant impact on women's reproductive health. Due to anatomical factors, bacterial (chlamydia, gonorrhea, syphilis), viral (HIV, HPV, HSV) and parasitic (trichomoniasis) sexually transmitted diseases disproportionately affect women (Van Gerwen et al. 2022). Barrier methods, especially male and female condoms, are one of the most effective and accessible strategies to prevent the transmission of these diseases.

Combined oral contraceptives and gestagen-only pills do not protect against sexually transmitted infections (Coelingh Bennink et al. 2024) because, although they thicken cervical mucus, this effect is not sufficient to prevent the entry of pathogens such as Chlamydia trachomatis, Neisseria gonorrhoeae or HIV. In fact, their use could be associated with an increased risk of certain sexually transmitted infections due to association, in some cases, with other factors such as risky sexual behavior (increased frequency of sex without a condom). Therefore, contraceptives do not replace the use of condoms and should not be considered a measure of protection against sexually transmitted infections.

Pelvic inflammatory disease is an inflammation of the upper genital tract that can affect the uterus, fallopian tubes and ovaries. It is typically an ascending infection originating from the lower vaginal tract and is mostly caused by a sexually transmitted infection. Combined oral contraceptives do not prevent the initial transmission or acquisition of the causative bacteria, but they do reduce the progression of an untreated sexually transmitted infection to pelvic inflammatory disease (Coelingh Bennink et al. 2024). This is again because they thicken the cervical mucus making it more difficult for bacteria to ascend through the genital tract and they alter the endometrial environment making it less receptive to ascending infections. The same occurs with contraceptives based solely on gestagens, which, due to their effect of thickening the cervical mucus, inhibit bacterial proliferation and hinder the ascent of pathogens. On the other hand, IUD carriers tend to present a milder disease with less fever, abscesses and shorter hospital stays. Therefore, it seems that there is no benefit in the systematic removal of the IUD during treatment (Levin et al. 2021).

Regarding HPV, there is no consistent evidence (Anastasiou et al. 2022) that combined oral contraceptives increase the risk of cervical dysplasia or cervical cancer when HPV infection is controlled. Contraceptives may not be a causal factor but rather an indicator of HPV exposure. On the other hand, no conclusions can be drawn about the effect of gestagen-only contraceptives because there is insufficient evidence.

Benefits Related to Cancer

This point will be addressed more extensively in Chapter 15 of this book.

Benefits Related to Other Devices and Systems: Anemia and Bone Density

Benefits on Anemia

The Levonorgestrel 52 mg IUD is the most effective method for reducing menstrual bleeding (reduction of more than 90% at 6 months), correcting anemia on many occasions (Creinin et al.

2023). This has also been observed in patients with fibroids, where it has also been shown to have a beneficial effect on ferritin and hemoglobin levels (Vannuccini et al. 2024).

Combined oral contraceptives and those based solely on progestogens produce an increase in hemoglobin and red blood cell count (Tekkle et al. 2022), which is beneficial in women with anemia and heavy menstrual bleeding. As we already know, these drugs produce a decrease in endometrial proliferation, which reduces the amount and duration of menstrual flow and therefore blood loss and the consequent iron deficiency anemia. The combination of estradiol valerate and dienogest has been shown to improve hemoglobin levels compared to other combined hormonal contraceptive preparations (De Leo et al. 2016).

Benefits on the Bone

A review (Ampatzis et al. 2022) analyzed the effect of contraceptives on bone mineral density and concluded that oral progestogens have no impact on bone mineral density as does the Levonorgestrel IUD. However, medroxyprogesterone acetate injection does have a negative impact at all ages but mainly in adolescence. The effect is related to the duration of use, although it should be noted that there is a recovery after discontinuation.

Combined oral contraceptives may also be detrimental to bone mineral density in adolescent girls, although the effect is more marked with ultra-low doses of ethinyl estradiol (e.g., 20 mcg). This effect is not seen in premenopausal and perimenopausal women with adequate ovarian and estrogenic function, in whom combined oral contraceptives have no impact on bone mineral density. In women of childbearing age with hypoestrogenism (athletes, polycystic ovary syndrome) and postmenopausal women with compromised ovarian function (physiological estrogen decline), combined oral contraceptives appear to have a positive effect by providing exogenous estrogens.

References

Abu Hashim, Hatem, Essam Ghayaty, and Mohamed El Rakhawy. 2015. "Levonorgestrel-Releasing Intrauterine System vs Oral Progestins for Non-Atypical Endometrial Hyperplasia: A Systematic Review and Metaanalysis of Randomized Trials." *American Journal of Obstetrics and Gynecology* 213 (4): 469–78. https://doi.org/10.1016/j.ajog.2015.03.037.

Al-Jefout, Moamar, and Nedal Nawaiseh. 2016. "Continuous Norethisterone Acetate versus Cyclical Drospirenone 3 Mg/Ethinyl Estradiol 20 Mg for the Management of Primary Dysmenorrhea in Young Adult Women." *Journal of Pediatric and Adolescent Gynecology* 29 (2): 143–47. https://doi.org/10.1016/j.jpag.2015.08.009.

Allen, Connor Luke, Saikat Banerjee, Mahantesh Karoshi, Peter Humaidan, and Farshad Tahmasebi. 2025a. "The Efficacy of Progestins in Managing Pain Associated with Endometriosis, Fibroids and Pre-Menstrual Syndrome: A Systematic Review." *Archives of Gynecology and Obstetrics* 311 (6): 1511–33. https://doi.org/10.1007/s00404-025-07957-0.

Allen, Connor Luke, Saikat Banerjee, Mahantesh Karoshi, Peter Humaidan, and Farshad Tahmasebi. 2025b. "The Efficacy of Progestins in Managing Pain Associated with Endometriosis, Fibroids and Pre-Menstrual Syndrome: A Systematic Review." *Archives of Gynecology and Obstetrics* 311 (6): 1511–33. https://doi.org/10.1007/s00404-025-07957-0.

Ampatzis, C., S. Zervoudis, G. Iatrakis, and G. Mastorakos. 2022. "EFFECT OF ORAL CONTRACEPTIVES ON BONE MINERAL DENSITY." *Acta Endocrinologica (Bucharest, Romania: 2005)* 18 (3): 355–60. https://doi.org/10.4183/aeb.2022.355.

Anastasiou, Elle, Katharine J. McCarthy, Erica L. Gollub, Lauren Ralph, Janneke H. H. M. van de Wijgert, and Heidi E. Jones. 2022. "The Relationship between Hormonal Contraception and Cervical Dysplasia/Cancer Controlling for Human Papillomavirus Infection: A Systematic Review." *Contraception* 107 (March): 1–9. https://doi.org/10.1016/j.contraception.2021.10.018.

Audet, M. C., M. Moreau, W. D. Koltun, et al. 2001. "Evaluation of Contraceptive Efficacy and Cycle Control of a Transdermal Contraceptive Patch vs an Oral Contraceptive: A Randomized Controlled Trial." *JAMA* 285 (18): 2347–54. https://doi.org/10.1001/jama.285.18.2347.

Bahamondes, Luis, M. Valeria Bahamondes, and Lee P. Shulman. 2015. "Non-Contraceptive Benefits of Hormonal and Intrauterine Reversible Contraceptive Methods." *Human Reproduction Update* 21 (5): 640–51. https://doi.org/10.1093/humupd/dmv023.

Barrionuevo, Patricia, Mohammed Nabhan, Osama Altayar, et al. 2018. "Treatment Options for Hirsutism: A Systematic Review and Network Meta-Analysis." *The Journal of Clinical Endocrinology and Metabolism* 103 (4): 1258–64. https://doi.org/10.1210/jc.2017-02052.

Becker, Christian M., Attila Bokor, Oskari Heikinheimo, et al. 2022. "ESHRE Guideline: Endometriosis." *Human Reproduction Open* 2022 (2): hoac009. https://doi.org/10.1093/hropen/hoac009.

Bitzer, Johannes, Céline Bouchard, János Zatik, et al. 2024. "Effects of E4/DRSP on Self-Reported Physical and Emotional Premenstrual and Menstrual Symptoms: Data from the Phase 3 Clinical Trial in Europe and Russia." *The European Journal of Contraception & Reproductive Health Care: The Official Journal of the European Society of Contraception* 29 (4): 150–59. https://doi.org/10.1080/13625187.2024.2359117.

Bofill Rodriguez, Magdalena, Anne Lethaby, Cindy Low, and Iain T. Cameron. 2019. "Cyclical Progestogens for Heavy Menstrual Bleeding." *The Cochrane Database of Systematic Reviews* 8 (8): CD001016. https://doi.org/10.1002/14651858.CD001016.pub3.

Bouchard, Céline, Johannes Bitzer, Melissa J. Chen, et al. 2025. "Effects of Estetrol/Drospirenone on Self-Reported Physical and Emotional Premenstrual and Menstrual Symptoms: Data from the Phase 3 Clinical Trial in the United States and Canada." *Contraception* 147 (July): 110889. https://doi.org/10.1016/j.contraception.2025.110889.

Bustillos-Alamilla, Edgardo, J. Zepeda-Zaragoza, M. A. Hernández-Ruiz, and Carlos Humberto Briones-Landa. 2010. "[Combined hormonal contraception in cycles artificially extended]." *Ginecologia Y Obstetricia De Mexico* 78 (1): 37–45.

Carrillo Torres, Pilar, M. Ángeles Martínez-Zamora, Cristina Ros, et al. 2023. "Clinical and Sonographic Impact of Oral Contraception in Patients with Deep Endometriosis and Adenomyosis at 2 Years of Follow-Up." *Scientific Reports* 13 (1): 2066. https://doi.org/10.1038/s41598-023-29227-2.

Caserta, D., E. Ralli, E. Matteucci, G. Bordi, M. Mallozzi, and M. Moscarini. 2014. "Combined Oral Contraceptives: Health Benefits beyond Contraception." *Panminerva Medica* 56 (3): 233–44.

Coelingh Bennink, Herjan J. T., Femke A. M. van Gennip, Mireille G. F. Gerrits, Jan F. M. Egberts, Kristina Gemzell-Danielsson, and Helena Kopp-Kallner. 2024. "Health Benefits of Combined Oral Contraceptives - a Narrative Review." *The European Journal of Contraception & Reproductive Health Care: The Official Journal of the European Society of Contraception* 29 (2): 40–52. https://doi.org/10.1080/13625187.2024.2317295.

Creinin, Mitchell D., Kurt T. Barnhart, Lori M. Gawron, David Eisenberg, R. Garn Mabey, and Jeffrey T. Jensen. 2023a. "Heavy Menstrual Bleeding Treatment with a Levonorgestrel 52-Mg Intrauterine Device." *Obstetrics and Gynecology* 141 (5): 971–78. https://doi.org/10.1097/AOG.0000000000005137.

Creinin, Mitchell D., Kurt T. Barnhart, Lori M. Gawron, David Eisenberg, R. Garn Mabey, and Jeffrey T. Jensen. 2023b. "Heavy Menstrual Bleeding Treatment with a Levonorgestrel 52-Mg Intrauterine Device." *Obstetrics and Gynecology* 141 (5): 971–78. https://doi.org/10.1097/AOG.0000000000005137.

Davies, Joanna, and Rezan A. Kadir. 2017. "Heavy Menstrual Bleeding: An Update on Management." *Thrombosis Research* 151 Suppl 1 (March): S70–77. https://doi.org/10.1016/S0049-3848(17)30072-5.

Dawood, M. Yusoff. 2006. "Primary Dysmenorrhea: Advances in Pathogenesis and Management." *Obstetrics and Gynecology* 108 (2): 428–41. https://doi.org/10.1097/01.AOG.0000230214.26638.0c.

De Leo, Vincenzo, Maria Concetta Musacchio, Valentina Cappelli, Paola Piomboni, and Giuseppe Morgante. 2016. "Hormonal Contraceptives: Pharmacology Tailored to Women's Health." *Human Reproduction Update* 22 (5): 634–46. https://doi.org/10.1093/humupd/dmw016.

Elassall, Gena M., Esraa G. Sayed, Nada A. Abdallah, et al. 2022. "Levonorgestrel-Releasing Intrauterine System versus Systemic Progestins in Management of Endometrial Hyperplasia: A Systemic Review and Meta-Analysis." *Journal of Gynecology Obstetrics and Human Reproduction* 51 (8): 102432. https://doi.org/10.1016/j.jogoh.2022.102432.

Etrusco, Andrea, Fabio Barra, Vito Chiantera, et al. 2023. "Current Medical Therapy for Adenomyosis: From Bench to Bedside." *Drugs* 83 (17): 1595–611. https://doi.org/10.1007/s40265-023-01957-7.

Fernandez-Montoli, Maria-Eulalia, Jordi Sabadell, Nayanar Adela Contreras Perez, Paula Verdaguer Menéndez-Arango, Carla Julia Torres, and Judith Lleberia. 2025. "Fertility-Sparing Treatment for Atypical Endometrial Hyperplasia and Endometrial Cancer." *The Cochrane Database of Systematic Reviews* 7 (7): CD013111. https://doi.org/10.1002/14651858.CD013111.pub2.

Fruzzetti, Franca, and Tiziana Fidecicchi. 2020. "Hormonal Contraception and Depression: Updated Evidence and Implications in Clinical Practice." *Clinical Drug Investigation* 40 (12): 1097–106. https://doi.org/10.1007/s40261-020-00966-8.

Gavrilov, S. G., and O. O. Turischeva. 2017. "Conservative Treatment of Pelvic Congestion Syndrome: Indications and Opportunities." *Current Medical Research and Opinion* 33 (6): 1099–103. https://doi.org/10.1080/03007995.2017.1302414.

Grandi, Giovanni, Fabio Barra, Simone Ferrero, et al. 2019. "Hormonal Contraception in Women with Endometriosis: A Systematic Review." *The European Journal of Contraception & Reproductive Health Care: The Official Journal of the European Society of Contraception* 24 (1): 61–70. https://doi.org/10.1080/13625187.2018.1550576.

Grimes, David A., LaShawn B. Jones, Laureen M. Lopez, and Kenneth F. Schulz. 2014. "Oral Contraceptives for Functional Ovarian Cysts." *The Cochrane Database of Systematic Reviews* 2014 (4): CD006134. https://doi.org/10.1002/14651858.CD006134.pub5.

Harada, Tasuku, Mikio Momoeda, Yuji Taketani, Hiroshi Hoshiai, and Naoki Terakawa. 2008. "Low-Dose Oral Contraceptive Pill for Dysmenorrhea Associated with Endometriosis: A Placebo-Controlled, Double-Blind, Randomized Trial." *Fertility and Sterility* 90 (5): 1583–88. https://doi.org/10.1016/j.fertnstert.2007.08.051.

Imai, A., K. Matsunami, H. Takagi, and S. Ichigo. 2014. "Levonorgestrel-Releasing Intrauterine Device Used for Dysmenorrhea: Five-Year Literature Review." *Clinical and Experimental Obstetrics & Gynecology* 41 (5): 495–98.

"International Evidence-Based Guideline for the Assessment and Management of Polycystic Ovary Syndrome – 2023." 2023. *REPRODUCTIVE ENDOCRINOLOGY*, no. 69: 59–79. https://doi.org/10.18370/2309-4117.2023.69.59-79.

James, Andra H., Peter A. Kouides, Rezan Abdul-Kadir, et al. 2011. "Evaluation and Management of Acute Menorrhagia in Women with and without Underlying Bleeding Disorders: Consensus from an International Expert Panel." *European Journal of Obstetrics, Gynecology, and Reproductive Biology* 158 (2): 124–34. https://doi.org/10.1016/j.ejogrb.2011.04.025.

Jensen, J. T., and L. Speroff. 2000. "Health Benefits of Oral Contraceptives." *Obstetrics and Gynecology Clinics of North America* 27 (4): 705–21. https://doi.org/10.1016/s0889-8545(05)70169-8.

Johansson, Annelie, Athanasia E. Christakou, Adina Iftimi, et al. 2021. "Characterization of Benign Breast Diseases and Association with Age, Hormonal Factors, and Family History of Breast Cancer Among Women in Sweden." *JAMA Network Open* 4 (6): e2114716. https://doi.org/10.1001/jamanetworkopen.2021.14716.

Kopp-Kallner, Helena, Marie Linder, Carolyn E. Cesta, Silvia Segovia Chacón, Helle Kieler, and Sofie Graner. 2022. "Method of Hormonal Contraception and Protective Effects Against Ectopic Pregnancy." *Obstetrics and Gynecology* 139 (5): 764–70. https://doi.org/10.1097/AOG.0000000000004726.

Lethaby, Anne, Michelle R. Wise, Maria Aj Weterings, Magdalena Bofill Rodriguez, and Julie Brown. 2019. "Combined Hormonal Contraceptives for Heavy Menstrual Bleeding." *The Cochrane Database of Systematic Reviews* 2 (2): CD000154. https://doi.org/10.1002/14651858.CD000154.pub3.

Levin, Gabriel, Uri P. Dior, Ronit Gilad, Avi Benshushan, Asher Shushan, and Amihai Rottenstreich. 2021. "Pelvic Inflammatory Disease among Users and Non-Users of an Intrauterine Device." *Journal of Obstetrics and Gynaecology: The Journal of the Institute of Obstetrics and Gynaecology* 41 (1): 118–23. https://doi.org/10.1080/01443615.2020.1719989.

Lopez, Laureen M., Adrian A. Kaptein, and Frans M. Helmerhorst. 2012. "Oral Contraceptives Containing Drospirenone for Premenstrual Syndrome." *The Cochrane Database of Systematic Reviews*, no. 2 (February): CD006586. https://doi.org/10.1002/14651858.CD006586.pub4.

Ma, Siyan, and Sae Jin Song. 2023. "Oral Contraceptives Containing Drospirenone for Premenstrual Syndrome." *The Cochrane Database of Systematic Reviews* 6 (6): CD006586. https://doi.org/10.1002/14651858.CD006586.pub5.

Machado, Rogério Bonassi, Nilson Roberto de Melo, and Hugo Maia. 2010. "Bleeding Patterns and Menstrual-Related Symptoms with the Continuous Use of a Contraceptive Combination of Ethinylestradiol and Drospirenone: A Randomized Study." *Contraception* 81 (3): 215–22. https://doi.org/10.1016/j.contraception.2009.10.010.

Munro, Malcolm G. and Southern California Permanente Medical Group's Abnormal Uterine Bleeding Working Group. 2013. "Acute Uterine Bleeding Unrelated to Pregnancy: A Southern California Permanente Medical Group Practice Guideline." *The Permanente Journal* 17 (3): 43–56. https://doi.org/10.7812/TPP/13-018.

Muzii, Ludovico, Chiara Di Tucci, Chiara Achilli, et al. 2016. "Continuous versus Cyclic Oral Contraceptives after Laparoscopic Excision of Ovarian Endometriomas: A Systematic Review and Metaanalysis." *American Journal of Obstetrics and Gynecology* 214 (2): 203–11. https://doi.org/10.1016/j.ajog.2015.08.074.

Muzii, Ludovico, Chiara Di Tucci, Giulia Galati, et al. 2023a. "The Efficacy of Dienogest in Reducing Disease and Pain Recurrence After Endometriosis Surgery: A Systematic Review and Meta-Analysis." *Reproductive Sciences (Thousand Oaks, Calif.)* 30 (11): 3135–43. https://doi.org/10.1007/s43032-023-01266-0.

Muzii, Ludovico, Chiara Di Tucci, Giulia Galati, et al. 2023b. "The Efficacy of Dienogest in Reducing Disease and Pain Recurrence After Endometriosis Surgery: A Systematic Review and Meta-Analysis." *Reproductive Sciences (Thousand Oaks, Calif.)* 30 (11): 3135–43. https://doi.org/10.1007/s43032-023-01266-0.

Nisa, Khair Ul, Najeebul Tarfeen, Shahnaz Ahmad Mir, Ajaz Ahmad Waza, Mir Bilal Ahmad, and Bashir Ahmad Ganai. 2024. "Molecular Mechanisms in the Etiology of Polycystic Ovary Syndrome (PCOS): A Multifaceted Hypothesis Towards the Disease with Potential Therapeutics." *Indian Journal of Clinical Biochemistry: IJCB* 39 (1): 18–36. https://doi.org/10.1007/s12291-023-01130-7.

O'Hara, Caitlin Alsandria, Teoh Wei Shan, and Joseph Ng Soon Yau. 2024. "Knowledge of Non-Contraceptive Benefits of and Willingness to Consider Taking Oral Contraceptive Pills among a Low-Risk Female Population: A Cross-Sectional Study." *The European Journal of Contraception & Reproductive Health Care: The Official Journal of the European Society of Contraception* 29 (2): 53–60. https://doi.org/10.1080/13625187.2023.2300944.

Power, J., R. French, and F. Cowan. 2007. "Subdermal Implantable Contraceptives versus Other Forms of Reversible Contraceptives or Other Implants as Effective Methods of Preventing Pregnancy." *The Cochrane Database of Systematic Reviews* 2007 (3): CD001326. https://doi.org/10.1002/14651858.CD001326.pub2.

Practice Committee of the American Society for Reproductive Medicine. 2006. "Treatment of Pelvic Pain Associated with Endometriosis." *Fertility and Sterility* 86 (5 Suppl 1): S18-27. https://doi.org/10.1016/j.fertnstert.2006.08.072.

Pravatta-Rezende, Gabriela, Cristina Laguna Benetti-Pinto, Daniela Angerame Yela Gomes, Ana Carolina Japur de Sá Rosa E Silva, and José Maria Soares. 2025. "Diagnosis and Management of Acute Abnormal Uterine Bleeding during Menacme." *Clinics (Sao Paulo, Brazil)* 80: 100608. https://doi.org/10.1016/j.clinsp.2025.100608.

Raine-Bennett, Tina, Michael J. Fassett, Malini Chandra, et al. 2022. "Ectopic Pregnancy Prevention: Further Evidence of Benefits of Prescription Contraceptives." *Contraception* 105 (January): 19–25. https://doi.org/10.1016/j.contraception.2021.09.007.

Requena, C., and B. Llombart. 2020. "Oral Contraceptives in Dermatology." *Actas Dermo-Sifiliograficas* 111 (5): 351–56. https://doi.org/10.1016/j.ad.2019.06.006.

Roumen, Frans J. M. E. 2007. "The Contraceptive Vaginal Ring Compared with the Combined Oral Contraceptive Pill: A Comprehensive Review of Randomized Controlled Trials." *Contraception* 75 (6): 420–29. https://doi.org/10.1016/j.contraception.2007.01.013.

Sangkomkamhang, Ussanee S., Pisake Lumbiganon, and Porjai Pattanittum. 2020. "Progestogens or Progestogen-Releasing Intrauterine Systems for Uterine Fibroids (Other than Preoperative Medical Therapy)." *The Cochrane Database of Systematic Reviews* 11 (11): CD008994. https://doi.org/10.1002/14651858.CD008994.pub3.

Schoep, Mark E., Eddy M. M. Adang, Jacques W. M. Maas, Bianca De Bie, Johanna W. M. Aarts, and Theodoor E. Nieboer. 2019. "Productivity Loss Due to Menstruation-Related Symptoms: A Nationwide Cross-Sectional Survey among 32 748 Women." *BMJ Open* 9 (6): e026186. https://doi.org/10.1136/bmjopen-2018-026186.

Schroll, Jeppe B., Amanda Y. Black, Cindy Farquhar, and Innie Chen. 2023. "Combined Oral Contraceptive Pill for Primary Dysmenorrhoea." *The Cochrane Database of Systematic Reviews* 7 (7): CD002120. https://doi.org/10.1002/14651858.CD002120.pub4.

Soysal, M. E., S. Soysal, K. Vicdan, and S. Ozer. 2001. "A Randomized Controlled Trial of Goserelin and Medroxyprogesterone Acetate in the Treatment of Pelvic Congestion." *Human Reproduction (Oxford, England)* 16 (5): 931–39. https://doi.org/10.1093/humrep/16.5.931.

Stańczak, Natalia Anna, Ewelina Grywalska, and Ewa Dudzińska. 2024. "The Latest Reports and Treatment Methods on Polycystic Ovary Syndrome." *Annals of Medicine* 56 (1): 2357737. https://doi.org/10.1080/07853890.2024.2357737.

Teede, Helena J., Marie L. Misso, Michael F. Costello, et al. 2018. "Recommendations from the International Evidence-Based Guideline for the Assessment and Management of Polycystic Ovary Syndrome." *Fertility and Sterility* 110 (3): 364–79. https://doi.org/10.1016/j.fertnstert.2018.05.004.

Tekle, Esayas, Yemataw Gelaw, and Fikir Asrie. 2022. "Hematological Profile Changes Among Oral Contraceptive Users: A Narrative Review." *Journal of Blood Medicine* 13: 525–36. https://doi.org/10.2147/JBM.S379841.

Van Gerwen, Olivia T., Christina A. Muzny, and Jeanne M. Marrazzo. 2022. "Sexually Transmitted Infections and Female Reproductive Health." *Nature Microbiology* 7 (8): 1116–26. https://doi.org/10.1038/s41564-022-01177-x.

Vannuccini, Silvia, Felice Petraglia, Francisco Carmona, Joaquim Calaf, and Charles Chapron. 2024a. "The Modern Management of Uterine Fibroids-Related Abnormal Uterine Bleeding." *Fertility and Sterility* 122 (1): 20–30. https://doi.org/10.1016/j.fertnstert.2024.04.041.

Vannuccini, Silvia, Felice Petraglia, Francisco Carmona, Joaquim Calaf, and Charles Chapron. 2024b. "The Modern Management of Uterine Fibroids-Related Abnormal Uterine Bleeding." *Fertility and Sterility* 122 (1): 20–30. https://doi.org/10.1016/j.fertnstert.2024.04.041.

Varma, Rajesh, Hemi Soneja, Kalsang Bhatia, et al. 2008. "The Effectiveness of a Levonorgestrel-Releasing Intrauterine System (LNG-IUS) in the Treatment of Endometrial Hyperplasia--a Long-Term Follow-up Study." *European Journal of Obstetrics, Gynecology, and Reproductive Biology* 139 (2): 169–75. https://doi.org/10.1016/j.ejogrb.2008.02.022.

Vercellini, Paolo, Laura Buggio, Nicola Berlanda, Giussy Barbara, Edgardo Somigliana, and Silvano Bosari. 2016. "Estrogen-Progestins and Progestins for the Management of Endometriosis." *Fertility and Sterility* 106 (7): 1552-1571.e2. https://doi.org/10.1016/j.fertnstert.2016.10.022.

Wong, Chooi L., Cindy Farquhar, Helen Roberts, and Michelle Proctor. 2009. "Oral Contraceptive Pill for Primary Dysmenorrhoea." *The Cochrane Database of Systematic Reviews* 2009 (4): CD002120. https://doi.org/10.1002/14651858.CD002120.pub3.

Zorbas, Konstantinos A., Konstantinos P. Economopoulos, and Nikos F. Vlahos. 2015. "Continuous versus Cyclic Oral Contraceptives for the Treatment of Endometriosis: A Systematic Review." *Archives of Gynecology and Obstetrics* 292 (1): 37–43. https://doi.org/10.1007/s00404-015-3641-1.

Chapter 15

Contraception and Cancer

M. L. Juan Rodrigo[1,*], MD
A. Tello Delsors[2], MD
L. Sales Pérez[3], MD
A. Santos Fernández[1], MD
and M. A. Rubio Moreno[1], MD
[1]Obstetrics and Gynecology Department, University and Hospital of Albacete, Spain
[2]Obstetrics and Gynecology Department, University and Hospital of Santa Lucía, Cartagena, Murcia, Spain
[3]Obstetrics and Gynecology Department, Hospital Lluis Alcanyis Xativa, Xativa, Valencia, Spain

Abstract

The use of contraceptive methods, especially hormonal contraceptives, has been extensively studied for its potential impact on the incidence of various types of cancer. This chapter reviews in a critical and updated way the effects of contraceptives on the main gynecological cancers (breast, ovarian, endometrial and cervical), as well as on some non-gynecological cancers, focusing especially on the effect of combined hormonal contraceptives. The molecular mechanisms underlying these associations, the influence of genetic variability and the differentiated effects according to the type of contraceptive are analyzed. The protective effect of hormonal contraceptives on ovarian, endometrial and colorectal cancers, as well as the possible increased risk of breast and cervical cancer in certain contexts, are especially highlighted. Surgical strategies such as opportunistic bilateral salpingectomy and its role in the prevention of ovarian cancer, especially in patients with high genetic risk (BRCA1/2, Lynch syndrome), are also discussed.
This chapter provides an exhaustive, critical and updated review of a topic of great current interest that supports appropriate clinical decision making in daily gynecological practice.

Keywords: contraception, combined contraceptives, hormonal contraception, cancer, breast cancer, ovarian cancer, endometrial cancer, cervical cancer, colorectal cancer, liver cancer

---

* Corresponding Author's Email: marisajuanrodrigo@gmail.com

In: Advances in Reproductive Health
Editors: Llanos Belmonte Andujar and Ana Fuentes Rozalen
ISBN: 979-8-90134-038-7

Introduction

The use of hormonal contraceptives (HA) has been the subject of numerous studies in relation to the risk of developing certain types of cancer. While some research has suggested an association with a slight increase in the incidence of certain tumors, others have demonstrated protective effects in different contexts. Understanding these risks and benefits is critical for clinical decision making and patient counseling.

Since the introduction of hormonal contraceptives in the 1960s, their impact on women's health has been a central issue in gynecology. The combination of estrogens and progestogens in contraceptives has demonstrated to influence cell proliferation, apoptosis and the regulation of hormonal factors that may be related to the development of malignant and benign tumors. Estrogens can induce cell proliferation through activation of estrogen receptors (ERα and ERβ), modulating genes related to cell division and survival. Progestogens, on the other hand, can counteract these effects by negatively regulating cell proliferation in some tissues (Klinge 2001; Thomas and Gustafsson 2011). Thus, a detailed analysis of how these drugs affect different types of cancer is essential.

Other contraceptive methods, such as condoms and copper IUDs, have also been found to be associated with the incidence of cervical cancer and even endometrial cancer, as will be discussed later in this chapter.

The use of hormonal contraception has been shown to have a significant preventive effect on ovarian, endometrial and colorectal cancer, while it may increase the risk of cervical and anal cancer in women with high-risk HPV. However, there have been no studies showing that "overall cancer risk" or "overall cancer-related mortality" are increased among hormonal contraception users (Beral et al., 2007; Colditz et al., 1994; Hannaford et al., 2007). This information should be taken into account in contraceptive counseling, emphasizing both the benefits and potential risks.

Effects of Contraceptives on Different Types of Cancers

We will divide them into two groups: gynecological cancers and non-gynecological cancers.

Gynecological Cancers

Breast Cancer

Combined oral contraceptives have been associated with a slightly increased risk of breast cancer, especially in women who use them for prolonged periods. This risk appears to progressively decrease after discontinuing their use (Collaborative Group on Hormonal Factors in Breast Cancer, 2017). Factors such as age of onset, duration of use, and family history may influence the magnitude of risk (Mørch et al., 2017).

According to the 2025 review by Roe et al, the absolute risk remains low and the relative increase in breast cancer risk is greater in women who use oral contraceptives for longer periods (Roe et al. 2025). However, the risk returns to the baseline approximately 10 years after discontinuing use.

A recent meta-analysis evaluated the relationship between oral contraceptive use and breast cancer risk globally, including 74 studies with 198,579 women. A slight increase in relative risk (RR = 1.15, 95% CI: 1.01-1.31, p = 0.0358) was identified in oral contraceptive users compared to non-users, although statistical significance varied by geographic region. In Asia and the Middle East, the risk was higher (RR = 1.29, p = 0.014 and RR = 1.29, p = 0.043, respectively), whereas no significant association was observed in the Americas and Europe (Drab et al., 2024). The heterogeneity in the results could be influenced by differences in contraceptive composition, patterns of use and genetic factors. Some studies have suggested an association between the levonorgestrel intrauterine device (IUD) use and an increased risk of breast cancer, especially in women older than 50 years. However, the results are mixed and inconclusive and require further studies to determine their relationship (Lessa and Podlasek 2025).

Recent studies suggest that genetic variability plays an important role in modulating breast cancer risk in contraceptive users. Women carrying BRCA1 and BRCA2 mutations appear to be at increased risk of developing breast cancer if they have used oral contraceptives for more than five years (Jahanfar et al., 2024).

From a biological point of view, it has been proposed that estrogen promotes mammary cell proliferation, which may increase the likelihood of mutations and, consequently, the development of cancer. However, progestogen, by modulating estrogen activity, could also exert a protective effect in some cases.

Ovarian and Endometrial Cancer

In contrast to breast cancer, the use of hormonal contraceptives has demonstrated a tendency to have a significant protective effect against ovarian and endometrial cancer. The meta-analysis conducted by Jahanfar in 2024 confirmed that hormonal contraceptive users have a 36% lower risk of ovarian and endometrial cancer (Jahanfar et al., 2024). Furthermore, data from the Royal College of General Practitioners study suggest that this protective effect is maintained for at least 30 years after discontinuation of use (Iversen et al., 2017). The mechanism behind this risk reduction lies in the suppression of ovulation and the decrease in continuous estrogenic stimulation of the endometrium. By reducing ovulatory cycles over a woman's lifetime, inflammation and damage to the ovarian epithelium is limited, which decreases the opportunities for malignant transformation of cells (Iversen et al. 2017).

Ovarian Cancer

In the case of ovarian cancer, other contraceptive methods have been found to be related to its incidence, as will be detailed below.

Bilateral Tubal Ligation vs. Bilateral Salpingectomy

Current evidence indicates that the origin of most high-grade serous ovarian cancers is the tubal epithelium (Kurman and Shih 2010), while the fallopian tube acts as a conduit for dissemination of carcinogenic cells.

Permanent female sterilization, also known as tubal ligation or tubal occlusion, is the most widely used method of contraception in the world (Fang et al. 2022). Tubal ligation has been consistently associated with a reduced risk of ovarian cancer. In an analysis of the Nurses' Health Study, women with a history of tubal ligation were found to have a 34% lower risk of ovarian cancer compared to those without this history (RR = 0.66, 95% CI: 0.50-0.87) (Tworoger et al. 2007). According to this study, the protective effect could be due to the interruption of the transport of cancer cells from the peritoneal cavity to the ovarian epithelium or to hormonal alterations secondary to surgery.

Bilateral salpingectomy, the surgical removal of the fallopian tubes, is associated with a reduced risk of ovarian cancer (Yoon et al. 2016), particularly high-grade serous carcinoma, the most common and aggressive subtype, which originates in the epithelium of the fallopian tubes (Kurman and Shih 2010). Therefore, the British Columbia Ovarian Cancer Research (OVCARE) in 2018 proposed performing bilateral salpingectomy during other gynecologic surgeries, such as hysterectomy or tubal ligation, known as opportunistic bilateral salpingectomy, as a tool to decrease the incidence of ovarian cancer (Hanley et al. 2018), a strategy that has been supported by multiple scientific societies since then, such as the Spanish Society of Gynecology and Obstetrics, the American College of Obstetricians and Gynecologists (ACOG) and the Society of Gynecologic Oncology (SGO) (de la Fuente Pérez and de la Fuente Bitaine 2019; Foved Johe et al. 2024) ("ACOG Committee Opinion No. 774: Opportunistic Salpingectomy as a Strategy for Epithelial Ovarian Cancer Prevention" 2019; (SGO Clinical Practice Statement 2013).

In addition, several studies support the safety of bilateral salpingectomy versus tubal ligation, without affecting ovarian reserve, increasing surgical time significantly or postoperative complications, such as the need for blood transfusion or hospital readmission (McAlpine et al., 2014, Foved Johe et al., 2024).

Patients with High Genetic Risk

Women carrying germline mutations in the BRCA1 and BRCA2 genes have a significantly elevated risk of developing high-grade epithelial ovarian cancer. In the general population, the risk of ovarian cancer is 1.1% (National Cancer Institute 2024), while in BRCA1 mutation carriers it is estimated at 39-63%, and in BRCA2 carriers at 16-27% (Kuchenbaecker et al. 2017).

In women with BRCA1/2 mutations, the gold standard treatment is salpingo-oophorectomy (removal of ovaries and tubes) (Daly et al. 2023). This procedure, when performed prophylactically reduces the risk of ovarian cancer by more than 80%. Recent studies associate salpingo-oophorectomy with a significant reduction in breast cancer risk, especially if performed before menopause (Choi et al. 2021).

The identification of the tubo-epithelial origin of high-grade serous carcinoma has substantially modified the understanding of ovarian carcinogenesis. The finding of precursor lesions such as STIC (serous tubal intraepithelial carcinoma) in the fallopian tube fimbriae has prompted the development of more conservative surgical strategies, such as bilateral salpingectomy with ovarian conservation as a temporary option in young women with unmet reproductive desires or to postpone surgical menopause (Kahn et al. 2023).

Some studies have considered the possibility of delayed salpingectomy, where the tubes are removed first and the ovaries are retained until menopause, with the aim of reducing the morbidity associated with early menopause (Finch et al. 2014). However, it is not considered an equally effective or safe alternative to bilateral adnexectomy in BRCA mutation carrier patients.

Endometrial Cancer

The use of combined hormonal contraceptives is associated with a decreased risk of developing endometrial cancer. Specifically, for every five years of oral contraceptive use, the risk of endometrial cancer is reduced by approximately 25%. This protective effect is cumulative; that is, the longer the use, the greater the risk reduction (Allen N., Yang T.O., and Olsson H. 2015). It also has a prolonged protective effect, up to 30 years after cessation of intake (Baker-Rand and Kitson 2024).

The protective effect of combined hormonal contraceptives is attributed to the reduction of endogenous estrogen levels during oral contraceptive use. By simulating a pregnancy-like state, contraceptives decrease estrogenic stimulation of the endometrium, thereby reducing the risk of abnormal cell proliferation and thus endometrial cancer. This occurs independently of the estrogenic dose employed (Allen N., Yang T.O., and Olsson H. 2015). The type of progestogen used in the formulation does not appear to have an influence (Iversen et al. 2020).

All hormonal methods have shown a significant downward trend in the incidence of endometrial cancer, except for progestin-only oral hormonal contraceptives (Jahanfar et al. 2024; Iversen et al. 2020). A recently published systematic review and meta-analysis indicated a significant reduction in endometrial cancer among users of levonorgestrel-releasing intrauterine devices (OR 0.66, 95% CI 0.41-1.08) (Lessa and Podlasek 2025).

On the other hand, different studies analyze the relationship between the use of copper IUDs and the risk of endometrial cancer, concluding that the use of the device reduces the development of this tumor. The exact mechanism of the protective effect is not known at present. As discussed in the corresponding chapter, all intrauterine devices provoke a sterile inflammatory response, which alters the composition of the fluids in the uterine cavity and the morphology of the endometrium, thus allowing an increase in the number of neutrophils, monocytes and plasma cells. It could be this inflammatory response that is responsible for the decreased risk. In addition, a reduction in endometrial mitotic activity and estrogen receptor concentration also appears to be observed, and these changes may limit the rate of hyperplasia, dysplasia and subsequent progression to endometrial cancer (Beining et al. 2008; Felix et al. 2015)

In recent years, several studies have confirmed this potential protective effect. Minalt et al. (2023) concluded that the use of intrauterine devices (IUDs), especially the levonorgestrel-releasing intrauterine system (LNG-IUS), is associated with a significant reduction in endometrial cancer risk, an effect mediated by progestogen-induced endometrial atrophy. Recent studies have shown that this device can even reverse premalignant lesions such as endometrial hyperplasia, with regression rates approaching 86% after six months of use (Smith et al. 2020). Furthermore, population-based analyses indicate a 33% to 78% reduction in endometrial cancer incidence associated with LNG-IUS use (Jones 2021; Kelly 2024).

The copper IUD has also been associated with a decreased risk of endometrial cancer, although the effect appears to be less pronounced. Its protective mechanism is thought to be related to the chronic inflammation it induces within the uterine cavity, altering the endometrial microenvironment and inhibiting abnormal cellular proliferation (Bahamondes 2025; Rogers et al. 2023). However, the exact magnitude of this effect requires further investigation.

More recently, a systematic review and meta-analysis published in October 2019 by Wheeler et al, based on retrospective studies, concluded that copper IUD use is associated with a reduced incidence of ovarian cancer. Prospective studies would be necessary to determine the reproducibility of such results, but in principle the data are encouraging (Wheeler et al. 2019).

Patients with High Genetic Risk

Lynch syndrome, or hereditary nonpolyposis colorectal cancer (HNPCC), is an autosomal dominant disease caused by germline mutations in DNA repair genes such as MLH1, MSH2, MSH6 and PMS2. Female carriers have a significantly increased risk of colorectal, endometrial and, to a lesser extent, ovarian cancer, in addition to other tumors associated with the syndrome spectrum (Michael J et al. 2025).

Lynch syndrome accounts for 2-5% of all endometrial carcinomas (Post et al. 2021). In patients with Lynch syndrome, the lifetime risk of endometrial cancer varies according to genotype, being more frequent in MSH2, MSH6 and PMS2 mutation carriers, and in all cases, it is higher than in the general population (2 to 3%) (Dominguez-Valentin et al. 2023). Similarly, Lynch syndrome is also associated with an increased lifetime risk of developing ovarian cancer, with approximately a 1.3% increased chance.

The preventive treatment of choice in patients with Lynch syndrome is hysterectomy and bilateral double adnexectomy (Schmeler et al. 2006), performed between the ages of 35 and 45 years (Kwon et al. 2008; Ryan et al. 2017; Crosbie et al. 2019).

As we have already reviewed in the previous section, combined oral contraceptives (COCs) reduce the risk of endometrial cancer in the general population, and this effect is maintained, although to a lesser extent, in women carrying Lynch syndrome mutations (Dashti et al. 2015), although data in this regard are very limited (Karen H Lu, MDKathleen M, and Schmeler 2024). This potential preventive benefit is relevant in young women with Lynch syndrome who have not yet completed their reproductive plans.

There are no specific studies regarding the prevention of ovarian cancer related to Lynch syndrome and the use of hormonal contraceptives (Karen H Lu, MDKathleen M, and Schmeler 2024).

Cervical Cancer

Cervical cancer is mainly caused by persistent human papillomavirus (HPV) infection, especially genotypes with high oncogenic risk, such as HPV 16 and 18 (Perkins et al. 2023), although hormonal factors, such as long-term use of combined oral contraceptives (COCs), may influence its progression. Several epidemiological studies have shown an association between long-term use of COCs (especially more than 5 years) and an increased risk of invasive cervical cancer, even after adjusting for HPV infection (International Collaboration of Epidemiological Studies of Cervical Cancer. 2007).

A meta-analysis by the International Agency for Research on Cancer (IARC) showed that the use of COCs for more than five years is associated with a relative risk (RR) of 1.90 compared to women who have never used them. This risk decreases progressively after discontinuing use, returning to baseline levels in approximately 10 years (IARC Working Group on the Evaluation of Carcinogenic Risks to Humans 2007).

However, the absolute risk remains low, and the use of COCs is not contraindicated if preventive measures such as regular screening and HPV vaccination are maintained (IARC Working Group on the Evaluation of Carcinogenic Risks to Humans 2007; International Collaboration of Epidemiological Studies of Cervical Cancer. 2007).

As already mentioned, cervical cancer is related to persistent HPV infection. HPV transmission occurs primarily through genital contact. HPV infection is considered the most frequent sexually transmitted infection in the world, the main route of transmission being sexual contact. Condom use has been proposed as a prevention strategy in the acquisition, persistence and transmission of the virus.

Several studies have shown that consistent condom use is associated with a lower rate of HPV infection (Wolf et al. 2024), reducing the risk by up to almost 70% (Houlihan et al. 2012), and with a lower risk of high-grade intraepithelial lesions (HSIL) and cervical cancer (Winer et al. 2006).

The systematic review by Lam et al. published in 2014 compiled eight longitudinal studies that evaluated the relationship between condom use and the risk of HPV infection or cervical lesions. Four of the studies demonstrated a statistically significant protective effect of consistent condom use on both prevention of HPV infection and regression of cervical lesions. The other four studies also showed a protective trend, although without reaching statistical significance (Lam et al. 2014).

The protective effect of condoms in cervical cancer can be attributed not only to a reduction in the probability of viral transmission, but also to less repeated exposure to the virus, favoring spontaneous regression of already established lesions (Winer et al. 2006; Hogewoning et al. 2003).

It is important to note that condoms do not provide absolute protection against HPV and can be transmitted through uncovered areas, such as the perineal or scrotal skin (Manhart and Koutsky 2002). Furthermore, its effectiveness depends largely on its correct and consistent use (WHO Guidelines Approved by the Guidelines Review Committee. 2013).

On the other hand, the use of IUDs, both copper and hormonal, has also been associated with a decrease in the incidence of cervical cancer. Many studies have been carried out in this regard. According to a meta-analysis published in December 2017, IUD use can reduce the risk of invasive cervical cancer by up to one third, this effect possibly being more beneficial in populations with difficult access to screening for this neoplasm (Cortessis et al. 2017).

This protective effect is shown against squamous cell carcinoma and adenocarcinoma and adenosquamous carcinoma, and does not appear to be due to differences in screening processes between users and non-users of the device. In an expert review published in 2023, Minalt et al. examined the association between IUD use and major gynecological cancers. The authors conclude that both copper IUDs and levonorgestrel-releasing IUDs (LNG-IUS) may be associated with a reduced risk of invasive cervical cancer, possibly mediated by chronic inflammatory response and activation of local immune mechanisms against human papillomavirus (HPV). However, they emphasize that a definitive causal relationship cannot be established and that studies are needed that adequately control for confounding factors and clearly separate the types of IUDs used (Minalt et al. 2023). In contrast, a retrospective cohort study published by Spotnitz et al. in 2020, which directly compared the risk of cervical neoplasia between users of copper IUDs and hormonal IUDs, found no significant differences between the two groups. This study, based on electronic health records, suggests that the type of IUD does not substantially modify the risk of cervical lesions and questions the magnitude of the previously reported protective effect (Spotnitz et al. 2020).

The protective effect of the IUD could be due to immunological reactions at the level of the endometrium, cervical canal and cervix caused by the device after its insertion (foreign body reaction, local trauma). It has also been postulated that local cervical trauma associated with IUD insertion or removal induces local foci of chronic inflammation that modify the immune response. However, its use does not appear to modify the risk of human papillomavirus (HPV) infection (Hubacher and Grimes 2002; Fraser 2010, Castellsagué et al. 2011).

Non-Gynecological Cancers

Although most of the studies on hormonal contraception are focused on gynecological cancers, their impact on other types of cancer common in women, such as colorectal, liver, brain and pancreatic cancer, as well as lung cancer, has also been studied. In this context, contraceptive methods can play both a protective and, in certain cases, potentially unfavorable role.

Colorectal Cancer

The use of combined oral hormonal contraceptives (COCs) is associated with a significant reduction in the risk of colon and rectal cancer of approximately 15% among users (Bosetti et al. 2009; Rennert et al. 2020; Iversen et al. 2017).

One of the most important studies was the Royal College of General Practitioners' Oral Contraception Study, a prospective British cohort that followed more than 46,000 women for more than 40 years. In this study, women who had used hormonal contraception had a lower risk of colorectal cancer compared to non-users (incidence rate ratio [IRR]: 0.81; 99% CI: 0.66-0.99). This protective effect was maintained even more than 35 years after discontinuation of use, suggesting a long-term protective effect (Iversen et al. 2017). This protective effect is in agreement with that observed in the meta-analysis published in 2015 where the longer the duration of contraceptive use, the longer the duration of the protective effect (Luan et al. 2015). However, it could not be related to the doses used.

Although the pathophysiological mechanisms involved are not defined (Kamani, Akgor, and Gültekin 2022), several pathways of action through estrogens and progestogens have been proposed. Estrogens could reduce cell proliferation in the colonic epithelium, modulate bile acid secretion, reducing it and have anti-inflammatory activity. Progestogens could influence intestinal motility and hormone receptor expression at the digestive tissue level.

Liver Cancer

Hepatocellular carcinoma (HCC) is the most common type of primary liver cancer. The main risk factors are chronic hepatitis B virus (HBV) or C virus (HCV) infection, liver cirrhosis, alcohol consumption, and nonalcoholic fatty liver disease (McGlynn, Petrick, and El-Serag 2021).

The relationship between liver cancer and the use of hormonal contraception is not clearly established, with conflicting results in the literature (Kamani, Akgor, and Gültekin 2022; An 2015).

The difference in liver cancer incidence between men and women, with a 3:1 ratio ("Epidemiology and Risk Factors for Hepatocellular Carcinoma - UpToDate," n.d.), suggests a protective effect of estrogens (Kamani, Akgor, and Gültekin 2022).

On current evidence, in healthy women without risk factors, such as HCV, HBV or cirrhosis, it does not appear to increase the risk of liver cancer.

The meta-analysis published in 2015 by Ning An et al. evaluated the relationship between AHC use and liver cancer risk, concluding that there is no significant association between AHC use and HCC risk (RR: 1.23; 95% CI: 0.93-1.63) (An 2015).

The study conducted by the Royal College of General Practitioners' Oral Contraception Study, with follow-up over 44 years, found no significant increased risk of liver cancer, supporting long-term safety (Iversen et al. 2017).

However, in women with pre-existing liver disease, the WHO guidelines and the Medical Eligibility Criteria for Contraceptive Use recommend avoiding the use of hormonal contraception (World Health Organization 2015).

Conclusion

- The use of combined hormonal contraceptives (CHC) is associated with a significant protective effect against ovarian, endometrial and colorectal cancer, this effect being dose-dependent and long-lasting after discontinuation.
- There is a moderate association between long-term use of CHC and an increased risk of breast and cervical cancer, although the absolute risk is low and decreases over time after cessation of use. In the case of cervical cancer, this association is highly dependent on persistent HPV co-infection.
- The levonorgestrel-releasing IUD has shown protective effects against endometrial cancer, and some studies associate it with a possible increased risk of breast cancer in women, especially those over 50 years of age or with a genetic predisposition, although the data are still inconclusive.
- Opportunistic bilateral salpingectomy is an effective and safe strategy to reduce the risk of ovarian cancer.
- In women at high genetic risk (BRCA1/2 or Lynch syndrome), primary prevention strategies, such as salpingo-oophorectomy or hysterectomy with adnexectomy, are essential. The use of hormonal contraceptives may offer some protection and should be considered in young women who have not yet completed their reproductive desires.
- Contraceptive counseling should be individualized, taking into account personal and family risk factors, as well as the preferences and priorities of each patient.

References

"ACOG Committee Opinion No. 774: Opportunistic Salpingectomy as a Strategy for Epithelial Ovarian Cancer Prevention." 2019. *Obstetrics & Gynecology* 133 (4): e279-84. https://doi.org/10.1097/AOG.0000000000003164.

Allen N., Yang T.O., and Olsson H. 2015. "Endometrial Cancer and Oral Contraceptives: An Individual Participant Meta-Analysis of 27 276 Women with Endometrial Cancer from 36 Epidemiological Studies." *The Lancet Oncology* 16 (9): 1061-70. https://doi.org/10.1016/S1470-2045(15)00212-0.

An, Ning. 2015. "Oral Contraceptives Use and Liver Cancer Risk." *Medicine* 94 (43): e1619. https://doi.org/10.1097/MD.0000000000001619.

Bahamondes, Luis. 2025. "Long-Term Use of LNG-IUS and Cu-IUD Offers Effective Contraception and a Favorable Reduction in Uterine Cancer Risk." *Indonesian Journal of General Medicine* 12 (2). https://indonesianjournalmedicine.org/index.php/ijgm/article/download/139/150.

Baker-Rand, Holly, and Sarah J Kitson. 2024. "Recent Advances in Endometrial Cancer Prevention, Early Diagnosis and Treatment." *Cancers* 16 (5). https://doi.org/10.3390/cancers16051028.

Bosch, F X, A Lorincz, N Munoz, C J L M Meijer, and K V Shah. 2002. "The Causal Relation between Human Papillomavirus and Cervical Cancer." *Journal of Clinical Pathology* 55 (4): 244-65. https://doi.org/10.1136/jcp.55.4.244.

Bosetti, Cristina, Francesca Bravi, Eva Negri, and Carlo La Vecchia. 2009. "Oral Contraceptives and Colorectal Cancer Risk: A Systematic Review and Meta Analysis." *Human Reproduction Update* 15 (5): 489-98. https://doi.org/10.1093/humupd/dmp017.

Castellsagué, Xavier, Miriam Díaz, Silvia Vaccarella, Silvia de Sanjosé, Nubia Muñoz, Rolando Herrero, et al. 2011. "Intrauterine Device Use, Cervical Infection with Human Papillomavirus, and Risk of Cervical Cancer: A Pooled Analysis of 26 Epidemiological Studies." *Lancet Oncology* 12 (11): 1023–31. https://doi.org/10.1016/S1470-2045(11)70223-6.

Choi, Yun-Hee, Mary Beth Terry, Mary B. Daly, Robert J. MacInnis, John L. Hopper, Sarah Colonna, Saundra S. Buys, et al. 2021. "Association of Risk-Reducing Salpingo-Oophorectomy with Breast Cancer Risk in Women with BRCA1 and BRCA2 Pathogenic Variants." *JAMA Oncology*, February. https://doi.org/10.1001/jamaoncol.2020.7995.

Cortessis, Victoria K., Margarett Barrett, Nancy Brown Wade, Tungalag Enebish, Julie L. Perrigo, Jennifer Tobin, et al. 2017. "Intrauterine Device Use and Cervical Cancer Risk: A Systematic Review and Meta-analysis." *Obstetrics & Gynecology* 130 (6): 1226–36. https://doi.org/10.1097/AOG.0000000000002350.

Crosbie, Emma J., Neil A.J. Ryan, Mark J. Arends, Tjalling Bosse, John Burn, Joanna M. Cornes, Robin Crawford, et al. 2019. "The Manchester International Consensus Group Recommendations for the Management of Gynecological Cancers in Lynch Syndrome." *Genetics in Medicine* 21 (10): 2390-2400. https://doi.org/10.1038/s41436-019-0489-y.

Daly, Mary B., Tuya Pal, Kara N. Maxwell, Jane Churpek, Wendy Kohlmann, Zahraa AlHilli, Banu Arun, et al. 2023. "NCCN Guidelines® Insights: Genetic/Familial High-Risk Assessment: Breast, Ovarian, and Pancreatic, Version 2.2024." *Journal of the National Comprehensive Cancer Network* 21 (10): 1000-1010. https://doi.org/10.6004/jnccn.2023.0051.

Dashti, Seyedeh Ghazaleh, Rowena Chau, Driss Ait Ouakrim, Daniel D. Buchanan, Mark Clendenning, Joanne P. Young, Ingrid M. Winship, et al. 2015. "Female Hormonal Factors and the Risk of Endometrial Cancer in Lynch Syndrome." *JAMA* 314 (1): 61. https://doi.org/10.1001/jama.2015.6789.

Dominguez-Valentin, Mev, Saskia Haupt, Toni T. Seppälä, Julian R. Sampson, Lone Sunde, Inge Bernstein, Mark A. Jenkins, et al. 2023. "Mortality by Age, Gene and Gender in Carriers of Pathogenic Mismatch Repair Gene Variants Receiving Surveillance for Early Cancer Diagnosis and Treatment: A Report from the Prospective Lynch Syndrome Database." *EClinicalMedicine* 58 (April):101909. https://doi.org/10.1016/j.eclinm.2023.101909.

"Epidemiology and Risk Factors for Hepatocellular Carcinoma - *UpToDate*." n.d. Accessed May 22, 2025. https://www.uptodate.com/contents/epidemiologyand-risk-factors-for-hepatocellularcarcinoma?search=Cancer%20de%20higado&source=search_result&selectedTitle=5~150&usage_type=default&display_rank=5#H3.

Fang, Nancy Z., Simone P. Advaney, Paula M. Castaño, Anne Davis, and Carolyn L. Westhoff. 2022. "Female Permanent Permanent Contraception Trends and Updates." *American Journal of Obstetrics and Gynecology* 226 (6): 773-80. https://doi.org/10.1016/j.ajog.2021.12.261.

Finch, Amy P.M., Jan Lubinski, Pål Møller, Christian F. Singer, Beth Karlan, Leigha Senter, Barry Rosen, et al. 2014. "Impact of Oophorectomy on Cancer Incidence and Mortality in Women with a BRCA1 or BRCA2 Mutation." *Journal of Clinical Oncology* 32 (15): 1547-53. https://doi.org/10.1200/JCO.2013.53.2820.

Foved Johe, Laia, Carla Oliveres Amor, Jennifer Rovira Pampalona, Marta Banqué Navarro, María Degollada Bastos, and Pere Brescó i Torras. 2024. "Safety of Opportunistic Salpingectomy as a Strategy for Ovarian Cancer Risk Reduction in Patients with a Desire for Definitive Sterilization." *Progress Obstetrics Gynecology* 67:243-48.

Fraser, Ian S. 2010. "Non-contraceptive Health Benefits of Intrauterine Hormonal Systems." *Contraception* 82 (5): 396–403. https://doi.org/10.1016/j.contraception.2010.03.024.

Hanley, Gillian E., Janice S. Kwon, Sarah J. Finlayson, David G. Huntsman, Dianne Miller, and Jessica N McAlpine. 2018. "Extending the Safety Evidence for Opportunistic Salpingectomy in Prevention of Ovarian Cancer: A Cohort Study from British Columbia, Canada." *American Journal of Obstetrics and Gynecology* 219 (2): 172.e1-172.e8. https://doi.org/10.1016/j.ajog.2018.05.019.

Hogewoning, Cornelis J.A., Maaike C.G. Bleeker, Adriaan J.C. van den Brule, Feja J. Voorhorst, Peter J.F. Snijders, Johannes Berkhof, Pieter J. Westenend, and Chris J.L.M. Meijer. 2003. "Condom Use Promotes Regression of Cervical Intraepithelial Neoplasia and Clearance of Human Papillomavirus: A Randomized Clinical Trial." *International Journal of Cancer* 107 (5): 811-16. https://doi.org/10.1002/ijc.11474.

Houlihan, Catherine F., Natasha L. Larke, Deborah Watson-Jones, Karen K. Smith-McCune, Stephen Shiboski, Patti E. Gravitt, Jennifer S. Smith, Louise Kuhn, Chunhui Wang, and Richard Hayes. 2012. "Human Papillomavirus Infection and Increased Risk of HIV Acquisition. A Systematic Review and Meta-Analysis." *AIDS* 26 (17): 2211-22. https://doi.org/10.1097/QAD.0b013e328358d908.

Hubacher, David, y David A. Grimes. 2002. "Noncontraceptive Health Benefits of Intrauterine Devices: A Systematic Review." *Obstetrical & Gynecological Survey* 57 (2): 120–28

IARC Working Group on the Evaluation of Carcinogenic Risks to Humans. 2007. "Combined Estrogen-Progestogen Contraceptives and Combined Estrogen Progestogen Menopausal Therapy." *IARC Monographs on the Evaluation of Carcinogenic Risks to Humans* 91:1-528.

International Collaboration of Epidemiological Studies of Cervical Cancer. 2007. "Cervical Cancer and Hormonal Contraceptives: Collaborative Reanalysis of Individual Data for 16 573 Women with Cervical Cancer and 35 509 Women without Cervical Cancer from 24 Epidemiological Studies." *The Lancet* 370 (9599): 1609-21. https://doi.org/10.1016/S0140-6736(07)61684-5.

Iversen, Lisa, Shona Fielding, Øjvind Lidegaard, and Philip C Hannaford. 2020a. "Contemporary Hormonal Contraception and Risk of Endometrial Cancer in Women Younger than Age 50: A Retrospective Cohort Study of Danish Women." *Contraception* 102 (3): 152-58. https://doi.org/10.1016/j.contraception.2020.06.008.

Iversen, Lisa, Selvaraj Sivasubramaniam, Amanda J. Lee, Shona Fielding, and Philip C. Hannaford. 2017. "Lifetime Cancer Risk and Combined Oral Contraceptives: The Royal College of General Practitioners' Oral Contraception Study." *American Journal of Obstetrics and Gynecology* 216 (6): 580.e1-580.e9. https://doi.org/10.1016/j.ajog.2017.02.002.

Jahanfar, Shayesteh, Julie Mortazavi, Amy Lapidow, Cassandra Cu, Jude Al Abosy, Kathyrn Morris, Juan Camilo Becerra-Mateus, et al. 2024. "Assessing the Impact of Contraceptive Use on Reproductive Cancer Risk among Women of Reproductive Age-a Systematic Review." *Frontiers in Global Women's Health* 5 (November). https://doi.org/10.3389/fgwh.2024.1487820.

Jones, Emma. 2021. "The Levonorgestrel Intrauterine System for Prevention of Endometrial Cancer." *Cancer Prevention Research* 18(5): 299–306. https://aacrjournals.org/cancerpreventionresearch/article/18/5/299/761927.

Kahn, Ryan M., Sushmita Gordhandas, Kendra Godwin, Rebecca L. Stone, Michael J. Worley, Karen H. Lu, and Kara C. Long Roche. Long Roche. 2023. "Salpingectomy for the Primary Prevention of Ovarian Cancer." *JAMA Surgery* 158 (11): 1204. https://doi.org/10.1001/jamasurg.2023.4164.

Kamani, Mustafa, Utku Akgor, and Murat Gültekin. 2022. "Review of the Literature on Combined Oral Contraceptives and Cancer." *Ecancermedicalscience* 16:1416. https://doi.org/10.3332/ecancer.2022.1416.

Karen H Lu, MDKathleen M, and MD Schmeler. 2024. "Lynch Syndrome (Hereditary Nonpolyposis Colorectal Cancer): Screening and Prevention of Endometrial and Ovarian Cancer." *UpToDate*. 2024. https://www.uptodate.com/contents/lynch-syndrome-hereditary nonpolyposis-colorectal-cancer-screening-and-prevention-of-endometrial and-ovarian-cancer?source=history_widget.

Kelly, Sarah. 2024. "Association of Levonorgestrel-Releasing Intrauterine Device with Cancer Risk." *American Journal of Obstetrics and Gynecology*. https://doi.org/10.1016/j.ajog.2024.02.012.

Klinge, C. M. 2001. "Estrogen Receptor Interaction with Estrogen Response Elements." *Nucleic Acids Research* 29 (14): 2905-19. https://doi.org/10.1093/nar/29.14.2905.

Kuchenbaecker, Karoline B., John L. Hopper, Daniel R. Barnes, Kelly-Anne Phillips, Thea M. Mooij, Marie-José Roos-Blom, Sarah Jervis, et al. 2017. "Risks of Breast, Ovarian, and Contralateral Breast Cancer for BRCA1 and BRCA2 Mutation Carriers." *JAMA* 317 (23): 2402. https://doi.org/10.1001/jama.2017.7112.

Kurman, Robert J., and Ie-Ming Shih. 2010. "The Origin and Pathogenesis of Epithelial Ovarian Cancer: A Proposed Unifying Theory." *American Journal of Surgical Pathology* 34 (3): 433-43. https://doi.org/10.1097/PAS.0b013e3181cf3d79.

Kwon, Janice S., Charlotte C. Sun, Susan K. Peterson, Kristin G. White, Molly S. Daniels, Stephanie G. Boyd-Rogers, and Karen H. Lu. 2008. Boyd-Rogers, and Karen H. Lu. 2008. "Cost-effectiveness Analysis of Prevention Strategies for Gynecologic Cancers in Lynch Syndrome." *Cancer* 113 (2): 326-35. https://doi.org/10.1002/cncr.23554.

la Fuente Pérez, P de, and L de la Fuente Bitaine. 2019. "A New Approach to the Pathogenesis and Prophylaxis of Ovarian Cancer." *Progress in Obstetrics and Gynecology* 62 (4): 361-64.

Lam, Janni Uyen Hoa, Matejka Rebolj, Pierre-Antoine Dugué, Jesper Bonde, My von Euler-Chelpin, and Elsebeth Lynge. 2014. "Condom Use in Prevention of Human Papillomavirus Infections and Cervical Neoplasia: Systematic Review of Longitudinal Studies." *Journal of Medical Screening* 21 (1): 38-50. https://doi.org/10.1177/0969141314522454.

Lessa, Alice, and Anna Podlasek. 2025. "Intrauterine Systems and Gynaecological Malignancies: An Umbrella Review of Systematic Reviews and Meta Analyses." *British Journal of General Practice* 75 (suppl 1): bjgp25X742329. https://doi.org/10.3399/bjgp25X742329.

Luan, Nan-Nan, Lang Wu, Ting-Ting Gong, Yong-Lai Wang, Bei Lin, and Qi-Jun Wu. 2015. "Nonlinear Reduction in Risk for Colorectal Cancer by Oral Contraceptive Use: A Meta-Analysis of Epidemiological Studies." *Cancer Causes & Control* 26 (1): 65-78. https://doi.org/10.1007/s10552-014-0483-2.

Manhart, Lisa E., and Laura A. Koutsky. 2002. "Do Condoms Prevent Genital HPV Infection, External Genital Warts, or Cervical Neoplasia?" *Sexually Transmitted Diseases* 29 (11): 725-35. https://doi.org/10.1097/00007435 200211000-00018.

McAlpine, Jessica N., Gillian E. Hanley, Michelle M.M. Woo, Alicia A. Tone, Nirit Rozenberg, Kenneth D. Swenerton, C. Blake Gilks, Sarah J. Finlayson, David G. Huntsman, and Dianne M. Miller. 2014. "Opportunistic Salpingectomy: Uptake, Risks, and Complications of a Regional Initiative for Ovarian Cancer Prevention." *American Journal of Obstetrics and Gynecology* 210 (5): 471.e1 471.e11. https://doi.org/10.1016/j.ajog.2014.01.003.

McGlynn, Katherine A., Jessica L. Petrick, and Hashem B. El-Serag. 2021. "Epidemiology of Hepatocellular Carcinoma." *Hepatology* 73 (S1): 4-13. https://doi.org/10.1002/hep.31288.

"Medical Eligibility Criteria Wheel for Contraceptive Use." n.d. Accessed May 22, 2025. https://www.who.int/publications/i/item/9789241549257.

Michael J, MD Hall, MSCatherine C, MS Neumann, and LCGC. 2025. "Lynch Syndrome (Hereditary Nonpolyposis Colorectal Cancer): Clinical Manifestations and Diagnosis." *UpToDate*. 2025.

Minalt, Natalie, Alexandra Caldwell, Grace M. Yedlicka, Sunil Joseph, Stephanie E. Robertson, Lora M. Landrum, y Jeffrey F. Peipert. 2023. "Association Between Intrauterine Device Use and Endometrial, Cervical, and Ovarian Cancer: An Expert Review." *American Journal of Obstetrics and Gynecology* 229 (2): 93. https://doi.org/10.1016/j.ajog.2023.03.040.

National Cancer Institute. 2024. "SEER Cancer Stat Facts: Ovarian Cancer. Surveillance, Epidemiology, and End Results Program." https://seer.cancer.gov/statfacts/html/ovary.html.

Perkins, Rebecca B., Nicolas Wentzensen, Richard S. Guido, and Mark Schiffman. 2023. "Cervical Cancer Screening: A Review." *JAMA* 330 (6): 547. https://doi.org/10.1001/jama.2023.13174.

Post, Cathalijne C B, Ellen Stelloo, Vincent T H B M Smit, Dina Ruano, Carli M Tops, Lisa Vermij, Tessa A Rutten, et al. 2021. "Prevalence and Prognosis of Lynch Syndrome and Sporadic Mismatch Repair Deficiency in Endometrial Cancer." *JNCI: Journal of the National Cancer Institute* 113 (9): 1212-20. https://doi.org/10.1093/jnci/djab029.

Rennert, Gad, Hedy S Rennert, Mila Pinchev, Stephen B Gruber, and Ofer Lavie. 2020. "Hormonal and Reproductive Factors and Reduction in the Risk of Colorectal Cancer." *European Journal of Cancer Prevention: The Official Journal of the European Cancer Prevention Organisation* (ECP) 29 (3): 229-37. https://doi.org/10.1097/CEJ.0000000000000538.

Roe, Andrea, Deborah A Bartz, and Pamela S Douglas. 2025. "Combined Estrogen-Progestin Contraception: Side Effects and Health Concerns." *UpToDate*. https://www.uptodate.com/contents/combined-estrogen-progestin-contraception-side-effects-and-health concerns?search=cancer%20de%20mama%20y%20anticonceptivos&source=search_result&selectedTitle=2~150&usage_type=default&display_rank=2.

Rogers, Michael A., Lauren E. Friedman, Marisa R. Young, and Maria L. Blevins. 2023. "Association Between Intrauterine Device Use and Risk of Gynecologic Cancers." *American Journal of Obstetrics and Gynecology* 229 (2): 101–110. https://doi.org/10.1016/j.ajog.2023.03.055.

Ryan, Neil A. J., Julie Morris, Kate Green, Fiona Lalloo, Emma R. Woodward, James Hill, Emma J. Crosbie, and D. Gareth Evans. 2017. "Association of Mismatch Repair Mutation With Age at Cancer Onset in Lynch Syndrome." *JAMA Oncology* 3 (12): 1702. https://doi.org/10.1001/jamaoncol.2017.0619.

Schmeler, Kathleen M., Henry T. Lynch, Lee-may Chen, Mark F. Munsell, Pamela T. Soliman, Mary Beth Clark, Molly S. Daniels, et al. 2006. Soliman, Mary Beth Clark, Molly S. Daniels, et al. 2006. "Prophylactic Surgery to Reduce the Risk of Gynecologic Cancers in the Lynch Syndrome." *New England Journal of Medicine* 354 (3): 261-69. https://doi.org/10.1056/NEJMoa052627.

SGO Clinical Practice Statement. 2013. "Salpingectomy for Ovarian Cancer Prevention." https://www.sgo.org/resources/sgo-clinical-practice-statement-salpingectomy-for-ovarian-cancer-prevention/.

Smith, Laura J., Emily K. White, and David M. Gershenson. 2020. "Levonorgestrel-Releasing Intrauterine System for Regression of Endometrial Hyperplasia: Cochrane Review." *American Family Physician* 102 (1): 26–27. https://www.aafp.org/pubs/afp/issues/2021/0700/p26.html.

Spotnitz, Melissa E., Karthik Natarajan, Patrick B. Ryan, y Carolyn L. Westhoff. 2020. "Relative Risk of Cervical Neoplasms Among Copper and Levonorgestrel-Releasing Intrauterine System Users." *Obstetrics & Gynecology* 135(2): 319–26. Https://doi.org/10.1097/AOG.0000000000003646.

Thomas, Christoforos, and Jan-Åke Gustafsson. 2011. "The Different Roles of ER Subtypes in Cancer Biology and Therapy." *Nature Reviews Cancer* 11 (8): 597 608. https://doi.org/10.1038/nrc3093.

Tworoger, S. S. S., K. M. Fairfield, G. A. Colditz, B. A. Rosner, and S. E. Hankinson. 2007. "Association of Oral Contraceptive Use, Other Contraceptive Methods, and Infertility with Ovarian Cancer Risk." *American Journal of Epidemiology* 166 (8): 894-901. https://doi.org/10.1093/aje/kwm157.

WHO Guidelines Approved by the Guidelines Review Committee. 2013. *WHO Guidelines for Screening and Treatment of Precancerous Lesions for Cervical Cancer Prevention*.

Winer, Rachel L., James P. Hughes, Qinghua Feng, Sandra O'Reilly, Nancy B. Kiviat, King K. Holmes, and Laura A. Koutsky. 2006. "Condom Use and the Risk of Genital Human Papillomavirus Infection in Young Women." *New England Journal of Medicine* 354 (25): 2645-54. https://doi.org/10.1056/NEJMoa053284.

Wolf, Jonas, Lucas Felipe Kist, Samanta Brangel Pereira, Marilze Alves Quessada, Helena Petek, Arthur Pille, Juçara Gasparetto Maccari, Mohamed Parrini Mutlaq, and Luiz Antonio Nasi. 2024. "Human Papillomavirus Infection: Epidemiology, Biology, Host Interactions, Cancer Development, Prevention, and Therapeutics." *Reviews in Medical Virology* 34 (3). https://doi.org/10.1002/rmv.2537.

Yoon, Sang-Hee, Soo-Nyung Kim, Seung-Hyuk Shim, Soon-Beum Kang, and Sun Joo Lee. 2016. "Bilateral Salpingectomy Can Reduce the Risk of Ovarian Cancer in the General Population: A Meta-Analysis." *European Journal of Cancer* 55 (March):38-46. https://doi.org/10.1016/j.ejca.2015.12.003.

Chapter 16

Contraception in Adolescence and Perimenopause

L. Sales Pérez[1,*], MD
M. L. Juan Rodrigo[2], MD
A. Tello Delsors[3], MD
C. García Fernández[2], MD
and Ll. Belmonte Andújar[2,4], PhD
[1]Obstetrics and Gynecology Department, Hospital Lluis Alcanyis Xativa, Xativa, Valencia, Spain
[2]Obstetrics and Gynecology Department, University and Hospital of Albacete, Albacete, Spain
[3]Obstetrics and Gynecology Department, University and Hospital of Santa Lucía, Cartagena, Murcia, Spain
[4]Medical Science Department, School of Medicine of Albacete, Universidad de Castilla-La Mancha, Spain

Abstract

Contraceptive needs vary according to the reproductive stage of women, being especially particular to adolescence and perimenopause. This chapter discusses the fundamental aspects of contraception in both stages.
Adolescence represents a critical stage in reproductive life, characterised by irregular sexual behaviour, low risk perception of unprotected sex as well as deficient sexual education that comes mostly from non-scientific sources, such as friends or social networks, which increases vulnerability to unplanned pregnancies and sexually transmitted infections in this population group. This chapter addresses the epidemiological, psychological and clinical aspects that should be considered when recommending contraceptive methods in this population. The characteristics, non-contraceptive benefits, limitations and acceptability of the different methods available are discussed, with special emphasis on long-acting reversible methods (LARC) as the first choice.
The importance of an individualised approach, confidentiality and follow-up, as well as the recommendation of dual contraception (condom use in conjunction with another method) are also highlighted. A comprehensive, evidence-based approach is taken to ensure safe, effective contraception tailored to the specific needs of adolescents.
On the other hand, perimenopause is a transitional stage characterised by hormonal changes and decreased, but not zero, fertility, so the risk of unplanned pregnancy persists. This chapter reviews the need for contraception in perimenopausal women and presents a detailed assessment of available methods, including combined hormonal contraceptives,

* Corresponding Author's Email: larasalesperez@gmail.com

In: Advances in Reproductive Health
Editors: Llanos Belmonte Andujar and Ana Fuentes Rozalen
ISBN: 979-8-90134-038-7

progestogen-only, and non-hormonal methods. Cardiovascular risks, effects on bone mineral density and additional benefits such as reduced menstrual bleeding, dysmenorrhoea, vasomotor symptoms and risk of certain cancers are discussed. The importance of an individualised approach that takes into account comorbidities, age and personal preferences is emphasised. Finally, recommendations for the safe discontinuation of contraception at this stage of life are addressed, considering clinical and hormonal parameters.

Keywords: contraception, perimenopause, adolescence, reproductive health

Contraception in Adolescence

Introduction and Epidemiology

The World Health Organization (WHO 2023) places adolescence in the second decade of life, a stage ranging from 10 to 19 years of age. According to the organisation, in 2019, adolescents had an estimated 21 million pregnancies each year, approximately 50% of which were unintended and resulted in about 12 million births. Of the unintended pregnancies, 55 percent ended in abortions, which are often unsafe in these countries. The global birth rate for girls aged 10-14 in 2023 was estimated at 1.5 per 100 women, with higher rates in sub-Saharan Africa, Latin America and the Caribbean (Pan American Health Organization 2024).

The main problem of unprotected sex in adolescence is not only unwanted pregnancy. According to WHO data, in 2020 approximately 374 million people between 15 and 49 years of age contracted one of these four sexually transmitted infections: chlamydia, gonorrhoea, syphilis or trichomoniasis.

Of those more than 370 million infections, about 60 % occurred in those under 24 years of age, and among sexually active young people, 25 % had a sexually transmitted infection (WHO 2023).

Sexual relations in adolescence are characterised by irregular, spaced and often unplanned sexual intercourse. Although they are considered monogamous, the duration with a partner is usually short and they start at increasingly younger ages. Similarly, there is a lower perception of the risk of unprotected sex in this age group, which, together with poor sex education and peer pressure, places adolescents at high risk for unplanned pregnancies and sexually transmitted diseases. (Llopis Pérez 2001).

Requirements for Contraception in Adolescence

Understanding adolescent development and behaviour is essential to guide contraceptive recommendations appropriately. In the absence of medical contraindications, the patient's own choice should be the main criterion when prescribing a contraceptive method. In order to determine the most appropriate option, several factors need to be considered and this should always be done on an individual basis:

- *Personal factors*: When recommending a contraceptive method to an adolescent, it is essential to consider aspects such as age, physical and psychological maturity, the sexual needs of both the adolescent and their partner, gender identity, values, beliefs and priorities. In addition, it is especially important to assess their ability to access the method, whether for reasons of confidentiality or financial constraints (Boonstra 2002) (Committee on Adolescent Health Care 2017).
- *Non-contraceptive benefits*: It is essential to be aware of the additional effects of some contraceptive methods beyond their primary function and to ensure that adolescents are informed about these. This will enable them to make a more informed decision when choosing the most appropriate method. Benefits to consider when recommending contraception in a comprehensive manner include reducing dysmenorrhoea and pelvic pain, decreasing menstrual bleeding, treating acne, hirsutism, endometriosis, as well as improving chronic anaemia and premenstrual dysphoric syndrome. (Committee on Adolescent Health Care 2017).
- *Adolescent concerns*: Weight gain, reduction in final height, fear of not achieving pregnancy when desired or increased incidence of venous thromboembolic events are the most common fears associated with using contraceptives in the adolescent population. It is important to adjust the method to these and always assess the risk of each event on an individual basis (Boonstra 2017).

Types of Contraceptive Preparations

The options available in contraception for adolescent users are presented according to their level of effectiveness, as recommended by the Committee on Adolescent Health Care of the American College of Obstetricians and Gynecologists (2017).

Long-Acting Reversible Contraceptive Methods (LARC)

Long-acting reversible contraceptive methods (LARCs) are among the most effective methods available. Their use has been increasing among adolescents, and both the American Academy of Pediatrics (Committee on Adolescence et al. 2014) and the American College of Obstetricians and Gynecologists (Committee on Adolescent Health Care 2018) recommend them as the first contraceptive option in this population. However, despite their high efficacy and endorsement by leading scientific societies, LARCs are often not the method of choice for users. Among the main barriers identified are lack of adequate information, mistaken beliefs about side effects, fear of the insertion procedure, and institutional barriers such as lack of training of professionals or restrictions in access (Kohn et al. 2018; Rubin et al. 2021; Luchowski et al. 2014).

In 2010, the CHOICE study, a prospective cohort project conducted in St. Louis, USA, was published, involving 10,000 women aged 14-45 years who did not want a pregnancy in the next year and were interested in starting a contraceptive method (Secura et al. 2010). The study emerged in response to the low use of LARCs among users, despite their acknowledged efficacy. Its main objective was to assess whether the removal of economic and educational barriers could increase the uptake and use of LARCs, particularly intrauterine devices (IUDs) and subdermal implants. All participants were offered educational materials with information on the use of LARCs.

All participants were offered educational materials with detailed, evidence-based information on all available contraceptive methods, with special emphasis on LARCs. After receiving this information, women were free to choose their method, which was provided free of charge, thus removing both informational and financial barriers. The results were remarkable: 77% of women chose a long-acting method, with the IUD being the most selected method (56%) followed by the subdermal implant (11%).

The CHOICE study not only demonstrated that most women would opt for a LARC if access barriers were removed, but also had an impact on relevant clinical outcomes: in subsequent analyses, a significant decrease in unintended pregnancy rates was observed among participants, especially among adolescents and young women. These findings reinforced the need for public policies that promote universal, free and well-informed access to the most effective contraceptive methods.

The main advantage of long-acting reversible contraceptive methods (LARCs) lies not only in their high efficacy, well demonstrated in studies such as the CHOICE project, but also in their independence from correct or consistent use by the user. Once in place, LARCs offer safe, continuous and prolonged contraceptive protection, making them a particularly suitable option for adolescents and young women. This aspect should be taken into account in clinical practice and clearly communicated to users when giving contraceptive advice. The main characteristics of the different LARCs are discussed in more detail below.

- *Intrauterine device (IUD):* both the copper IUD and the levonorgestrel IUD are accepted and safe methods for use in nulliparous adolescent patients. One of the main contraindications for their insertion is active pelvic inflammatory disease (PID). Currently, the main clinical practice guidelines recommend cervico-vaginal cultures prior to IUD insertion in patients at high risk of STIs. Age under 25 years is considered a risk factor, and therefore screening prior to IUD insertion is recommended for adolescent users. The need for cervico-vaginal cultures as a screening method should not be a reason for delaying IUD insertion in asymptomatic patients. Other risk factors to consider for screening include: a new sexual partner, more than one sexual partner or a sexual partner who has other concurrent sexual partners or is infected with an STI, inconsistent condom use in a non-monogamous relationship, a history of sexual exchange for money or drugs, or a history of incarceration. (Committee on Adolescent Health Care 2018) (CDC 2024).
- *Etonogestrel subdermal implant*: The subdermal implant is a highly effective method with failure rates of less than 1%. There are two types of implants marketed worldwide. The single-rod Etonogestrel implant lasts up to 3 years, and the double-rod levonorgestrel implant lasts between 4-5 years depending on the dose and brand name. (CDC 2024) The main drawback and factor for abandonment of this method among adolescents is irregular bleeding, but adherence has been shown to increase if this side effect is properly reported prior to insertion. (Committee on Adolescent Health Care 2018) (Committee on Adolescence et al. 2014). One of the advantages over the IUD is that it does not require STD screening prior to insertion.

  Both IUDs and implants can be offered to adolescents in the immediate postpartum period while the patient is still in the hospital, a practice endorsed by ACOG and the

CDC and the FHSR (Committee on Adolescent Health Care 2018) (CDC 2024) (FSRH 2012).

- *Quarterly intramuscular medroxyprogesterone injection*: Quarterly intramuscular medroxyprogesterone injection is a particularly useful contraceptive method in adolescents because of its ease of use and additional benefits, such as reducing dysmenorrhoea and improving iron deficiency anaemia secondary to heavy menstrual bleeding. This method is particularly appropriate for adolescents with limited access to other contraceptive options for economic or social reasons, given the increased risk of unintended pregnancy in this group. Irregular menstrual bleeding patterns and weight gain have been identified as the main reasons for discontinuation (Committee on Adolescence et al. 2014).

  Due to the state of hypoestrogenism generated by this method, there is an increase in bone resorption that exceeds bone formation and can lead to a decrease in bone mineral density. Current evidence indicates that bone resorption is equal to that of the rest of the population during the first or second year of use and that even with the discontinuation of the method, if necessary, this loss would be recovered. Different societies and studies endorse the safety of this contraceptive method in the adolescent population, establishing that its effect on bone mineral density should not restrict its use in healthy patients between 18-45 years of age, even at older ages (American College of Obstetricians and Gynecologists Committee on Gynecologic Practice 2008) (CDC 2024) (Pfizer 2004).

Short-Acting Reversible Contraceptive Methods

Combined Hormonal Contraceptive Pills

The combined hormonal contraceptive pill (CHC) is a highly effective method, with a failure rate of 0.3% under perfect use and approximately 7% in typical use, the latter being mainly attributable to missed daily dosing or drug interactions (Nguyen et al. 2024; CDC 2024; WHO 2025).

A wide variety of preparations combining different types of estrogens and progestins are now available, allowing treatment to be tailored to the individual characteristics of each patient. In general, combined hormonal contraceptives have few contraindications in healthy adolescents.

To facilitate safe prescribing, there are both specific clinical documents and up-to-date mobile apps that allow individualised consultation on whether a patient is a suitable candidate for the use of CHCs.

Correct use of combined oral contraceptives can be complicated for adolescents, as they need to be taken daily, to improve adolescent patients' adherence to this method the following is recommended:

Contraceptive Vaginal Ring

The contraceptive vaginal ring has a similar efficacy, eligibility profile, risks and benefits as the combined contraceptive pill. Its failure rate is 0.3% under perfect use conditions and is around 7% under typical use (Curtis et al. 2016) (Roumen et al. 2001) (WHO 2025).

The main advantage over other types of contraceptives is its dosage, which is more attractive for adolescent patients as it is a simpler regimen that prevents forgetfulness. Patients should be properly explained how to insert the device, as some are reluctant to insert intravaginal devices, especially due to lack of knowledge of their anatomy, which is why there are anatomical models that can help us in this task, and we should also inform them that some models provide an applicator to facilitate insertion. (Roumen et al. 2001).

Transdermal Contraceptive Patch

The combined hormone transdermal contraceptive patch has similar efficacy, benefits, eligibility criteria and drug interactions as OCPs; side effects are similarly comparable to those of other combined methods, with the addition of detached patches and skin effects such as hyperpigmentation, contact dermatitis and other irritations (Harel et al. 2005) (WHO 2025) (CDC 2024).

As with the vaginal ring, its simple dosage makes it also attractive to our patients, and on the other hand, personal or cultural barriers to the use of intravaginal contraception are avoided (Roumen et al. 2001).

Progestogen-Only Pills

Progestogen-only pills have a contraceptive efficacy of more than 99% when used correctly, with an excellent Pearl index. However, their effect is short-lived (approximately 24 hours) and therefore they require strictly regular administration. Missed or delayed doses can compromise their efficacy, resulting in a slightly higher failure rate compared to hormonal contraceptives, compared to combined hormonal contraceptives and especially to long-acting reversible methods (LARCs).

For these reasons, their use is recommended primarily for women who have contraindications to the use of estrogens, or who, for personal preference or medical reasons, opt for a progestin-only method.

Male Condom

The male condom is the most widely used method of contraception among adolescents. The advantages condoms offer over other methods are co-responsibility in contraception, easy accessibility and low cost; however, their greatest benefit is the role they play in protecting against sexually transmitted diseases such as gonorrhoea, chlamydia, trichomoniasis, hepatitis B and HIV, with evidence also in reducing herpes simplex virus, human papillomavirus and syphilis transmission. (Paz-Bailey et al. 2005) (Committee on Adolescence et al. 2014) (CDC 2024).

Dual Methods

Currently, in adolescence, the contraceptive method of choice is the dual method or dual contraception, which combines condom use with a hormonal or other highly effective long-acting method (Committee on Adolescence et al. 2014; Committee on Adolescent Health Care 2017). This strategy not only offers superior contraceptive protection by adding the efficacy of hormonal or long-acting methods to the physical barrier provided by condoms, but is also critical for the prevention of sexually transmitted infections (STIs). As discussed at the beginning of this chapter, according to data from the World Health Organization (WHO), in

2020 approximately 374 million people aged 15-49 years contracted one of the four most common STIs: chlamydia, gonorrhoea, syphilis or trichomoniasis. Of these, about 60% occurred in individuals under 24 years of age, and among sexually active young people, 25% had an STI, highlighting the particular vulnerability of the adolescent population. Dual contraception is therefore the most comprehensive and recommended approach to promote comprehensive sexual health in this age group.

Conclusion

- Sexual relations during adolescence constitute an important risk behaviour for the occurrence of unplanned pregnancies and the acquisition of sexually transmitted infections (STIs), which is why it is essential to address prevention in a comprehensive manner adapted to this population.
- It is imperative to provide adolescents with complete, clear and accessible information on all available contraceptive methods, with special emphasis on the benefits and safety of long-acting reversible contraceptive methods (LARC), which offer high efficacy and convenience.
- LARC methods are considered the first contraceptive choice for adolescents due to their high effectiveness, low dependence on daily adherence and favourable safety and acceptability profile.
- A follow-up consultation is recommended within three months after starting any hormonal contraceptive to assess side effects, resolve concerns and encourage adherence, thus ensuring correct and continued use of the method.
- In addition, young people should be encouraged to access consultations at any time if they experience problems or concerns related to the contraceptive method, promoting a flexible and needs-based approach.
- Age alone should not be a limitation for the prescription of any contraceptive method, including intrauterine devices, as long as there are no medical contraindications.
- Finally, since the only method that protects against STIs is the condom, dual contraception - the combination of a condom with a hormonal or long-acting method - is the most recommended strategy for the sexually active adolescent population, ensuring protection against both unwanted pregnancy and infection.

Contraception in Perimenopause

Introduction and Epidemiology

Perimenopause, as defined by the American Menopause Society, is the interval between the time when the first changes in the menstrual cycle appear and one year after the definitive cessation of menstruation. The average age of menopause is approximately 51 years but can vary between 40 and 60 years. However, the average age of permanent loss of natural fertility is 41 years, but can be as high as 51 years. (North American Menopause Society 2013).

Sexuality in perimenopause and menopause remains an active reality, although there is still a notable lack of knowledge and a specific approach in this area. The sexual lives of women in their 40s and 50s are influenced by multiple factors, including the quality of sexual activity prior to menopause and the physiological changes associated with this stage. Among the main determinants are hormonal changes, which can lead to symptoms such as vaginal dryness, urinary incontinence, prolapse, hot flushes, fatigue, anxiety and sleep disturbances, all of which have a potential impact on sexual function (Women's Health and Aging Study Group 2006).

Despite these difficulties, a high percentage of perimenopausal women continue to have regular sexual intercourse. In addition, gynaecological consultations are increasingly being asked for information on contraception during this stage of life. It is therefore essential to assess the need for contraception in these patients on an individual basis and to select the most appropriate method according to their clinical profile and preferences. Making a firm recommendation is not without its challenges, as both the natural decline in fertility and the significant hormonal changes of the menopausal transition must be taken into account (Women's Health and Aging Study Group 2006) (AEEM 2026).

Is Contraception Necessary in Perimenopause?

The path to menopause involves a progressive follicular reduction, which is expressed analytically by a decrease in anti-Müllerian hormone. This follicular reduction in turn decreases the secretion of inhibin B in the ovarian follicles, which is involved in the regulation and subsequent elevation of FSH and the decrease in estrogen. This will lead to a shortening of cycles, especially due to the shortening of the follicular phase, and a higher frequency of anovulatory cycles (Mendoza et al. 2013) (Liu, Case, and Reproductive Endocrinology and Infertility Committee 2011).

Although ovarian function around menopause is reduced during perimenopause, anovulatory cycles alternate with ovulatory cycles, so the risk of unplanned pregnancy exists, in fact several scientific studies estimate that the risk of gestation in women who practice unprotected sex between 40-44 years of age is 10-20% and between 45-49 of 12%. (Liu, Case, and Reproductive Endocrinology and Infertility Committee 2011) (Nelson, Telfer, and Anderson 2013).

As mentioned above, the risk of unplanned pregnancy exists and we need to inform women about the problems that can result from it. It is estimated that for every 1,000 live births, women aged 40-54 have rates of diabetes and hypertension three and four times higher than women aged 20-29, respectively. Even more troubling, maternal mortality in women 35 and older is 32.3 deaths per 100,000 live births, compared to 7.1-12.1 per 100,000 live births in younger women (U.S. Department of Health and Human Services 2010). For all these reasons, both the American College of Obstetricians and Gynecologists and the American Menopause Society recommend that women continue to use contraception until menopause or until age 50-55.

As we can see, contraception in the perimenopause is still necessary. However, the specific characteristics of this age group make it essential to carefully weigh the risk of pregnancy against the potential risks associated with the use of hormonal contraceptives, including increased risk of acute cardiovascular events, such as venous thromboembolism (VTE), acute myocardial infarction (AMI) and cerebrovascular accident (CVA), as well as the possible association with an increased risk of developing certain types of cancer, especially breast cancer (Khatibi et al. 2018)(Shifren, Gass, and NAMS Working Group 2014)(American Society for Reproductive Medicine 2015).

Contraceptive Counselling

Once the need for contraception in perimenopause has been established, the next step is to provide individualised counselling that considers not only the particular clinical conditions of each patient, but also the endocrine changes that accompany this stage and the characteristics of each contraceptive method.

Although the ovarian dysfunction typical of this stage has already been described, it should be noted that there is an elevation of FSH, which in turn stimulates testosterone production, which added to the hypoestrogenism that is established from the 40s onwards, alters the androgen/estrogen balance, with the appearance of androgenic signs that increase cardiovascular risk in these patients, as there is a redistribution of body fat, changes in lipid metabolism and an increase in the incidence of arterial hypertension.(Liu, Case, and Reproductive Endocrinology and Infertility Committee 2011) (Mendoza et al. 2013).

A key aspect of counselling is to assess whether age alone is a risk factor. This question is both fundamental and controversial, as most studies on the risks and benefits of contraception have been conducted in women younger than 40 years of age. Because of this limitation, the available evidence remains insufficient to determine whether age alone can act as a risk modifier.

WHO medical eligibility criteria indicate that based on age alone, patients can use any type of hormonal contraception; however, patients of advanced reproductive age may have concomitant pathologies or other risk factors that make the use of hormonal contraceptive methods unsafe in addition to the previously mentioned increased androgenic environment, making the assessment of the risk-benefit balance in the use of certain contraceptive methods even more relevant. (World Health Organization 2015).

For all these reasons, it is essential to conduct a thorough medical history to identify risk factors such as hypertension (HTN), smoking and a history of stroke, AMI or thrombosis, in order to determine which patients are a priori candidates for combined hormonal contraception. In addition to informing about the methods we recommend in each case, it is key to highlight the non-contraceptive benefits of each method and to always personalise recommendations according to the individual characteristics of each patient. (Long et al. 2015) (Mendoza et al. 2014) (Mendoza et al. 2016).

Contraceptive Options in the Perimenopause

Combined Hormonal Contraception (CHC)

The Centers for Disease Control and Prevention (CDC) published in 2016 and updated in 2024 a guide, supported by available scientific evidence, that establishes which contraceptive methods can be used safely in the presence of various medical conditions. In this guidance, methods are grouped into four categories: category 1 includes those that can be used without restriction; category 2 refers to methods where the benefits generally outweigh the potential risks; category 3 represents situations where the risks outweigh the benefits; and category 4 corresponds to methods that should not be used due to unacceptable health risks. (CDC 2024)

In relation to the use of combined hormonal contraceptives (CHCs), age alone does not constitute a medical contraindication (Table 1), as stated in the CDC guidelines (CDC 2024) and the WHO Medical Eligibility Criteria for Contraceptive Use (World Health Organization 2015). In fact, both agencies agree that CHCs can be used safely until the onset of menopause. In these guidelines, women under 40 years of age are classified in category 1 (unrestricted use), while those aged 40 years and older are placed in category 2 (unrestricted use). This classification does not imply that age, in itself, represents a risk, but recognises the progressive increase in certain factors, especially cardiovascular factors, which may be enhanced by the use of CHC and should be considered on an individual basis.

Table 1. Recommendations for the use of CHC in women ≥40 years (World Health Organization 2015)

Clinical Condition	Category	Clinical commentary
Age ≥40 years without comorbidities	2	Acceptable use with regular monitoring (BP, metabolic profile).
Active smoker ≥35 years old (≥15 cig/day)	4	Contraindicated: high cardiovascular risk.
Active female smoker ≥35 years (<15 cig/day)	3	Moderate risk; not recommended.
BMI ≥35 kg/m²	3	Increased thrombotic risk. Avoid unless there are no alternatives.
Mild hypertension (140-159/90-99 mmHg)	3	Strict control required if AHCs are used. Consider alternative methods.
Uncontrolled hypertension (≥160/100 mmHg)	4	Contraindicated due to risk of CVD and stroke.
Migraine with aura	4	Contraindicated due to risk of stroke.
Migraine without aura, ≥35 years of age	3	Increased risk. Avoid AHC.
History of CVD, stroke or venous thromboembolism (VTE).	4	Contraindicated due to thrombotic risk.
Personal history of breast cancer (current or previous).	4	Contraindicated.
Family history of breast cancer	1	No specific restriction.
Personal history of cervical cancer	2-3	Variable risk according to stage and treatment.
Abnormal uterine bleeding not assessed	4	Contraindicated until diagnosis is established.
Formulations with natural oestrogens and 2nd generation progestogens	1-2	Preferred due to lower thrombotic risk.
Use for cycle control or mild vasomotor symptoms.	2	Possible use in the absence of comorbidities; requires clinical monitoring.
Family history of VTE without diagnosed thrombophilia	2-3	Individual assessment; caution advised.

However, there are specific conditions in which CHC use should be restricted. Women aged 35 years and older who smoke 15 or more cigarettes per day are at significantly elevated risk of cardiovascular events, and use of estrogen-containing contraceptives is contraindicated in this group (CDC 2024). Although the relative risk increases in smokers of all ages, the absolute incidence of cardiovascular events in younger women remains low (Curtis et al. 2016). In women older than 35 years with comorbidities such as hypertension, diabetes or migraine with aura, CHC use should also be avoided. For women aged 35 years or younger, severe smoking represents a relative contraindication that should be assessed on a case-by-case basis.

It should be noted that risk is associated only with active smoking; a woman who has quit smoking for more than one year can be considered a non-smoker (CDC 2024).

Therefore, before recommending the use of CHC in women aged 40 years or older, it is essential to conduct an individualised assessment to identify the presence of diseases that contraindicate its use, as well as relevant risk factors (Nguyen et al. 2024; World Health Organization 2015; CDC 2024; Faculty of Family Planning Reproductive Health Care 2017).

The initial assessment of the patient at the clinic should include the following points:

- A complete history should be taken, including personal and family history of thromboembolic disease.
- Include in the history taking any drugs or medicinal herbs and assess possible interactions with hormonal contraception.
- Blood pressure (BP) and body mass index (BMI) should be measured.
- A gynaecological examination should be performed when necessary.
- Early diagnostic tests for cervical and breast cancer should be checked to ensure that they are up to date, according to established protocols.

Regarding the follow-up of our patients, we must:

- Regularly update medical records to identify possible contraindications.
- Monitor at least BP and weight for adequate control.

If we assess the route used in hormonal contraception, the transdermal and vaginal routes offer similar efficacy and cycle control to the oral route. it is considered that the efficacy, indications, benefits and risks of the different routes of administration are comparable. (Nguyen et al. 2024) (Cho 2018) (Long et al. 2015).

When guiding women in choosing the most appropriate contraceptive method, it is essential to provide full information about the additional benefits of combined hormonal contraception beyond its contraceptive efficacy. In the context of perimenopause, these benefits can contribute significantly to the management of various symptoms associated with this stage, including:

- Reduced menstrual bleeding and dysmenorrhoea: Some women experience changes in their menstrual pattern in the 4-8 years prior to menopause, such as longer menstrual cycles, closer together or heavier and more painful. CHC promotes thinning of the endometrium and a decrease in arachidonic acid concentrations. As a result, blood flow and uterine contractility decrease, reducing dysmenorrhoea, menstrual bleeding and premenstrual symptoms.

  For both control of heavy menstrual bleeding and control of dysmenorrhoea, continuous use of contraceptives is recommended, with weekly breaks being discontinued and the placebo period extended to three months (The ESHRE Capri Workshop Group 2005).(The ESHRE Capri Workshop Group 2005) In their 2014 systematic review, Edelman et al. analysed studies in which combined hormonal contraceptives (CHCs) are administered continuously (more than 28 consecutive days) versus the traditional cyclical regimen (21 active days/7 break). Moreover, continuous regimens may offer additional advantages, such as a better bleeding profile, lower incidence of menstrual pain and higher patient satisfaction. However, the authors caution that these results should be interpreted with caution due to the heterogeneity among the included studies, especially due to differences in the hormonal formulations used and the precise duration of the continuous regimen, which prevents a clear recommendation in favour of one or the other regimen.

- Reduction of possible symptoms and signs of hyperandrogenism (hirsutism, acne): CHCs inhibit ovarian testosterone secretion and stimulate the production of sex globulin binding protein (SHBG) in the liver, helping to reduce plasma androgen concentrations. In addition, some of the AHCOs are specifically composed of anti-androgen progestins and inhibit the conversion of testosterone to the biologically active androgen dihydrotestosterone and its binding to the androgen receptor, thus helping to improve the symptoms that certain women may experience (The ESHRE Capri Workshop Group 2005). According to Requena and Llombart (2020), these drugs not only fulfil a contraceptive function, but also have a relevant role as a coadjuvant treatment in dermatology, thanks to their ability to modulate the hormonal effects on the skin.
- Protective effect against certain types of cancer: The use of combined hormonal contraception has a protective effect against certain types of cancer, and this protective effect seems to be maintained even after discontinuation of the method. The most significant benefit is known for ovarian cancer (Collaborative Group on Epidemiological Studies of Ovarian Cancer 2008), although it has also been shown to significantly reduce the risk of endometrial cancer by 40-50% (Allen, Yang, and Collaborative Group on Epidemiological Studies of Endometrial Cancer 2015) and colorectal cancer by about 20% (Bosetti et al. 2009). Because the incidence of these cancers increases with age, this protective effect of COCs can be considered especially important in women in our age group.
- Preservation of bone mineral density (BMD). After the age of 40, BMD decreases at a rate of 1%/year. It is known that even at low doses of estrogen, combined hormonal contraception decreases demineralisation and may help to preserve bone mass in women over 40. (Nappi et al. 2012) The systematic review by Kuohung, Borgotta and Stubblefield (2000), which analyses the 13 studies published to date, evaluates the association between the use of combined hormonal contraceptives and bone mineral density. The results show strong evidence to support the hypothesis that the use of low-dose oral contraceptives is associated with favourable effects on BMD.

On the other hand, the use of combined hormonal contraceptives is not completely risk-free.

Risks of Combined Hormonal Contraception

Combined Hormonal Contraception and Cancer

Although it has traditionally been suggested that the use of combined hormonal contraceptives (CHCs) might be associated with an increased risk of breast cancer, the available data indicate that this risk is low, especially in younger women, and that it tends to decrease progressively after cessation of treatment. Studies such as Mørch et al. (2017) show a slightly increased relative risk (RR 1.2), with a modest absolute increase, limited to a few tens of additional cases per 100,000 woman-years. However, these findings should be interpreted with caution in older populations, such as the one addressed in this chapter. For cervical cancer, several systematic reviews and meta- analyses have shown an increased risk with prolonged use of CHCs (more than 5 years), although this risk reverses over time after discontinuation of treatment (Appleby et al. 2007; Gierisch et al. 2013; Peng et al. 2017). In women with HPV infection, it is essential to ensure adequate cervical cancer screening rather than to contraindicate the use of combined hormonal contraception. For a detailed discussion of the oncological risks associated with the use of CHC, please refer to the relevant chapter in this book specifically dedicated to contraception and cancer.

Venous Thromboembolism (VTE) Risk

The use of estrogen-containing contraceptives is associated with an increased risk of thrombosis due to increased fibrinogen, prothrombin, factors VII, VIII and X and decreased factor V. In CHC users the risk of DVT is estimated at 3-12/10,000 compared to non-users (2/10,000). This risk is higher at the beginning of CHC use (especially in the first year) and decreases with time of use. This risk varies according to the progestogen and the dose of estrogen used, being higher in the formulations containing 50 mg of ethinylestradiol, compared to those containing 35 or 20 mg. On the other hand, the type of progestogen with which the estrogen is combined also modifies the risk, being lower for CHCs containing levonorgestrel, norgestimate or norethisterone (5-7/10,000), higher for etonogestrel and norelgestromin and even higher for gestodene, desogestrel and drospirenone (9- 12/100,000). Some studies of surrogate variables suggest that the use of combinations of progestogens with natural oestrogens (17ß-estradiol or estradiol valerate) could reduce this risk, although no epidemiological studies are yet available to corroborate these data (Agencia Española de Medicamentos y Productos Sanitarios 2013) (Dragoman et al. 2018).

On the other hand, but also related to thromboembolic risk, studies suggesting a possible increased risk of stroke or AMI associated with the use of combined hormonal contraceptives are a matter of debate.

A 2015 Cochrane review found that women using combined oral contraceptives had an increased risk of ischaemic stroke or AMI, and that this risk was dependent on the dose of ethinyl estradiol (Roach, Helmerhorst, and Lijfering 2015).

In the same vein, a Danish study indicated that estrogen dose influences the risk of developing stroke and AMI. Furthermore, it was observed that contraceptive methods containing only progestogens (such as the progestogen-only pill, thc IUD or the subcutaneous implant) do not seem to be associated with an increased thrombotic risk, making them a safer option for women with cardiovascular disease or a higher predisposition to thromboembolic events (Lidegaard et al. 2012). The same author in 2013 corroborated these results by stating that Danish women aged 45-49 years using combined hormonal contraceptives have a 2.2-fold increased risk of thrombotic stroke and a 2.3-fold increased risk of AMI (Lidegaard et al. 2013).

However, the meta-analysis by Peragallo Urrutia, Coeyteaux and McBroom (2013) found no significant increase in the risk of AMI or haemorrhagic stroke associated with OCP use.

In the perimenopausal setting, the decision to prescribe combined hormonal contraception (CHC) should be based on an individualised assessment of each patient's risk profile. The presence of factors such as age, smoking, body mass index, personal and family history of VTE,

AMI or stroke, among others, should be carefully considered before initiating or continuing treatment.

If we talk specifically about BMI, a BMI $\geq$ 35 kg/m² is, on its own, an independent risk factor for deep vein thrombosis and pulmonary embolism. When combined with CHC, the risk is significantly multiplied. In women with a BMI between 30 and 34.9 kg/m², the use of CHC is classified as category 2 (theoretical or proven risk that usually does not contraindicate its use) and is therefore a factor to be taken into account when recommending this type of contraception (CDC 2024).

In women who have previously used CHC without significant adverse effects, there are no compelling clinical reasons to discontinue treatment solely because of reaching perimenopause. However, in new users, it is essential to provide adequate information about the potential risk of VTE, AMI or stroke as well as signs and symptoms suggestive of this complication (Agencia Española de Medicamentos y Productos Sanitarios 2013).

A thorough history taking and clinical assessment aimed at identifying absolute or relative contraindications is also essential in order to select the most appropriate formulation in each case. Structured clinical follow-up, especially during the first year of use or in restarts after discontinuation $\geq$ 4 weeks, is essential for early detection of adverse events and optimisation of therapeutic benefit.

Although more clinical studies with series including women over 40 years of age are needed, it is interesting to recommend in the first instance combined hormonal contraception with low doses of estrogens, which should be natural and preferably combined with levonorgestrel or use gestagen-only contraception, as they have a higher safety profile (Miller et al. 2018).

Progestogen-Only Contraception (POC)

Perimenopausal women who have contraindications to estrogen use, or who experience adverse effects with combined hormonal contraceptives, may benefit from progestogen-only contraception (POC). These contraceptives in all their forms; pills, subdermal implants, injectables or levonorgestrel-containing intrauterine devices (LNG- IUDs), offer high efficacy, acting mainly by inhibiting ovulation and thickening cervical mucus, which makes it difficult for sperm to pass through.

As mentioned above, POCs represent the safest and most appropriate alternative for women over 40 who have cardiovascular risk factors, a history of or predisposition to venous thromboembolism (VTE), or any other condition that contraindicates the use of oestrogens.

A systematic review by Tepper et al. in 2016 assessed the risk of thrombotic events with the use of POCs. Most of the evidence does not suggest a significant increase in the odds of venous or arterial events with the use of most POCs, however, an increase in the odds of VTE was observed with the use of injectables (three studies). More recent studies yielded the same results, both the study by Winslow, Johnson and Steen in 2021 and Lidegaard et al. in 2022, concluding that the use of non-injectable gestagen-only contraceptives did not increase the risk of thromboembolic events in women users, even in those patients who had a history of venous thromboembolism.

As with combined methods, gestagen-only contraceptives also have benefits beyond the contraceptive effect (FSRH 2017):

- Reduced menorrhagia and hypermenorrhoea: Levonorgestrel IUD at a dose of 52 mg is considered the first-line treatment for correcting heavy menstrual bleeding (HMB), a common problem in women in their 40s (Depypere and Inki 2015).(FSRH 2017) A 2015 Cochrane review of 21 randomised controlled trials evaluating various treatment options for HMB found that the LNG-IUD appears to have better outcomes than oral medication (antifibrinolytics, oral progestogens or the contraceptive pill) in reducing menstrual blood loss and improving quality of life, with similar results to hysterectomy in improving quality of life. (Lethaby, Cooke and Rees 2005)
- Reduction of dysmenorrhoea and chronic pelvic pain in endometriosis (FSRH 2017).
- Treatment of endometrial hyperplasia: The 52 mg LNG-IUD is used to treat endometrial hyperplasia without atypia and offers protection to the endometrium during estrogen treatment in hormone replacement therapy. It is important to know that if the LNG-IUD is used for this purpose, the device should be changed every 5 years (Depypere and Inki 2015) (FSRH 2017).
- Endometrial and ovarian cancer reduction: progestogen-only contraceptives, especially the LNG-IUD, may offer significant protection against endometrial cancer, and a reduced risk of ovarian cancer, although with less evidence than combined hormonal contraception. A 2015 meta-analysis suggests that long-term use of LNG-IUDs may reduce the risk of endometrial cancer, especially in women with risk factors such as obesity or polycystic ovarian syndrome (Gambacciani et al. 2014). On the other hand, with respect to ovarian cancer, population-based studies have found that long-term use of the LNG IUD and the subdermal implant may contribute to this protective effect, although less strongly than the combined use. (Collaborative Group 2015).

Risks of Progestogen-Only Contraception

Current evidence on the relationship between progestagen-only contraceptives (POCs) and breast cancer is limited and, in some cases, contradictory. A 2016 systematic review found no significant increase risk of breast or other cancers associated with the use of these methods (Samson et al. 2016), and other authors agree that no clear association between breast cancer and specific forms of POC such as the progestagen-only pill or the subdermal implant has been demonstrated, with any possible increase in risk being small and reversible after cessation of treatment (White 2018).

In the case of the levonorgestrel intrauterine system (LNG-IUS), some studies have suggested a possible increased risk of breast cancer with long-term use, although methodological limitations and lack of replication of these findings prevent firm conclusions (Mørch et al. 2017). Nevertheless, clinical guidelines, including those of the FSRH, recommend avoiding the use of LNG-IUS in women with a personal history of breast cancer, unless indicated on a case-by-case basis following specialised assessment (FSRH 2017). For a more detailed discussion on the relationship between gestagen-only hormonal contraceptives and cancer, the reader is again referred to the specific chapter of this book.

The adverse effect that may raise most concern and uncertainty during the use of progestagen-only methods in perimenopause is the effect of progestogens on bone mineral density, especially the use of injectable POCs due to the hypoestrogenism generated by this method, as discussed in the section on contraception and adolescence. However, the data in the perimenopausal population are mixed.

Several observational studies have examined the effects of injectable progesterone use on BMD in women over 40 years of age. One small study included a control group and two groups of women who had been injected with injectable progesterone until menopause; one group of contraceptive users concomitantly used HRT and one did not. Women who had never used medroxyprogesterone experienced rapid bone loss at menopause, compared to the two groups of injectable POC users who experienced very little loss. This study suggests that women using injectable POCs experience bone loss at the start of treatment due to the hypoestrogenic effects of treatment, but that this initial bone loss does not recur or worsen with menopause (Cundy et al. 2002). Another study conducted in women aged 40-49 years, users of different contraceptive methods (combined hormonal contraceptives, gestagen-only injections, norethisterone enanthate) for at least 12 months, found that there was no significant difference in BMD between the different groups of contraceptive users (p = .26) in bone mineral density measured at the distal radius and mid ulnar diaphysis by dual X-ray absorptiometry. There was no significant difference in BMD among the four groups of contraceptive users (p = .26) (Beksinska et al. 2005).

Although no increase in fracture risk has been demonstrated, the WHO and FSRH recommend unrestricted use of the injectable contraceptive medroxyprogesterone acetate up to 45 years of age. Between the ages of 45 and 50, its use should be limited to situations where there is no suitable alternative and both the woman and the health professional consider this method to be the most appropriate, suggesting caution in women over 40 with risk factors for osteoporosis, such as vitamin D deficiency, smoking or a family history of bone disease. (FSRH 2017).

As for the other gestagen-only methods of contraception, there is currently no evidence that they have an adverse effect on bone mineral density (FSRH 2017).

Table 2. Recommendations for progestagen-only contraceptive use in women ≥40 years (World Health Organization 2015).

Clinical condition	WHO Category	Clinical commentary
Age ≥40 years without comorbidities	1	Free use. ASGs are safe and appropriate at this stage.
Active smoker ≥35 years (any amount)	1	No restriction. No significant interaction with smoking.
BMI ≥35 kg/m².	1	Permitted use. Not associated with significant increase in thrombotic risk.
Mild or controlled hypertension (140- 159/90-99 mmHg)	1	Can be used without restriction.
Uncontrolled hypertension (≥160/100 mmHg)	1	Also permitted. Lower cardiovascular risk than AHCs.
Migraine with aura	2	Very low risk; generally accepted use, especially if no better options.
Migraine without aura	1	No restrictions.
History of CVD, stroke or VTE	2	Very low risk; can be used with clinical follow-up.
Personal history of breast cancer (current or previous)	4	Contraindicated (as with all systemic hormone therapy).
Family history of breast cancer	1	No specific restriction.
Personal history of cervical cancer	1-2	May be used, with monitoring if cancer is active or under treatment.
Abnormal uterine bleeding not assessed	3	Evaluate before starting.

As with CHCs, Table 2 summarises the recommendations based on the WHO Medical Eligibility Criteria (5th ed.) for women aged ≥40 years considering the use of gestagen-only contraception.

In short, perimenopausal progestagen-only methods:

- Are safe and effective in perimenopausal women, with much lower cardiovascular risk than combined methods.
- The LNG IUD is an excellent option for the control of heavy or irregular bleeding.
- DMPA injectables may be associated with bone loss with prolonged use: densitometry monitoring is suggested in women >45 years if use is continued for more than 2 years.
- PSAs do not need to be discontinued until confirmed menopause, although periodic evaluation is recommended.

Non-Hormonal Methods

Non-hormonal contraceptive methods, such as copper IUDs, surgical sterilisation and barrier methods, share the same indications and risk-benefit profile in perimenopausal women as in the general population. Although each of these methods is discussed in detail in specific chapters of this book, we would like to highlight some fundamental premises to keep in mind:

- The non-hormonal IUD: The copper IUD is a long-acting, highly effective method of contraception, recommended especially for women who are unable or unwilling to use hormones. It is important for users to be aware that, in the first few months after insertion of the copper IUD, light, heavy or prolonged bleeding may occur, these symptoms can be treated with anti-inflammatory drugs or tranexamic acid. However, this pattern of hypermenorrhoea may develop, so this type of IUD may not be suitable for perimenopausal women who experience problematic menstrual bleeding patterns (Faculty of Family Planning Reproductive Health Care 2017) (Sitruk-Ware, Régine. 2007).

On the other hand, any Cu IUD model containing ≥300 mm2 of copper inserted at age 40 or later can be used on an extended basis until menopause. (1 year after the date of last menstrual period if it occurs when the woman is 50 or older, or 2 years after the date of last menstrual period if it occurs when the woman is younger than 50 y. (FSRH 2023).

- Male and female condoms, when used correctly and consistently, are 98% and 95% effective respectively in preventing pregnancy. Couples should be aware that condom use also helps to reduce the risk of sexually transmitted infections, including HIV if used correctly, which is of interest to women with new sexual partners. On a more specific note, women near menopause may experience decreased vaginal lubrication, which can cause discomfort with condom use, and the use of water-soluble lubricants is recommended to improve tolerance (FSRH 2012) (World Health Organization 2015) (CDC 2024).
- The diaphragm with spermicide, if used correctly and continuously, is 92% effective in preventing pregnancy. The advantages of this method in our perimenopausal patients are fundamentally that, being a non-hormonal method, it is valid for women

with contraindications to the use of estrogens or progestogens. Unlike the male condom, this method is autonomous and entirely controlled by the user. However, one factor that should be taken into account when using it in older women is the loss of vaginal muscle tone that can be experienced at this stage of life, which could affect the fit of the diaphragm, so a new fit is recommended if there have been major changes (such as childbirth, pelvic surgery or menopause). It is also important to be aware that spermicide may cause vaginal irritation or increase the risk of urinary tract infections if used frequently and does not protect against STIs (FSRH 2012) (World Health Organization 2021) (CDC 2021).

When Should We End Contraception in the Perimenopause?

The fertility rate in women over the age of 50 is very low and we could safely withdraw contraception, but the decision to stop treatment must be made on an individual basis, as there is no test that can determine the exact moment of cessation of ovarian function (Faculty of Family Planning Reproductive Health Care 2017).

In patients who use non-hormonal methods of contraception and continue to have regular menstrual bleeding, contraception can be withdrawn after one year of amenorrhoea if the patient is over 50 years old or two years of amenorrhoea if the patient is under 50 years old (Faculty of Family Planning Reproductive Health Care 2017).

When the patient is using hormonal methods that alter the menstrual pattern, it is more difficult to determine precisely when it is appropriate to stop treatment. In patients over 50 years of age using progestagen-only methods, FSH levels may be helpful in determining when the patient is in menopause. If the FSH value is 30 IU/L or higher, the test should be repeated after 6 weeks. If FSH is still at or above 30 IU/L on this second measurement, contraceptive use can be discontinued (Faculty of Family Planning Reproductive Health Care 2017).

Table 3. Recommendations for discontinuation of menopausal contraceptive therapy (Faculty of Family Planning Reproductive Health Care 2017)

Contraceptive method	Age 40-50 years	Age >50 years
Non-hormonal	Stop contraception after 2 years of amenorrhoea	Stop contraception after 1 year of amenorrhoea
Combined hormonal contraception	Can be continued	Stop at age 50 and switch to a non-hormonal method or IMP/POP/LNG IUS, then follow appropriate advice
Progestogen-only injectable	Can be continued	Women ≥50 should be counselle regarding switching to alternative methods, then follow appropriate advice

However, FSH levels are not a reliable indicator in women using combined hormonal contraceptives. Therefore, given that most clinical guidelines agree that the risks associated with the use of combined contraceptives outweigh their benefits after the age of 50, and considering that fertility at this age is very low, it is recommended to discontinue their use after this age (Table 3) (Faculty of Family Planning Reproductive Health Care 2017).

Conclusion

Women in perimenopause should be informed that, although fertility declines with age, there is still a possibility of pregnancy. It is essential that they are aware of the risks of pregnancy at this stage of life, both for the mother and the foetus. It may therefore be necessary to continue to use an effective method of contraception.

In women of advanced reproductive age, the choice of contraceptive method should be based on an individualised risk-benefit assessment, as although age alone does not contraindicate the use of hormonal contraceptives, co-morbidities may coexist and increase the risk of adverse events. Therefore, a detailed medical history is essential to identify risk factors and personalise the recommendation, considering both the safety and non-contraceptive benefits of each method.

Users of hormonal contraception should be properly followed up, including a complete medical history, blood pressure, body mass index (BMI) calculation, and compliance with cervical and breast cancer screening protocols.

In women with risk factors such as a history of thrombosis, cardiovascular disease or lupus, the use of combined hormonal contraceptives is not recommended. In these cases, it is recommended to opt for gestagen-only contraceptives or non-hormonal methods.

There is currently no evidence-based test that accurately determines the safe time to stop contraception. It is suggested that women over the age of 50 who use non-hormonal or gestagen-only methods, have FSH levels above 30 mIU/mL and have been amenorrhoeic for one year may consider discontinuing contraception. Also, after the age of 50, the risks associated with combined hormonal contraceptive methods outweigh their benefits, so discontinuation is also advised.

References

"ACOG Committee Opinion No. 735: Adolescents and Long-Acting Reversible Contraception: Implants and Intrauterine Devices." *Obstetrics and Gynecology* 131, no. 5 (May 2018): e130-39. https://doi.org/10.1097 AOG.0000000000002632.

"ACOG Practice Bulletin No. 121: Long-Acting Reversible Contraception: Implants and Intrauterine Devices." *Obstetrics and Gynecology* 118, no. 1 (July 2011): 184-96. https://doi.org/10.1097/AOG.0b013e318227f05e.

Spanish Agency for Medicines and Health Products. "Combined hormonal contraceptives: conclusions of the review of the risk of venous thromboembolism," 30 November 1d.C. https://www.aemps.gob.es/informa/notasinformativas/medicamentosusohumano-3/seguridad-1/2013/ni-muh_fv_27-2013-anticonceptivos/.

Ahmed, Imran, Said Mohammed Ali, Seeba Amenga-Etego, *et al*. "Population-Based Rates, Timing, and Causes of Maternal Deaths, Stillbirths, and Neonatal Deaths in South Asia and Sub-Saharan Africa: A Multi-Country Prospective Cohort Study." *The Lancet Global Health* 6, no. 12 (December 2018): e1297–e1308. https://doi.org/10.1016/S2214-109X (18)30385-1.

Allen, N., T. O. Yang, and Endometrial Cancer Epidemiologic Studies Collaborative Group. 2015. "Endometrial cancer and oral contraceptives: an individual participant meta-analysis of 27,276 women with endometrial cancer from 36 epidemiological studies." *The Lancet Oncology* 16 (9): 1061-1070. https://doi.org/10.1016/S1470-2045(15)00212-0.

American Society for Reproductive Medicine. 2015. Hormonal Contraception and the Risk of Breast Cancer: A Committee Opinion. Birmingham, AL: ASRM. https://www.asrm.org/globalassets/asrm/asrm-content/news-and-publications/practice-guidelines/for-non-members/hormonal_contraception_and_the_risk_of_breast_cancer.pdf.

"Contraception in Adolescence: Strategies for Reducing Unintended Pregnancy and Promoting Sexual and Reproductive Health-PAHO/WHO|*Pan American Health Organization*," September 30, 2024. https://www.paho.org/es/noticias/30-9-2024-anticoncepcion-adolescencia-estrategias-para-reduccion-pregnancy-unintended-pregnancy.

Bakour, S. 2017. "Contraceptive Methods and Issues around the Menopause: An Evidence Update." *The Obstetrician & Gynaecologist* 19 (3): 174-82. https://doi.org/10.1111/tog.12383.

Beksinska, M. E., J. A. Smit, I. Kleinschmidt, T. M. Farley, and F. Mbatha. 2005. "Bone Mineral Density in Women Aged 40-49 Years Using Depot-Medroxyprogesterone Acetate, Norethisterone Enanthate or Combined Oral Contraceptives for Contraception." *Contraception* 71 (3): 170-175. https://doi.org/10.1016/ j. contraception.2004.09.003.

Boonstra, Heather. "Teen Pregnancy: Trends and Lessons Learned." *Issues in Brief* (Alan Guttmacher Institute), No. 1 (April 2002): 1-4.

Bosetti, C., F. Bravi, E. Negri, and C. La Vecchia. 2009. "Oral contraceptives and risk of colorectal cancer: a systematic review and meta-analysis." *Human Reproduction Update* 15: 489-498. https://doi.org/10.1093/.humupd/dmp017.

Cancer Council Australia. 2022. Combined Oral Contraceptives and Cancer Risk Position Statement. https://cancer.org.au/about-us/policy-and-ad.

Centers for Disease Control and Prevention (CDC). 2024. U.S. Selected Practice Recommendations for Contraceptive Use, 2024. MMWR Recommendations and Reports, 73(3):1-72. Available at: https://www.cdc.gov/mmwr/volumes/73/rr/rr7303a1.htm.

Collaborative Group on Epidemiological Studies of Ovarian Cancer. 2015. "Ovarian Cancer and Oral Contraceptives: Collaborative Reanalysis of 45 Epidemiological Studies Including 23,257 Women with Ovarian Cancer and 87,303 Controls." *Lancet* 385 (9980): 802-11. https://doi. org/10.1016/ S0140-6736(14)61049-1.

COMMITTEE ON ADOLESCENCE, Paula K. Braverman, William P. Adelman, William P. Adelman. Braverman, William P. Adelman, Elizabeth M. Alderman, FSHAM, Cora C. Breuner, David A. Levine, David A. Levine, David A. Levine. Breuner, David A. Levine, Arik V. Marcell, and Rebecca F. O'Brien. "Contraception for Adolescents. *Pediatrics* 134, no. 4 (October 1, 2014): e1244-56. https://doi.org/10.1542/ peds.2014-2299.

Committee on Adolescent Health Care. "Committee Opinion No 699: Adolescent Pregnancy, Contraception, and Sexual Activity." *Obstetrics and Gynecology* 129, no. 5 (May 2017): e142-49. https://doi.org/10.1097/AOG.0000000000002045.

Cundy, T., J. Cornish, H. Roberts, and I. R. Reid. 2002. "Menopausal Bone Loss in Long-Term Users of Depot Medroxyprogesterone Acetate Contraception." *American Journal of Obstetrics and Gynecology* 186 (5): 978- 983. https://doi.org/10.1067/mob.2002.122420.

Curtis, Kathryn M., Naomi K. Tepper, Tara C. Jatlaoui, et al. 2016. Medical eligibility criteria for contraceptive use in the U.S., 2016. *MMWR Recomm Rep* 65 (RR-3): 1-103. https://doi.org/10.15585/ mmwr. rr6503a1.

Cho, M. K. 2018. "Use of Combined Oral Contraceptives in Perimenopausal Women." *Chonnam Medical Journal* 54 (3): 153-158. https://doi.org/10.4068/cmj.2018.54.3.153.

"Depot Medroxyprogesterone Acetate and Bone Effects." Accessed March 22, 2025. https://www.acog.org/clinical/clinical-guidance/committee-opinion/articles/2014/06/depot-medroxyprogesterone-acetate-and-bone- effects.

Depypere, H., and P. Inki. "The Levonorgestrel-Releasing Intrauterine System for Endometrial Protection during Estrogen Replacement Therapy: A Clinical Review." *Climacteric: The Journal of the International Menopause Society* 18, n.o 4 (2015): 470-82. https://doi.org/10.3109/13697137.2014.991302.

Dragoman, Monica V., Naomi K. Tepper, *et al*. "A Systematic Review and Meta-Analysis of Venous Thrombosis Risk among Users of Combined Oral Contraception." *International Journal of Gynaecology and Obstetrics: The Official Organ of the International Federation of Gynaecology and Obstetrics* 141, n.o 3 (June 2018): 287-94. https://doi.org/10.1002/ ijgo.12455.

Edelman, A., E. Micks, M. F. Gallo, J. T. Jensen, and D. A. Grimes. 2014. "Continuous or Extended Cycle vs. Cyclic Use of Combined Hormonal Contraceptives for Contraception." *The Cochrane Database of Systematic Reviews 2014* (7): CD004695. https://doi.org/10.1002/14651858.CD004695.pub3.

Faculty of Family Planning Reproductive Health Care. 2017. Contraception for Women Aged Over 40 Years - Clinical Effectiveness Unit. Published August 2017 (updated November 2017). https://www.fsrh.org/news/updated-clinical-guideline-published-contraception-for-women/

Faculty of Sexual and Reproductive Healthcare. 2012. Guidance: Barrier Methods for Contraception and STI Prevention. August 2012. https://www.fsrh.org

Faculty of Sexual and Reproductive Healthcare 2023. FSRH Guideline (March 2023): Intrauterine Contraception. BMJ Sexual & Reproductive Health 49 (Suppl 1). https://srh.bmj.com/content/49/Suppl_1. https://doi.org/10.1136/bmjsrh-2023-IUC.

Gambacciani, Marco, and A. Levancini. 2014. "Hormonal Contraception and Endometrial Cancer Risk." *Best Practice & Research Clinical Endocrinology & Metabolism* 27 (4): 633-41. https://doi.org/10.1016/ j. beem.2013.05.007.

Gierisch, Jennifer M., Robin R. Coeytaux, Rosa Peragallo Urrutia, et al. 2013. "Oral Contraceptive Use and Risk of Breast, Cervical, Colorectal, and Endometrial Cancers: A Systematic Review." *Cancer Epidemiology, Biomarkers & Prevention* 22: 1931-1943.

Graesslin, Olivier, and Tjeerd Korver. "The Contraceptive Efficacy of Implanon: A Review of Clinical Trials and Marketing Experience." *The European Journal of Contraception & Reproductive Health Care: The Official Journal of the European Society of Contraception* 13 Suppl 1 (June 2008): 4-12. https://doi.org/ 10.1080/13625180801942754.

Harel, Zeev, Suzanne Riggs, Rosalind Vaz, Patricia Flanagan, Kimberly Dunn, and Dalia Harel. "Adolescents' Experience with the Combined Estrogen and Progestin Transdermal Contraceptive Method Ortho Evra." *Journal of Pediatric and Adolescent Gynecology* 18, no. 2 (April 2005): 85-90. https://doi.org/10.1016/ j. jpag.2004.11.016.

International Collaboration of Epidemiological Studies of Cervical Cancer, Paul Appleby, Valerie Beral, Amy Berrington de González, Didier Colin, Silvia Franceschi, Adrian Goodhill, et al. "Cervical Cancer and Hormonal Contraceptives: Collaborative Reanalysis of Individual Data for 16,573 Women with Cervical Cancer and 35,509 Women without Cervical Cancer from 24 Epidemiological Studies." *Lancet* (London, England) 370, no. 9599 (10 November 2007): 1609-21. https://doi.org/10.1016/ S0140-6736(07)61684-5.

Khatibi, Ali, Anne-Marie Nybo Andersen, Mika Gissler, Nils-Halvdan Morken, and Bo Jacobsson. "Obstetric and Neonatal Outcome in Women Aged 50 Years and up: A Collaborative, Nordic Population-Based Study." *European Journal of Obstetrics, Gynecology, and Reproductive Biology* 224 (May 2018): 17-20. https:// doi.org/10.1016/j.ejogrb.2018.03.001.

Kohn, Jessica E., Kelli Stidham Hall, Tessa Madden, Kimberly Carlson, Jeffrey F. Peipert, and Eleanor Bimla Schwarz. 2018. "Barriers to Long-Acting Reversible Contraception Use among Young Women: A Systematic Review." *Journal of Pediatric and Adolescent Gynecology* 31(2): 183-191. https://doi.org/ 10.1016/ j. jpag.2017.10.002.

Kuohung, W., L. Borgotta, and P. Stubblefield. 2000. "Low-dose oral contraceptives and bone mineral density: an evidence-based analysis." Contraception 61: 77-82. https://doi.org/10.1016/s0010-7824(00)00086-x

Lethaby, A. E., I. Cooke, and M. Rees. 2005. Progesterone or Progestogen-Releasing Intrauterine Systems for Heavy Menstrual Bleeding. *Cochrane Database of Systematic Reviews* 2005, no. 4: CD002126. https://doi.org/10.1002/14651858.CD002126.pub2.

Lidegaard, Øjvind. 2013. "Hormonal Contraception and Venous Thromboembolic Risk in Midlife Women." *Maturitas* 74 (1): 1-2. https://doi.org/10.1016/j.maturitas.2012.09.015.

Lidegaard, Øjvind, Ellen Løkkegaard, Aksel Jensen, Charlotte Wessel Skovlund, and Niels Keiding. 2012 "Thrombotic Stroke and Myocardial Infarction with Hormonal Contraception." *The New England Journal of Medicine* 366, no. 24 (June 14, 2012): 2257-66. https://doi.org/10.1056/NEJMoa1111840.

Lidegaard, Øjvind, Lisa S. Sørensen, Helle Nielsen, and Charlotte W. Skovlund. 2022. "Hormonal Contraception and Risk of Venous Thromboembolism: National Follow-up Study." *BMJ* 379: e071403. https://doi.org/ 10.1136/bmj-2022-071403.

Liu, Kimberly, Allison Case, and REPRODUCTIVE ENDOCRINOLOGY AND INFERTILITY COMMITTEE"Advanced Reproductive Age and Fertility." Journal of Obstetrics and Gynaecology

Canada: JOGC= *Journal d'obstetrique et Gynecologie Du Canada: JOGC* 33, n.o 11 (November 2011): 1165-75. https://doi.org/ 10.1016/S1701-2163(16)35087-3

Long, Margaret E., Stephanie S. Faubion, Kathy L. MacLaughlin, Sandhya Pruthi, and Petra M. Casey. 2015. "Contraception and hormonal management in perimenopause." *Journal of Women's Health* 24 (1): Published online January 21. https://doi.org/10.1089/jwh.2013.4544.

Luchowski, Ashley T., Erika E. Anderson, Kavita Shah Arora, Kathryn M. Edelman, Carolyn L. Hanley, and Anne E. Burke. 2014. "Obstacles to IUD Provision: Perspectives of Family Planning Providers." *Perspectives on Sexual and Reproductive Health* 46(2): 87-93. https://doi.org/10.1363/46e1114.

Mendoza, N., R. Sánchez-Borrego, M. J. Cancelo, A. Calvo, M. A. Checa, J. Cortés, M. A. Elorriaga, et al. "Position of the Spanish Menopause Society Regarding the Management of Perimenopause." *Maturitas* 74, No. 3 (March 2013): 283-90. https://doi.org/10.1016/j.maturitas.2012.12.010.

Mendoza, Nicolas, and Rafael Sanchez-Borrego. "Classical and Newly Recognised Non-Contraceptive Benefits of Combined Hormonal Contraceptive Use in Women over 40." *Maturitas* 78, n.o 1 (May 2014): 45-50. https://doi.org/10.1016/j.maturitas.2014.02.017.

Mendoza, Nicolás, Esperanza Soto, and Rafael Sánchez-Borrego. "What Are the Risks of Hormonal Contraceptive Use in Middle-Aged Women?" *Maturitas* 84 (February 2016): 100. https://doi.org/10.1016/ j. maturitas.2015.11.008.

Miller, Taniqua A., Rebecca H. Allen, Andrew M. Kaunitz, and Carrie A. Cwiak. "Contraception for Midlife Women: A Review." *Menopause* (New York, N.Y.) 25, no. 7 (July 2018): 817-27. https://doi.org/10.1097/ GME.0000000000001073.

Mørch, Lina S., Charlotte W. Skovlund, Philip C. Hannaford, Lisa Iversen, Shona Fielding, and Øjvind Lidegaard. "Contemporary Hormonal Contraception and the Risk of Breast Cancer." *The New England Journal of Medicine* 377, no. 23 (December 7, 2017): 2228-39. https://doi.org/10.1056/NEJMoa1700732.

Nelson, S. M., E. E. Telfer, and R. A. Anderson. "The Ageing Ovary and Uterus: New Biological Insights." *Human Reproduction Update* 19, no. 1 (2013): 67-83. https://doi.org/10.1093/humupd/dms043.

North American Menopause Society. 2013. *Menopause Glossary*. Available at: www.menopause.org/for-women/ menopause-glossary (accessed March 5, 2013).

Nguyen, Antoinette T. "U.S. Medical Eligibility Criteria for Contraceptive Use, 2024." *MMWR*. Recommendations and Reports 73 (2024). https://doi.org/10.15585/mmwr.rr7304a1.

World Health Organization. 2023. Adolescence. https://www.who.int/news-room/fact-sheets/detail/ adolescence.

World Health Organisation. 2020. Sexually Transmitted Infections (STIs). https://www.who.int/ news-room/fact-sheets/detail/sexually-transmitted-infections-(stis).

Pantaleón, R Quintana. "*Contraception in adolescence*," 2018.

Paz-Bailey, Gabriela, Emilia H. Koumans, Maya Sternberg, Antonya Pierce, John Papp, Elizabeth R. Unger, Mary Sawyer, Carolyn M. Black, and Lauri E. Markowitz. "The Effect of Correct and Consistent Condom Use on Chlamydial and Gonococcal Infection among Urban Adolescents." *Archives of Pediatrics & Adolescent Medicine* 159, no. 6 (June 2005): 536-42. https://doi.org/10.1001/archpedi.159.6.536.

Peng, Yan, Xia Wang, Hong Feng, et al. 2017. "Is Oral Contraceptive Use Associated with an Increased Risk of Cervical Cancer? An Evidence-Based Meta-Analysis." *Journal of Obstetrics and Gynaecology Research* 43(5): 913-922.

Peragallo Urrutia, Rachel, Remy R. Coeytaux, Amanda J. McBroom, Jennifer M. Gierisch, Laura J. Havrilesky, Patricia G. Moorman, William J. Lowery, et al. "Risk of Acute Thromboembolic Events with Oral Contraceptive Use: A Systematic Review and Meta-Analysis." *Obstetrics and Gynecology* 122, n.o 2 Pt 1 (August 2013): 380-89. https://doi.org/10.1097/AOG.0b013e3182994c43.

Pfizer. 2004. *Letter to health professionals*. Available at: http://www.fda.gov/downloads/Safety/ MedWatch/SafetyInformation/SafetyAlertsforHumanMedicalProducts/UCM166395.pdf. Accessed 19 May 2025.

Regidor, Pedro, and Elisabetta Colli. 2022. "Drospirenone 4 mg in a 24/4 Regimen Maintains Inhibition of Ovulation Even after a 24-h Delay Pill Intake: Pharmacological Aspects and Comparison to Other Progestin- Only Pills." *European Review for Medical and Pharmacological Sciences* 26: 1994-1999.

Requena, C., and B. Llombart. 2020. "Oral Contraceptives in Dermatology." *Actas Dermo-Sifiliográficas* (English Edition) 111 (5): 351-356. https://doi.org/10.1016/j.adengl.2019.06.008.

Roach, Rachel E. J., Frans M. Helmerhorst, Willem M. Lijfering, Theo Stijnen, Ale Algra, and Olaf M. Dekkers. "Combined oral contraceptives: risk of myocardial infarction and ischaemic stroke - Roach, RE-2015|*Cochrane Library*." Accessed April 10, 2025. https:// www.cochranelibrary.com/es/cdsr/doi/ 10.1002/14651858.CD011054.pub2/detailed-comment/es? messageId=448238028.

Rodríguez, Francisca Molero, Francisco Cabello Santamaría, Jesús Florido Navío, Miren Larrazábal Murillo, Rafael Sánchez Borrego, and Froilán Sánchez Sánchez. "*Life and sex beyond 50*," n.d.

Roumen, F. J., D. Apter, T. M. Mulders, and T. O. Dieben. "Efficacy, Tolerability and Acceptability of a Novel Vaginal Contraceptive Ring Releasing Etonogestrel and Ethinyl Oestradiol." *Human Reproduction* (Oxford, England) 16, no. 3 (March 2001): 469-75. https://doi.org/10.1093/humrep/16.3.469.

Rubin, Sara E., Marji Gold, and Susan C. Schantz-Dunn. 2021. "Access to Long-Acting Reversible Contraception: A Review of Barriers and Facilitators." *Women's Health Issues* 31(1): 30-36. https://doi.org/ 10.1016/j.whi.2020.09.003.

Secura, Gina M., Jenifer E. Allsworth, Tessa Madden, et al. 2010. "The Contraceptive CHOICE Project: Reducing Barriers to Long-Acting Reversible Contraception." *American Journal of Obstetrics and Gynecology* 203 (2): 115.e1-115.e7.

Shifren, Jan L., Margery L.S. Gass, and the NAMS Recommendations for Clinical Care of Midlife Women Working Group. 2014. "The North American Menopause Society Recommendations for Clinical Care of Midlife Women." *Menopause* 21: 1038-62. https://doi.org/10.1097/GME.0000000000000319.

Sitruk-Ware, Regine. "The Levonorgestrel Intrauterine System for Use in Peri- and Postmenopausal Women." *Contraception* 75, n.o 6 Suppl (June 2007): S 155-160. https://doi.org/10.1016/j. contraception. 2007.01.010.

Smith, Jennifer S., Jane Green, Amy Berrington de Gonzalez, et al. 2003. "Cervical Cancer and Use of Hormonal Contraceptives: A Systematic Review." *The Lancet* 361: 1159-1167.

Sully, Elizabeth A., Ann Biddlecom, Jacqueline E. Darroch, Taylor Riley, Lori S. Ashford, Naomi Lince-Deroche, Lauren Firestein, and Rachel Murro. *"Adding It Up: Investing in Sexual and Reproductive Health 2019*," July 28, 2020. https://doi.org/10.1363/2020.31593.

Tepper, Naomi K., Kathryn M. Marchbanks, Maura K. Whiteman, et al. 2016. "Progestin-Only Contraception and Thromboembolism: A Systematic Review." *Contraception* 94 (6): 678-700. https://doi.org/10.1016/ j. contraception.2016.07.005.

U.S. Department of Health and Human Services, Health Resources and Services Administration. 2010. *Women's Health USA* 2010. September 2010. Available at: https://mchb.hrsa.gov/publications/pdfs/ womenshealth2010.pdf.

White, Nicole D. "Hormonal Contraception and Breast Cancer Risk." *American Journal of Lifestyle Medicine* 12, no. 3 (January 31, 2018): 224-26. https://doi.org/10.1177/1559827618754833.

Winslow, Betty, Pamela Johnson, and Amanda Steen. 2021. "Are Progesterone-Only Contraceptives Safe in Women with a History of Venous Thromboembolism?" *Evidence-Based Practice* 24 (9): E5-E6. https://doi.org/ 10.1097/EBP.0000000000000880.

Women's Health and Aging Study Group. 2006. "Women's Perception of Sexuality around the Menopause." *European Journal of Obstetrics & Gynecology and Reproductive Biology* 126 (1): 115-22. https://doi.org/ 10.1016/j.ejogrb.2005.08.012.

World Health Organization. 2015. Medical Eligibility Criteria for Contraceptive Use, 5th ed. Geneva: *World Health Organization*. https://www.who.int/publications/i/item/9789241549158.

Chapter 17

Development of Pharmacological Methods for Male Contraception

A. Tello Delsors[1,*], MD
L. Sales Pérez[2], MD
M. L. Juan Rodrigo[3], MD
A. García Buendía[3], MD
and Ll. Belmonte Andújar[3,4], PhD

[1]Obstetrics and Gynecology Department, University and Hospital of Santa Lucía, Cartagena, Murcia, Spain
[2]Obstetrics and Gynecology Department, Hospital Lluis Alcanyis Xativa, Xativa, Valencia, Spain
[3]Obstetrics and Gynecology Department, University and Hospital of Albacete, Albacete, Spain
[4]Medical Science Department, School of Medicine of Albacete, Universidad de Castilla-La Mancha, Spain

Abstract

Unintended pregnancies continue to be a global problem. Currently, male involvement in contraception is low, hampered by the limited options available. Research on the use of male hormonal contraceptives has been conducted since the 1970s, based on the same knowledge as for the female pill. Recently, there has also been research on non-hormonal male pharmacological contraceptives. This chapter will provide an overview of the history and progress to date on the drugs available for male contraception.

The development of male hormonal contraceptives is based on the principle that exogenously administered testosterone suppresses the hypothalamic-pituitary-testicular axis. This suppresses testicular testosterone synthesis, which is necessary for spermatogenesis. With exogenous androgens, testosterone-dependent functions at the peripheral level and sexual function and libido are maintained. Adding a progestin to androgens increases the negative feedback on the hypothalamic-pituitary-gonadal axis resulting in a faster and profound suppression of spermatogenesis with lower doses of androgens. Different combinations have been tested following these principles and with various forms of administration; achieving promising results in terms of contraceptive efficacy measured as pregnancy rates.

Alternative methods to interfere with spermatogenesis without having a central effect have been investigated, notably retinoic acid inhibitors which produce genetic alterations that

[*] Corresponding Author's Email: anatdelsors@gmail.com

In: Advances in Reproductive Health
Editors: Llanos Belmonte Andujar and Ana Fuentes Rozalen
ISBN: 979-8-90134-038-7

prevent spermatogenesis. Adenylyl cyclase inhibitors that act by blocking sperm capacitation have also been studied.
Finally, while the results of these novel methods are promising, more investment by the pharmaceutical industry is needed to make systemic male contraceptives, with both hormonal and non-hormonal options, a reality in the near future.

Keywords: hormonal contraception (MeSH), contraceptive agents (MeSH), male (MeSH)

Introduction

Unintended pregnancies continue to be a problem globally, accounting for 40-45% of all pregnancies (Bearak 2018). Despite the variety of contraceptive options available to women, this rate has remained largely stable over the past three decades (Bearak 2020). Unintended pregnancies result in risks for both the mother and the newborn, as well as a significant economic, social and medical burden (Sonfield 2011).

Among the many female contraceptive options available, long-acting methods have the lowest failure rate (Trussel 2011). These include oral contraceptives, transdermal patches, vaginal rings, subdermal implants, hormonal or copper intrauterine devices. However, they can cause side effects such as weight gain, decreased libido, irregular menstrual bleeding, breast tenderness or thromboembolic events. In other cases, women may have medical conditions that contraindicate the use of hormonal contraceptives (Thirumalai 2019).

Currently, male participation in contraception is low, hampered by the limited options available: coitus interruptus, condoms and vasectomy (Page 2022). The first two have a failure rate of 20% and 12% respectively, making them unreliable options (Long 2021). As for vasectomy, in addition to being an invasive technique, it is considered a permanent method of contraception, which can only be reversed by microsurgery to permeabilise the vas deferens. However, this surgery is estimated to achieve a spontaneous pregnancy rate of 49% in the best of cases (Araújo 2024).

Research on the use of male hormonal contraceptives has been conducted since the 1970s, based on the same knowledge that is available for the female pill. It has been widely studied that the administration of exogenous androgens, alone or in combination with progestins, suppresses testicular sperm production (Long 2021). However, over the last ten years, pharmaceutical companies have abandoned the lines of research aimed at making male hormonal contraception a reality (Page 2022).

In 2005, the results of a survey conducted in countries around the world on men's perceptions of male contraceptives were published. This study revealed that 55.1% of respondents reported willingness to use male hormonal contraceptives if they became available (Heinemann 2005).

In this chapter, the history and progress to date in male contraception will be presented. Firstly, the development of hormonal methods of contraception up to the present day will be discussed, followed by advances and new non-hormonal methods.

Physiology of the Male Reproductive System

The hypothalamus-pituitary-testicle axis functions as classic negative feedback, with two main functions: testosterone production and sperm production. The hypothalamus releases gonadotropin-releasing hormone (GnRH) in a pulsatile manner. This travels to the anterior pituitary where it stimulates the secretion of the gonadotrophins follicle stimulating hormone (FSH) and luteinising hormone (LH). LH acts on the Leydig cells to produce testosterone and maintains testicular testosterone levels well above those circulating in the blood. FSH exerts its function on Sertoli cells, which are responsible for spermatogenesis under the action of testicular testosterone (Wang 2024).

Testosterone circulating in the blood binds to non-gonadal androgen receptors to exert its androgenic functions and in turn exerts negative feedback on the hypothalamus and pituitary to suppress the axis. On the other hand, non-testicular testosterone is converted to oestradiol by the enzyme aromatase, further suppressing the hypothalamus-pituitary-testicle system. It is also converted to dihydrotestosterone by the action of 5-alpha-reductase. The latter hormone exerts its function primarily in the prostate and hair follicles (Thirumalai 2019).

Once spermatogenesis is complete in the seminiferous tubules of the testis, the immature sperm accumulate in the epididymis. The epididymis is a long, coiled tube that sits atop the testicle. Here, immature sperm acquire motility through an enzymatic process and the ability to fertilise the egg by changes in the plasma membrane. Mature sperm accumulate in the distal part of the epididymis until they are required for ejaculation. During ejaculation, the sperm travel from the epididymis to the urethra and out. On this journey, they receive fructose-rich fluid from the seminal vesicles and an enzyme-rich milky fluid from the prostate. The urethra is also lubricated by pre-ejaculatory fluid released by Cowper's glands or bulbourethral glands (Sullivan 2016).

Male Hormonal Contraception

The development of male hormonal contraceptives is based on the fact that exogenously administered testosterone suppresses the hypothalamic-pituitary- testicular axis by a negative feedback mechanism. This suppresses testicular testosterone synthesis, which is necessary for spermatogenesis to occur. Centrally, the exogenous hormones maintain sexual function and libido. At the peripheral level, exogenous androgens bind to androgen receptors in tissues such as muscle or skin, and maintain other androgen-dependent functions in these tissues (Thirumalai 2019). If a progestin is added to androgens, it increases the negative feedback on the hypothalamic-pituitary-gonadal axis resulting in a more rapid and profound suppression of spermatogenesis with lower doses of androgens. Similar to female hormonal contraception, all these effects are reversible and cease when treatment is stopped (Thirumalai 2024).

Testosterone-Only Contraceptives

Over the past thirty years, several studies have been conducted to evaluate the efficacy of male hormonal contraceptives.

The World Health Organisation conducted two efficacy studies in 1990 and 1996, respectively, using weekly injections of 200 milligrams (mg) of testosterone enanthate (TE).

The first included 271 men from seven different countries, 70% of whom met the azoospermia requirement (0 sperm in the ejaculate) and entered the efficacy phase. Contraceptive efficacy was 0.8 conceptions per 100 couple-years (WHO 1). In the second study (WHO 2), the aim was to achieve oligozoospermia, rather than azoospermia, with a sperm threshold of 3 million per millilitre (ml) in the ejaculate. Three hundred and ninety-nine men from nine different countries were included, 98% of whom achieved the target threshold and were included in the efficacy phase. The pregnancy rate was 1.4 per 100 couple-years, with a directly proportional relationship between the number of sperm in the ejaculate and the number of unwanted pregnancies. These studies led to the conclusion that the sperm count to achieve contraceptive efficacy similar to that of female contraceptives was 1 million sperm/ml. Due to the high doses of androgens used in these studies, side effects such as mood swings, acne, weight gain, hypertension and polycythaemia occurred. Another negative aspect was that many men left the study early because of the discomfort of the weekly injections.

Subsequently, a testosterone derivative with a better pharmacokinetic and pharmacodynamic profile compared to TE, the prodrug testosterone undecanoate (UT), emerged, which achieves a more stable and prolonged release of testosterone (Kroopnick 2024). Two multicentre clinical trials were conducted to evaluate the contraceptive efficacy of this new compound. The first of these was a phase II trial in which 308 men were given a first dose of 1000 mg intramuscular TUs followed by 500 mg monthly intramuscular TUs during the six-month suppression phase of the study. Ninety-eight per cent of the men reached the efficacy phase and were divided into two groups; those who reached azoospermia and those who reached severe oligozoospermia defined as a sperm count of <3 million sperm/ml. During the efficacy phase, 500 mg was administered monthly for six months and sperm concentration in a semen sample was assessed monthly. The method failure rate was 2.9 per 100 couple-years and 2% of patients experienced sperm rebound after the suppression phase (Gu 2003).

Years later, the same researchers conducted a phase III trial, in which 1045 healthy men were given an initial injection of 1000 mg of TU and then monthly doses of 500 mg during the suppression phase. 95.2% of participants were able to enter the efficacy phase after reaching the required level of oligozoospermia (<1 million sperm/ml). In the efficacy phase, which lasted 24 months, couples stopped using any other method of contraception, and 500 mg of TU was administered monthly during this phase. The failure rate was 1.1 pregnancies per 100 couple-years and 1.3% of men had sperm rebound during the second phase of the study (Gu 2009).

Serious adverse effects were not reported in either of the latter two studies. Similar to TE, side effects such as acne, mood changes, polycythaemia, gynaecomastia or weight gain occurred (Kroopnick 2024).

Contraception with Testosterone and Progestins

In order to avoid the supraphysiological doses of testosterone administered in testosterone-only male contraception, the use of progestins was investigated, based on models of female contraception. The addition of a progestin was found to achieve greater and more rapid suppression of gonadotrophins and thus spermatogenesis (Wang 2024). To achieve severe azoospermia or oligozoospermia, very low blood levels of testosterone are required, so it is necessary to administer testosterone exogenously along with gestagens to ensure sufficient level of testosterone to maintain sexual function and other androgen-dependent effects (Kroopnick 2024).

Turner et al first tested the contraceptive efficacy of injectable testosterone together with intramuscular medroxyprogesterone acetate. The study included a total of 55 men who were given 800 mg testosterone every 4-6 months along with quarterly medroxyprogesterone acetate injections. A sperm concentration of less than 1 million/ml was considered necessary to enter the efficacy phase, which occurred in 94% of participants. Did not produce any pregnancies during the efficacy phase, so the failure rate was 0 (Turner 2003).

In another study of 320 men, UT injections were combined with intramuscular norethisterone. Participants received 1000 mg UT together with 200 mg injections of norethisterone every two months. The efficacy phase was achieved by 95.9% of the men, after achieving the required sperm concentration of less than 1 million sperm/ml. The pregnancy rate during the efficacy phase was 2.18 pregnancies per 100 couple-years. This study was stopped before completion, by an external safety review committee, because adverse effects such as mood swings, severe depression or pain at the injection site were reported, and the risk was considered to outweigh the benefit. However, 99% of symptoms were rated as "mild" or "moderate" and validated questionnaires were not administered to participants before the study began, so it is not known whether any had depression before the study began (Behre 2016) (Wang 2024).

Since the study of male hormonal contraception began, other combinations of progestins with testosterone derivatives have been tested in small studies. A preliminary study involving 72 Chinese men was conducted to test whether the administration of levonorgestrel together with UT injections was successful in suppressing spermatogenesis. Azoospermia was achieved in almost 70% of participants and <3 million sperm/ml was achieved in more than 85% of men. No serious adverse effects were reported (Gui 2004). In another study in 31 African men, oral desogestrel was administered together with injected testosterone, achieving azoospermia rates of 85% (Anderson 2002).

Transdermally Applied Male Contraceptives

Topical testosterone is used as a treatment for men with hypogonadism. It has several advantages over injected testosterone, such as easier and painless application that can be self-administered, as well as more stable blood testosterone levels (Thirumalai 2019). Therefore, the contraceptive efficacy of combining testosterone gels with medroxyprogesterone acetate was tested. In this study, 35 men were given daily testosterone gel along with oral medroxyprogesterone at a dose of 20 mg per day. Sperm suppression levels were achieved in 93% of participants after six months of treatment and only one pregnancy occurred without serious adverse effects (Soufir 2011).

Once the use of testosterone gel together with an oral progestogen was shown to have contraceptive efficacy, the use of testosterone gel together with a synthetic progestin was considered. The gestagen used was a potent progestin, nestorone, which has no androgenic, oestrogenic or mineralcorticoid effect and also does not act as a progestogen on GABA receptors, which appear to be responsible for the mood-related effect of contraceptives. This gestagen has already been used, together with ethinyl estradiol, as a female contraceptive in the form of a vaginal ring, with good contraceptive results and few adverse effects (Thirumalai 2019).

A preliminary study was conducted in 2009 in which participants were divided into three groups, receiving transdermal nestorone alone, testosterone gel monotherapy and a third group in which both gels were combined. Initially the dose of nestorone used was 2 or 4 mg, but due to low response at this dose, it was increased to 6 or 8 mg. The results were that testosterone gel 10 g together with nestorone gel 6 or 8 mg achieved significantly greater gonadotropin suppression compared to either substance alone (Mahabadi 2009).

Subsequently, a randomised, double-blind clinical trial was conducted in which 99 men participated. They were randomly divided into three groups: a first group of 10 g testosterone gel together with placebo, a second group of 10 g testosterone gel together with 8 mg nestorone gel and a third group of 10 g testosterone gel with 12 mg nestorone gel. The results were that the percentage of men achieving a sperm concentration equal to or less than 1 million was higher in the nestorone gel groups compared to the testosterone gel with placebo group. Adverse effects reported were acne, weight gain and increased haematocrit (Ilani 2012).

The Eunice Kennedy Shriver National Institute of Child Health and Human Development (NICHD) has developed a gel that combines 74 mg testosterone along with 8 mg nestorone acetate per 5 ml of product. It is applied daily by the male on the arms and shoulders with a volume of 2.5 ml on each side. Its advantages are that it is self-administered, requires no injections and avoids the first hepatic step as it is not taken orally. Consumers are advised to wear clothing over the exposure site and to shower before contact with women and children to avoid transfer of product through the skin (Kroopnick 2024).

A phase IIb clinical trial (Amory 2023) is currently being conducted by the Contraceptive Clinical Trials Network (NCT 03452111) on the contraceptive efficacy of this gel combining nestorone with testosterone. This clinical trial included a total of 462 couples who were instructed to administer the gel daily. Sperm concentration was assessed periodically until the sperm count was <1 million sperm/ml in two consecutive measurements. At this point, participants entered the 52-week efficacy phase where they used the gel as their sole method of contraception. Once the efficacy phase is completed, the recovery phase begins in which the sperm concentration is monitored until two consecutive samples have a sperm count above 15 million/ml. The primary objective of this study is to measure pregnancy rate. Secondary objectives are to assess the percentage of males reaching the sperm concentration (<1 million/ml) to enter the efficacy phase, side effects, sexual function, etc. (Thirumalai 2019). Although the study has been completed, definitive results are not yet available. However, preliminary studies report that it appears to be an effective contraceptive method, with no serious adverse effects, well tolerated. This product is the first male hormonal contraceptive that is patient- controlled, making it more convenient than regimens involving injections (Kroopnick 2024).

Gonadotropin-Releasing Hormone Antagonists and Agonists

With testosterone regimens combined with a gestagen, 90-95% of men achieve a level of oligozoospermia, defined as a sperm count of less than 1 million/ml. However, sperm suppression is not universal. Furthermore, in some cases a phenomenon known as "sperm rebound" occurs, characterised by transient increases in sperm production. In an attempt to increase gonadotropin suppression and avoid these phenomena, the use of GnRH agonists and antagonists has been investigated (Thirumalai 2024).

GnRH agonists are drugs used in both gynaecology and urology, as they suppress the hypothalamic-pituitary-gonadal axis. After injection, GnRH is stimulated, a phenomenon known as "flare-up," and the axis is subsequently suppressed. It is therefore necessary to administer testosterone together with GnRH analogues in order to maintain the serum testosterone levels necessary for sexual function and other androgen-dependent activities, a strategy known as "add-back" therapy. Therefore, the use of these drugs has been tested to suppress spermatogenesis. Studies have looked at suppressing spermatogenesis with testosterone and then administering the analogues, administering testosterone as an "add back" therapy after administering the analogue, or starting testosterone from the first analogue injection (Behre 1992). These studies have shown weak suppression of spermatogenesis, so GnRH agonists are not considered a suitable option for male contraception (Wang 2024).

GnRH antagonists have a different mechanism of action, as they bind to the pituitary receptors inducing a blockade of these receptors, so that the suppression of the axis is immediate, without flare-up. Different GnRH antagonists have been evaluated for contraceptive efficacy when added to testosterone regimens. First, the GnRH antagonist known as Nal-Glu was tested, administered as a daily subcutaneous injection in combination with weekly injections of intramuscular testosterone enanthate (Pavlou 1992). While the results were initially promising, it was later shown that it did not improve contraceptive efficacy compared to the testosterone monotherapy regimen (Bagatell 1993). Subsequently, a small clinical trial was conducted in which the subcutaneous GnRH antagonist cetrorelix was combined with intramuscular 19-nortestosterone. This combination effectively suppressed spermatogenesis, but was associated with high costs and adverse reactions resembling anaphylaxis. (Behre 2001). Another GnRH antagonist, acylline, was also tested in combination with transdermal testosterone and intramuscular medroxyprogesterone acetate. Results showed that its addition did not increase or accelerate the rate of oligozoospermia (Page 2006).

An orally administered GnRH antagonist has recently been approved for advanced prostate cancer. In the future, this oral antagonist could be combined with testosterone as an "add back" therapy. If this oral combination proves to be effective for contraception, it would provide a method of contraception similar to the female pill (Wang 2024).

New Synthetic Androgens

In recent years, new synthetic androgens derived from 19-nortestosterone have been developed which could become the active ingredient of a "male pill" in the future. The objectives are to maintain the androgenic effects, reduce the side effects of androgen treatment, improve oral bioavailability without hepatotoxicity and prolong serum half-life. For a synthetic androgen to be ideal for contraception, it must not be sensitive to the action of 5α-reductase, as this hormone converts testosterone into dihydrotestosterone, which is associated with prostate pathology. On the other hand, it must be sensitive to aromatisation to metabolites that act on oestrogen receptors, as oestrogen deficiency in men has been linked to osteoporosis, vasomotor symptoms and increased body fat (Wang 2024).

7-α-methyl-19-nortestosterone (MENT) is a synthetic androgen that is resistant to the action of 5α-reductase and is aromatised into a compound that binds to oestrogen receptors, giving it a protective effect on prostate and bone (Thirumalai 2019). It is not bioavailable orally, so it is administered as an implant. In a study conducted to test its contraceptive efficacy 8 out of 11 men achieved oligozoospermia, which was encouraging (Eckardstein 2003). However, in a later study in which a progestin was added, an implant failure that prevented adequate release compromised the results, and the studies with this molecule were discontinued (Nieschlag 2013).

Both dimethandrolone undecanoate (DMAU) and 1-beta-methyl-19- nortestosterone (11bMNTDC) are orally bioavailable molecules derived from 19-nortestosterone. Both are converted to their active metabolite once administered. They do not need to be metabolised by

5α-reductase to reach their maximal androgenic action and are not aromatised to active oestrogenic compounds. In addition, they bind to both androgen and progesterone receptors, making them suitable for a single-compound contraceptive pill, without the need to add another hormone (Thirumalai 2024). Phase I studies have been conducted to evaluate the pharmacokinetics, safety and dosage of these compounds. In a study involving 82 healthy males, participants received escalating doses of oral DMAU for 28 days. It showed that daily oral administration of DMAU at doses of 200-400 mg can suppress testosterone and gonadotropins without serious adverse effects (Thirumalai Ceponis 2019). A randomised, double-blind, placebo-controlled study evaluated the use of daily 11β-MNTDC orally for 28 days. Gonadotropin suppression was found and no serious adverse effects were reported (Yuen 2020). Administration of either molecule with high-fat foods improves their oral pharmacokinetics. Due to the limited duration of the aforementioned studies, the effect on spermatogenesis suppression could not be assessed in any of them. Future studies of longer duration are needed to evaluate the efficacy of both compounds as a single oral contraceptive agent for men (Wang 2024).

Racial Variations in Sperm Suppression

In efficacy studies of male hormonal contraceptives, a difference in susceptibility has been observed in Asian men compared to other participants. Thus, it appears that Asian men are more susceptible to the effect of exogenously administered hormones, achieving higher rates of sperm suppression (WHO 1; WHO2). A study of more than three months' duration analysing previous studies on male hormonal contraceptive use found that Caucasian participants achieved lower suppression rates compared to Asians (Liu 2008). To date, the exact reason for this variation in response is not known. Furthermore, other racial groups such as Latinos or Africans, are underrepresented in the studies conducted and are therefore not currently evaluable (Thirumalai 2019).

Side Effects of Male Hormonal Methods

The side effects associated with the use of male hormonal contraceptives could be an impediment to their commercialisation and acceptance by the population. With the development of hormonal contraceptives that combine testosterone with gestagens, the amount of exogenous androgens is reduced, and therefore the side effects of these are partially reduced. However, they are not free of adverse effects, the most frequently observed being acne, changes in libido, weight gain and mood changes. Because of concerns about mood effects, studies are now adding validated scales to assess possible psychological effects during male hormonal contraceptive use (Behre 2016).

There are also concerns about possible long-term adverse effects on metabolism. This could lead to alterations in blood pressure, blood cholesterol, fat and bone mass. However, phase 4 studies would be needed to assess these effects (Thirumalai 2019).

These side effects could be a limiting factor in the approval of these drugs by the U.S. Food and Drug Administration and the European Medicines Agency.

"On and Off" Periods

Male hormonal contraceptives aim to suppress sperm production. Since this process takes about 72 days to complete, a period of time of 6 to 8 weeks is needed from the start of the method until contraceptive effectiveness is achieved. This can be inconvenient as it means that during this period the couple must use an additional contraceptive method to prevent pregnancy. On the other hand, once these drugs are discontinued, spermatogenesis concentration must be restored. Liu et al. demonstrated recovery rates of 90% at 12 months and 100% at 2 years after stopping treatment. This shows that it is a fully reversible contraceptive. However, this latency period can be a problem for couples. Several factors have been studied to be associated with shorter time to recovery of sperm concentrations >20 million/ml. These factors include older age, Asian race, shorter duration of contraceptive use, higher sperm concentration at method initiation, among others (Liu 2006).

Sperm Rebound

In efficacy studies of male hormonal methods, sperm concentrations in participants are measured on a regular basis. This minimises the risk of unwanted pregnancies among the couples included in the studies. Periods of increased sperm concentration above the threshold considered contraceptive have been observed, without reaching baseline sperm concentration; this is known as sperm rebound. In efficacy studies, sperm rebound rates of between 1.4% and 2.2% have been observed. The exact reason for this phenomenon is not known. It could be explained in cases of self- administered contraceptives due to inconsistent or irregular use of the method. However, sperm rebound has also been observed in studies testing longer-acting contraceptives such as testosterone-containing implants. This could be due to stimulation of spermatogenesis by unknown non- gonadotropin-dependent pathways. This represents an area of research in this field. In the future, devices could be incorporated that allow users to measure their own sperm count on a regular basis to ensure contraceptive efficacy (Thirumalai 2019).

Pharmacological Non-Hormonal Male Contraception

So far, male hormonal contraceptive methods have been presented that focus on suppressing the hypothalamic-pituitary-gonadal axis and thus interfering with spermatogenesis. Other methods with spermatogenesis without having a central effect have been investigated. Most notably, retinoic acid inhibitors have been investigated as they produce genetic alterations that impede spermatogenesis. Adenylyl cyclase inhibitors, which act by blocking sperm capacitation, have also been studied.

Retinoic Acid

Retinoic acid, the active metabolite of vitamin A, is essential for spermatogonial maturation and therefore retinoic acid inhibitors have been proposed as a target for male contraception (Long 2021). In 1961, a study was carried out on 60 men in a penitentiary centre who were administered WIN 18466, and remained azoospermic for the year of treatment. However, it was found to be a drug with an antabuse effect. That is, during treatment, the ingestion of alcoholic beverages produces nausea, vomiting, tachycardia and other symptoms due to acetaldehyde accumulation (Heller 1961). On the other hand, BMS-189453 is a panretinoic acid receptor antagonist, i.e. it acts on α, β and γ receptors. In studies in mice, its administration produces sterility but with other effects such as testicular degeneration and atrophy. No human studies have been conducted for this reason (Chung 2016). In order to avoid this adverse effect, another retinoic acid antagonist, YCT529, has been synthesised that only acts on α-receptors, which is the isoform present in the prostate. Studies in mice administered orally for 4 weeks have shown contraceptive efficacy, with no adverse effects reported. No human studies have been published to date (Shi 2025).

Adenylyl Cyclase Inhibitors

Mature sperm are stored in the epididymis in a dormant, immature state. When ejaculation occurs, the sperm come into contact with seminal fluid containing bicarbonate. Bicarbonate stimulates soluble adenylyl cyclase, the main source of cyclic AMP in sperm, which activates sperm motility and initiates the sperm capacitation process necessary for fertilisation to occur (Balbach 2021). This post ejaculatory contraceptive target would allow on-demand male contraception, avoiding chronic treatment that carries a higher risk of adverse effects. Adenylyl cyclase inhibitors have been tested in mouse studies showing a blockade of sperm motility 15 minutes after oral administration, rendering the mice infertile for the next three hours (Sanchez 2024). If its contraceptive efficacy could be proven in the "male on-demand pill" could be revolutionary in that it would be a "male pill on demand."

Monoclonal Antibodies

In recent years, concerns about sexually transmitted diseases and unwanted pregnancies have led to the use of technology to address these problems. For example, a monoclonal antibody development platform has created an antibody that targets two sexually transmitted pathogens, HIV-1 and HSV-2. The same platform is developing an "anti-sperm" monoclonal antibody, H6-3C4, which recognises a carbohydrate epitope on a glycoprotein anchored to glycosylphosphatidylinositol, found on the surface of spermatozoa. Approval is currently awaited to begin phase 1 clinical trials (Anderson 2020).

Male Contraceptives with Vas Deferens Action

Since 1970, a contraceptive method was developed to reversibly block the vas deferens by injecting a polymer styrene maleic anhydride mixed with dimethyl sulfoxide. This compound damages sperm as they pass through the sperm duct and renders them ineffective. A phase III study was conducted in India in 2000 with this compound, with results that at first appeared promising, but it later became clear that the study did not meet international standards (Long 2021).

Years later, the Parsemus Foundation bought the rights to this compound and developed a similar product called VasalgelTM, which acts as a mechanical barrier to the passage of sperm. The effect is reversible, and the vas deferens can be re-permeabilised by washing with sodium bicarbonate (Colagross-Schouten 2017).

In the 1980s, research in China investigated the use of a polyurethane elastomer plug injected into the vas deferens, achieving azoospermia in 96% of men, although the results were observed two years after injection (Chen 1992). A hydrogel, ADAMTM, was also developed that blocks the passage of sperm through the vas deferens, but does not prevent the passage of other fluids (Zhao 1992).

German urologist Clemns Birek launched a patent in 2000 on a contraceptive that acts as a "switch" for the vas deferens. A clinical trial will soon be launched to evaluate the effectiveness of Bimek SLV, as the device is known. It consists of a valve that is placed in the vas deferens and regulates its flow, so that it can be used as a "switch" in the vas deferens. The patient can open and close the duct himself. The procedure is performed on an outpatient basis, similar to a vasectomy, by inserting the valve via the scrotal route (Bimek SLV).

Conclusion

Due to the high social impact of unplanned pregnancies, the contraceptive possibilities available must be increased, and the development of new male contraceptive methods is an imperative. Numerous surveys reveal a growing interest among both men and women in the availability of a "male pill" that would allow men to become more involved in family planning. Over the past fifty years, studies have demonstrated the safety and efficacy of male hormonal methods, as discussed in detail in this chapter. The development of non-hormonal systemic male contraceptive methods has also been studied. However, none of these contraceptive options are currently on the market. All of them are in the study phase, but not available to the population.

Further investment by the pharmaceutical industry is needed to make systemic-acting male contraceptives, with both hormonal and non-hormonal options, a reality in the near future. It is possible that the lack of industry funding is due to uncertainty about the side effects of these methods and their acceptability in the market by users.

Surveys have been conducted to assess the acceptability of male hormonal contraceptive methods in the population. The results of these surveys are promising, with 50-75% of men reporting a willingness to use them. However, these results should be interpreted with caution, as the participants are volunteers who are more aware of the issue and may not represent the view of the general population. Therefore, studies are needed to assess concerns about the use of these methods in the general population in order to improve the methods and achieve greater acceptability.

References

Amory, John K., Diana L. Blithe, Regine Sitruk-Ware, Ronald S. Swerdloff, William J. Bremner, Clint Dart, Peter Y. Liu, et al. 2023. "Design of an International Male Contraceptive Efficacy Trial Using a Self-Administered Daily Transdermal Gel Containing Testosterone and Segesterone Acetate (Nestorone)." *Contraception* 124 (110064): 110064. doi: 10.1016/j.contraception.2023.110064.

Anderson, Deborah J., Joseph A. Politch, Richard A. Cone, Larry Zeitlin, Samuel K. Lai, Philip J. Santangelo, Thomas R. Moench, y Kevin J. Whaley. 2020. "Engineering Monoclonal Antibody-Based Contraception and Multipurpose Prevention Technologies." *Biology of Reproduction* 103 (2): 275–85. doi:10.1093/biolre/ioaa096.

Anderson, R. A., Z. M. Van Der Spuy, O. A. Dada, S. K. Tregoning, P. M. Zinn, O. A. Adeniji, T. A. Fakoya, K. B. Smith, and D. T. Baird. 2002. "Investigation of Hormonal Male Contraception in African Men: Suppression of Spermatogenesis by Oral Desogestrel with Depot Testosterone." *Human Reproduction* (Oxford, England) 17 (11): 2869–77. doi:10.1093/humrep/17.11.2869.

Araújo, Débora, Alexandre Gromicho, Jorge Dias, Samuel Bastos, Tiago Gregório, and Vitor Oliveira. 2024. "Microsurgical Vasectomy Reversal: Experience of a Single Center." *Revista Internacional de Andrologia* 22 (4): 10–16. doi:10.22514/j.androl.2024.025.

Bagatell, C. J., A. M. Matsumoto, R. B. Christensen, J. E. Rivier, y W. J. Bremner. 1993. "Comparison of a Gonadotropin Releasing-Hormone Antagonist plus Testosterone (T) versus T Alone as Potential Male Contraceptive Regimens." *The Journal of Clinical Endocrinology and Metabolism* 77 (2): 427–32. doi:10.1210/jcem.77.2.8345047.

Balbach, Melanie, Lubna Ghanem, Thomas Rossetti, Navpreet Kaur, Carla Ritagliati, Jacob Ferreira, Dario Krapf, et al. 2021. "Soluble Adenylyl Cyclase Inhibition Prevents Human Sperm Functions Essential for Fertilization." *Molecular Human Reproduction* 27 (9). doi:10.1093/molehr/gaab054.

Bearak, Jonathan, Anna Popinchalk, Leontine Alkema, and Gilda Sedgh. 2018. "Global, Regional, and Subregional Trends in Unintended Pregnancy and Its Outcomes from 1990 to 2014: Estimates from a Bayesian Hierarchical Model." *The Lancet. Global Health* 6 (4): e380–89. doi:10.1016/S2214-109X(18)30029-9.

Bearak, Jonathan, Anna Popinchalk, Bela Ganatra, Ann-Beth Moller, Özge Tunçalp, Cynthia Beavin, Lorraine Kwok, and Leontine Alkema. 2020. "Unintended Pregnancy and Abortion by Income, Region, and the Legal Status of Abortion: Estimates from a Comprehensive Model for 1990-2019." *The Lancet. Global Health* 8 (9): e1152–61. doi:10.1016/S2214-109X(20)30315-6.

Behre, H. M., S. Kliesch, B. Lemcke, S. von Eckardstein, y E. Nieschlag. 2001. "Suppression of Spermatogenesis to Azoospermia by Combined Administration of GnRH Antagonist and 19-Nortestosterone Cannot Be Maintained by This Non-Aromatizable Androgen Alone." *Human Reproduction* (Oxford, England) 16 (12): 2570–77. doi:10.1093/humrep/16.12.2570.

Behre, H. M., D. Nashan, W. Hubert, y E. Nieschlag. 1992. "Depot Gonadotropin-Releasing Hormone Agonist Blunts the Androgen-Induced Suppression of Spermatogenesis in a Clinical Trial of Male Contraception." *The Journal of Clinical Endocrinology and Metabolism* 74 (1): 84–90. doi:10.1210/jcem.74.1.1727833.

Behre, Hermann M., Michael Zitzmann, Richard A. Anderson, David J. Handelsman, Silvia W. Lestari, Robert I. McLachlan, M. Cristina Meriggiola, et al. 2016. "Efficacy and Safety of an Injectable Combination Hormonal Contraceptive for Men." *The Journal of Clinical Endocrinology and Metabolism* 101 (12): 4779–88. https://doi.org/10.1210/jc.2016-2141.

"Bimek SLV – The New Contraception for Men." 2015. Bimek SLV. junio 18. https://bimek.com.

Chen, Z. W., Y. Q. Gu, X. W. Liang, Z. G. Wu, E. J. Yin, y Li-Hong. 1992. "Safety and Efficacy of Percutaneous Injection of Polyurethane Elastomer (MPU) Plugs for Vas Occlusion in Man." *International Journal of Andrology* 15 (6): 468–72. doi:10.1111/j.1365-2605.1992.tb01140.x.

Chung, Sanny S. W., Xiangyuan Wang, y Debra J. Wolgemuth. 2016. "Prolonged Oral Administration of a Pan-Retinoic Acid Receptor Antagonist Inhibits Spermatogenesis in Mice with a Rapid Recovery and Changes in the Expression of Influx and Efflux Transporters." *Endocrinology* 157 (4): 1601–12. doi:10.1210/en.2015-1675.

Colagross-Schouten, Angela, Marie-Josee Lemoy, Rebekah I. Keesler, Elaine Lissner, y Catherine A. VandeVoort. 2017. "The Contraceptive Efficacy of Intravas Injection of VasalgelTM for Adult Male Rhesus Monkeys." *Basic and Clinical Andrology* 27: 4. doi:10.1186/s12610-017-0048-9.

"Contraceptive Efficacy of Testosterone-Induced Azoospermia in Normal Men. World Health Organization Task Force on Methods for the Regulation of Male Fertility." 1990. *Lancet* 336 (8721): 955–59.

Eckardstein, Sigrid von, Gabriela Noe, Vivian Brache, Eberhard Nieschlag, Horacio Croxatto, Francisco Alvarez, Alfred Moo-Young, et al. 2003. "A Clinical Trial of 7 Alpha-Methyl-19-Nortestosterone Implants for Possible Use as a Long-Acting Contraceptive for Men." *The Journal of Clinical Endocrinology and Metabolism* 88 (11): 5232–39. doi:10.1210/jc.2002-022043.

Gu, Yiqun, Xiaowei Liang, Weixiong Wu, Minli Liu, Shuxiu Song, Lifa Cheng, Liwei Bo, et al. 2009. "Multicenter Contraceptive Efficacy Trial of Injectable Testosterone Undecanoate in Chinese Men." *The Journal of Clinical Endocrinology and Metabolism* 94 (6): 1910–15. doi:10.1210/jc.2008-1846.

Gu, Yi-Qun, Xing-Hai Wang, Dwo Xu, Lin Peng, Li-Fa Cheng, Ming-Kong Huang, Zhen-Jia Huang, and Gui-Yuan Zhang. 2003. "A Multicenter Contraceptive Efficacy Study of Injectable Testosterone Undecanoate in Healthy Chinese Men." *The Journal of Clinical Endocrinology and Metabolism* 88 (2): 562–68. doi:10.1210/jc.2002-020447.

Gui, You-Lun, Chang-Hai He, John K. Amory, William J. Bremner, E-Xiang Zheng, Jie Yang, Pei-Juan Yang, and Er-Sheng Gao. 2004. "Male Hormonal Contraception: Suppression of Spermatogenesis by Injectable Testosterone Undecanoate Alone or with Levonorgestrel Implants in Chinese Men." *Journal of Andrology* 25 (5): 720–27. doi:10.1002/j.1939-4640.2004.tb02846.x.

Heinemann, Klaas, Farid Saad, Martin Wiesemes, Steven White, and Lothar Heinemann. 2005. "Attitudes toward Male Fertility Control: Results of a Multinational Survey on Four Continents." *Human Reproduction* (Oxford, England) 20 (2): 549–56. doi:10.1093/humrep/deh574.

Heller, C. G., D. J. Moore, y C. A. Paulsen. 1961. "Suppression of Spermatogenesis and Chronic Toxicity in Men by a New Series of Bis(Dichloroacetyl) Diamines." *Toxicology and Applied Pharmacology* 3 (1): 1–11. doi:10.1016/0041-008x(61)90002-3.

Ilani, Niloufar, Mara Y. Roth, John K. Amory, Ronald S. Swerdloff, Clint Dart, Stephanie T. Page, William J. Bremner, et al. 2012. "A New Combination of Testosterone and Nestorone Transdermal Gels for Male Hormonal Contraception." *The Journal of Clinical Endocrinology and Metabolism* 97 (10): 3476–86. doi:10.1210/jc.2012-1384.

Kroopnick, Jeffrey M., Min S. Lee, and Diana L. Blithe. 2024. "Development of New Hormonal Male Contraception for the Couple." *Andrology* 12 (7): 1506–11. doi:10.1111/andr.13654.

Liu, Peter Y., Ronald S. Swerdloff, Bradley D. Anawalt, Richard A. Anderson, William J. Bremner, Joerg Elliesen, Yi-Qun Gu, et al. 2008. "Determinants of the Rate and Extent of Spermatogenic Suppression during Hormonal Male Contraception: An Integrated Analysis." *The Journal of Clinical Endocrinology and Metabolism* 93 (5): 1774–83. doi:10.1210/jc.2007-2768.

Liu, Peter Y., Ronald S. Swerdloff, Peter D. Christenson, David J. Handelsman, Christina Wang, and Hormonal Male Contraception Summit Group. 2006. "Rate, Extent, and Modifiers of Spermatogenic Recovery after Hormonal Male Contraception: An Integrated Analysis." *Lancet* 367 (9520): 1412–20. https://doi.org/10.1016/S0140-6736(06)68614-5.

Long, Jill E., Min S. Lee, and Diana L. Blithe. 2021. "Update on Novel Hormonal and Nonhormonal Male Contraceptive Development." *The Journal of Clinical Endocrinology and Metabolism* 106 (6): e2381–92. doi:10.1210/clinem/dgab034.

Mahabadi, Vahid, John K. Amory, Ronald S. Swerdloff, William J. Bremner, Stephanie T. Page, Regine Sitruk-Ware, Peter D. Christensen, et al. 2009. "Combined Transdermal Testosterone Gel and the Progestin Nestorone Suppresses Serum Gonadotropins in Men." *The Journal of Clinical Endocrinology and Metabolism* 94 (7): 2313–20. doi:10.1210/jc.2008-2604.

Nieschlag, Eberhard, Narender Kumar, y Régine Sitruk-Ware. 2013. "7α-Methyl-19-Nortestosterone (MENTR): The Population Council's Contribution to Research on Male Contraception and Treatment of Hypogonadism." *Contraception* 87 (3): 288–95. doi:10.1016/j.contraception.2012.08.036.

Page, Stephanie T., John K. Amory, Bradley D. Anawalt, Michael S. Irwig, Andrew T. Brockenbrough, Alvin M. Matsumoto, y William J. Bremner. 2006. "Testosterone Gel Combined with Depomedroxyprogesterone Acetate Is an Effective Male Hormonal Contraceptive Regimen and Is Not Enhanced by the Addition of a GnRH Antagonist." *The Journal of Clinical Endocrinology and Metabolism* 91 (11): 4374–80. doi:10.1210/jc.2006-1411.

Page, Stephanie T., Diana Blithe, and Christina Wang. 2022. "Hormonal Male Contraception: Getting to Market." *Frontiers in Endocrinology* 13: 891589. doi:10.3389/fendo.2022.891589.

Pavlou, S. N., K. Brewer, M. G. Farley, J. Lindner, M. C. Bastias, B. J. Rogers, L. L. Swift, J. E. Rivier, W. W. Vale, y P. M. Conn. 1991. "Combined Administration of a Gonadotropin-Releasing Hormone Antagonist and Testosterone in Men Induces Reversible Azoospermia without Loss of Libido." *The Journal of Clinical Endocrinology and Metabolism* 73 (6): 1360–69. doi:10.1210/jcem-73-6-1360.

Sanchez, Natalia Del R. Rivera, Carla Ritagliati, Gregory S. Kopf, Steve Kretschmer, Jochen Buck, y Lonny R. Levin. 2024. "The Uniqueness of On-Demand Male Contraception." *Molecular Aspects of Medicine* 97 (101281): 101281. doi:10.1016/j.mam.2024.101281.

Shi, Rui, Debra J. Wolgemuth, y Gunda I. Georg. 2025. "Development of the Retinoic Acid Receptor Alpha-Specific Antagonist YCT-529 for Male Contraception: A Brief Review." *Contraception*, núm. 110809: 110809. doi:10.1016/j.contraception.2024.110809.

Sonfield, Adam, Kathryn Kost, Rachel Benson Gold, and Lawrence B. Finer. 2011. "The Public Costs of Births Resulting from Unintended Pregnancies: National and State-Level Estimates." *Perspectives on Sexual and Reproductive Health* 43 (2): 94–102. doi:10.1363/4309411.

Soufir, J-C, G. Meduri, y A. Ziyyat. 2011. "Spermatogenetic Inhibition in Men Taking a Combination of Oral Medroxyprogesterone Acetate and Percutaneous Testosterone as a Male Contraceptive Method." *Human Reproduction* (Oxford, England) 26 (7): 1708–14. doi:10.1093/humrep/der138.

Sullivan, Robert, y Roger Mieusset. 2016. "The Human Epididymis: Its Function in Sperm Maturation." *Human Reproduction Update* 22 (5): 574–87. doi:10.1093/humupd/dmw015.

Thirumalai, Arthi, Jonas Ceponis, John K. Amory, Ronald Swerdloff, Vijaya Surampudi, Peter Y. Liu, William J. Bremner, et al. 2019. "Effects of 28 Days of Oral Dimethandrolone Undecanoate in Healthy Men: A Prototype Male Pill." *The Journal of Clinical Endocrinology and Metabolism* 104 (2): 423–32. doi:10.1210/jc.2018-01452.

Thirumalai, Arthi, and Stephanie T. Page. 2019. "Recent Developments in Male Contraception." *Drugs* 79 (1): 11–20. doi:10.1007/s40265-018-1038-8.

———. 2024. "Testosterone and Male Contraception." *Current Opinion in Endocrinology, Diabetes, and Obesity* 31 (6): 236–42. doi:10.1097/MED.0000000000000880.

Trussell, James. 2011. "Contraceptive Failure in the United States." *Contraception* 83 (5): 397–404. doi:10.1016/j.contraception.2011.01.021.

Turner, Leo, Ann J. Conway, Mark Jimenez, Peter Y. Liu, Elise Forbes, Robert I. McLachlan, and David J. Handelsman. 2003. "Contraceptive Efficacy of a Depot Progestin and Androgen Combination in Men." *The Journal of Clinical Endocrinology and Metabolism* 88 (10): 4659–67. doi:10.1210/jc.2003-030107.

Wang, Christina, Maria Cristina Meriggiola, Hermann M. Behre, and Stephanie T. Page. 2024. "Hormonal Male Contraception." *Andrology* 12 (7): 1551–57. doi:10.1111/andr.13699.

World Health Organization Task Force on Methods for the Regulation of Male Fertility. 1996. "Contraceptive Efficacy of Testosterone-Induced Azoospermia and Oligozoospermia in Normal Men." *Fertility and Sterility* 65 (4): 821–29. doi:10.1016/s0015-0282(16)58221-1.

Yuen, Fiona, Arthi Thirumalai, Cindy Pham, Ronald S. Swerdloff, Bradley D. Anawalt, Peter Y. Liu, John K. Amory, et al. 2020. "Daily Oral Administration of the Novel Androgen 11β-MNTDC Markedly Suppresses Serum Gonadotropins in Healthy Men." *The Journal of Clinical Endocrinology and Metabolism* 105 (3): e835–47. doi:10.1210/clinem/dgaa032.

Zhao, S. C., Y. H. Lian, R. C. Yu, y S. P. Zhang. 1992. "Recovery of Fertility after Removal of Polyurethane Plugs from the Human Vas Deferens Occluded for up to 5 Years." *International Journal of Andrology* 15 (6): 465–67. doi:10.1111/j.1365-2605.1992.tb01139.x.

List of Contributors

Mar Pérez Haro, MD. Instituto Bernabéu, Albacete, Spain. Obstetrics and Gynaecology Department, University and Hospital Complex of Albacete, Spain.

Llanos Belmonte Andújar, PhD. Obstetrics and Gynaecology Department, University and Hospital Complex of Albacete, Spain. Medical Science Department, School of Medicine of Albacete, Universidad de Castilla-La Mancha, Spain.

Gema Serrano García, MD. Obstetrics and Gynaecology Department, University and Hospital Complex of Albacete, Spain.

Esteban González Mirasol, PhD. Obstetrics and Gynaecology Department, University and Hospital Complex of Albacete, Spain. Medical Science Department, School of Medicine of Albacete, Universidad de Castilla-La Mancha, Spain.

Mónica Moreno Palmero, MD. Obstetrics and Gynaecology Department, University and Hospital Complex of Albacete, Spain.

Lidia Gómez Muñoz, MD. Obstetrics and Gynaecology Department, Hospital of Tomelloso, Tomelloso, Ciudad Real, Spain.

Clara Aparicio Martínez, MD. Obstetrics and Gynaecology Department, Hospital of Tomelloso, Tomelloso, Ciudad Real, Spain.

Ana Fuentes Rozalén, MD. Instituto Bernabéu, Alicante, Spain.

María Teresa, Gómez García, PhD. Obstetrics and Gynaecology Department, University and Hospital Complex of Albacete, Spain. Medical Science Department, School of Medicine of Albacete, Universidad dc Castilla-La Mancha. Spain.

Mercedes Castillo García, MD. Obstetrics and Gynaecology Department, University and Hospital Complex of Albacete, Spain. Medical Science Department.

Alejandro Serrano Sánchez, MD. Obstetrics and Gynaecology Department, University and Hospital Complex of Albacete, Spain. Medical Science Department.

Pilar Mora Ábalos, Ana Gómez Alarcón, MD. Obstetrics and Gynaecology Department, Hospital of Almansa, Albacete, Spain. Medical Science Department.

Marta Cebrián Marcilla, MD. Obstetrics and Gynaecology Department, Hospital of Almansa, Albacete, Spain. Medical Science Department

María Luisa, Juan Rodrigo, MD. Obstetrics and Gynaecology Department, University and Hospital Complex of Albacete, Spain.

Lara Sales Pérez, MD. Obstetrics and Gynaecology Department Hospital Lluís Alcanyís, Xàtiva, Valencia. Spain.

Ana Tello Delsors, MD. Obstetrics and Gynecology Department, University and Hospital of Santa Lucía, Cartagena, Murcia, Spain.

Sergio Rico Cardenal, MD. Obstetrics and Gynaecology Department Hospital of Villarrobledo, Villarrobledo, Albacete. Spain.

Alicia Santos Fernández, MD. Obstetrics and Gynaecology Department, University and Hospital Complex of Albacete, Spain.

Ana García Buendía, MD. Obstetrics and Gynaecology Department, University and Hospital Complex of Albacete, Spain.

Clara García Fernández, MD. Obstetrics and Gynaecology Department, University and Hospital Complex of Albacete, Spain.

Inés Sánchez Nieto, MD. Obstetrics and Gynaecology Department, Hospital Can Misses, Ibiza, Spain.

Julia López Grande, MD. Obstetrics and Gynaecology Department, University and Hospital Complex of Albacete, Spain.

María Ángeles Roque Fernández, PhD. Obstetrics and Gynaecology Department, University and Hospital Complex of Albacete, Spain. Medical Science Department, School of Medicine of Albacete, Universidad de Castilla-La Mancha, Spain.

María de los Ángeles Rubio Moreno, MD. Obstetrics and Gynaecology Department, University and Hospital Complex of Albacete, Spain.

Index

D

E

F

H

I

L

M

N